EPILEPSY
Patient and Family Guide

SECOND EDITION

ORRIN DEVINSKY, MD
Director, Comprehensive Epilepsy Center
New York University
Professor of Neurology, Neurosurgery,
and Psychiatry
New York University School of Medicine
New York, New York

Director, Saint Barnabas Institute of Neurology
Livingston, New Jersey

F. A. DAVIS COMPANY • Philadelphia

F. A. Davis Company
1915 Arch Street
Philadelphia, PA 19103
www.fadavis.com

Printed in Canada

Last digit indicates print number: 10 9 8 7 6 5

Acquisitions Editor: Margaret M. Biblis
Developmental Editor: Bernice M. Wissler
Production Editor: Jack Brandt
Designer: Melissa Walters
Cover Designer: Louis J. Forgione

Cover art: *Sunflowers*, Vincent van Gogh. © Philadelphia Museum of Art: The Mr. and Mrs. Carroll S. Tyson, Jr. Collection.

Color plates were provided by *Physicians' Desk Reference,* 55th edition, year 2001, published November 2000.

As new scientific information becomes available through basic and clinical research, recommended treatments and drug therapies undergo changes. The author(s) and publisher have done everything possible to make this book accurate, up to date, and in accord with accepted standards at the time of publication. The authors, editors, and publisher are not responsible for errors or omissions or for consequences from application of the book, and make no warranty, expressed or implied, in regard to the contents of the book. Any practice described in this book should be applied by the reader in accordance with professional standards of care used in regard to the unique circumstances that may apply in each situation. The reader is advised always to check product information (package inserts) for changes and new information regarding dose and contraindications before administering any drug. Caution is especially urged when using new or infrequently ordered drugs.

Library of Congress Cataloging-in-Publication Data
Devinsky, Orrin.
    Epilepsy : patient and family guide / Orrin Devinsky.—2nd ed.
        p. cm.
    Previously published as: A guide to understanding and living with epilepsy.
    Includes bibliographical references and index.
    ISBN 0-8036-0498-X
    1. Epilepsy–Popular works. I. Devinsky, Orrin. Guide to understanding and living with epilepsy. II. Title.

RC372 .D48 2001
616.8'53—dc21

2001037243

Acknowledgments

The information and thoughts that fill these pages are a collective effort. They reflect data from my colleagues' research, observations and anecdotes from the people I help care for, and my own views on epilepsy and its care. Several colleagues have generously donated their time and helped ensure a broader and more accurate perspective. Many thanks to Greg Barkley, Blaise Bourgeois, Carol and Peter Camfield, Joyce Cramer, Shawna Cutting, Hank Chesbrough, Alan Ettinger, John Gates, Jeff Katz, Shawn Masia, Cecilia McCarton, Tad Walczak, and Lauren Westbrook.

BJ Hessie and Bernice Wissler provided outstanding editorial suggestions and help. Very special thanks go to Ann Scherer, Margaret Calvano, and others at the Epilepsy Foundation for their valuable information and advice.

My deepest appreciation goes to my wife, Deborah, and my daughters, Janna and Julie, who have always supported my passions and tolerated my disappearances into the study to write.

Foreword

If you are someone who faces the challenge of epilepsy, either person-ally or with a loved one, you know it is a daily battle for control in many areas of life. Epilepsy seeks to rob the individual of power, the ability to choose and shape the future. It is not only the seizures themselves that cause momentary loss of control, but the range of implications they bring to everything, from employment and driving to dating and mar-riage. At times it seems that epilepsy seeks to invade every aspect of life, right to the core of personal self-esteem.

One of the best weapons with which to arm yourself in this battle with epilepsy is knowledge. Knowledge is power—the power to take back control of your life. Knowledge will enable you to work in a close partnership with your health care professionals to determine the op-timum medical treatments and to advocate for your rights in education, employment, transportation, or any other aspect of life. Perhaps most importantly, knowledge will enable you to enlighten those around you. Sharing your personal knowledge about epilepsy with family, friends, and coworkers helps to reduce the ignorance that leads to fear and the resulting stigma. Sharing your knowledge is like dropping a stone in a pond—the ripple effect spreads out in an ever-widening circle.

The Epilepsy Foundation believes strongly in the power of knowledge, and we are especially pleased to welcome this second edition of *Epilepsy: Patient and Family Guide*. Like its predecessor, it is an excellent source of accurate information on the medical aspects of epilepsy. Medical knowl-edge is no longer the sole province of health care professionals. It is people who are informed about their health, working in partnership with their health care professionals, who will achieve the best results. This new edition offers a wealth of information, from details of how the brain works to the specific medications used to treat seizures. It also rec-ognizes that certain populations have unique medical issues and needs, and it provides information on epilepsy for women and the elderly.

However, epilepsy is not solely a medical condition, and this book, like the Epilepsy Foundation, recognizes that the social aspects of epi-lepsy are often the most difficult challenge for individuals and families. This edition of *Epilepsy: Patient and Family Guide* provides information on employment, insurance, driving, and legal issues—all areas of concern for adults with epilepsy. Importantly, it also recognizes the unique challenges faced by parents caring for a child with epilepsy who must deal with school pressures as well as seizures. Perhaps more than any other group, parents must be knowledgeable about the spectrum of medical and social issues surrounding epilepsy to ensure a full life for children with seizures and to allay the fear and guilt that all parents face.

Reviewing this book, and comparing it with the first edition, published in 1994, is a reminder of the enormous progress that has been made in treatment options for people with epilepsy. This edition describes new medications and devices that were barely envisioned just a few years ago. It is also a sobering reminder of areas where things have not yet improved. We wish that the section on insurance could have been dropped on the basis that by now everyone with epilepsy has access to affordable, comprehensive medical care. Sadly, that is not yet the case. In fact, the availability of insurance and access to care described in this second edition has deteriorated from that earlier, unacceptable level.

While *Epilepsy: Patient and Family Guide* is both comprehensive and authoritative, no single book will provide all the information to empower you to win the battle against epilepsy. We encourage you to talk with your health care professionals. Use emerging technology, especially the World Wide Web. If you don't have access at home, it is free at the public library. But be careful; just because it is on the Web doesn't mean it is true. Experts suggest that 70% of health information on the Web is inaccurate or misleading, so rely on sites you trust. A good place to start is www.epilepsyfoundation.org. Take full advantage of literature available from your doctor and health organizations like the Epilepsy Foundation. Above all, never accept that something is "too technical" for you to understand; it just means it needs a better explanation—the kind of explanation you will find in these pages.

The Epilepsy Foundation would like to recognize and thank Dr. Orrin Devinsky for donating the proceeds from this book to the Epilepsy Foundation and to New York University for research. We believe that with an expanded commitment to research, a future with no seizures and no side effects is possible for the next generation. The Epilepsy Foundation will commit our very best to the goal that one day there will be no more need for books—however excellent—on living with epilepsy.

Eric R. Hargis
President and CEO
Epilepsy Foundation
June 14, 2000

Preface

Vincent Van Gogh's *Sunflowers* appears on the cover of this book because that great artist is an example of a person who fulfilled his potential in spite of epilepsy. Because we often fear the unknown, the uncertainties created by a diagnosis of epilepsy may give individuals more difficulty than do the seizures themselves. The main goal of this book is to help people with epilepsy—whether they have a new diagnosis or have been living with epilepsy for years—to understand the disorder and learn about the nature and diversity of seizures, the psychological and social implications of seizures and the diagnosis of epilepsy, the educational and vocational effects, and the medical and surgical therapies for seizures. My real motivation for writing this book, however, was to empower people with epilepsy with knowledge that will remove the fears fueled by misinformation. I want to encourage these people to assume a greater role in their medical care, help them to understand the importance of independence and self-esteem, and give them information that will assist in their efforts to achieve a better quality of life.

The world views epilepsy through the eyes of those who are most directly touched by it. Many patients and families are embarrassed and fearful about epilepsy and try to hide it. It provokes discomfort in them and lowers self-esteem. These attitudes become self-fulfilling and magnified in the outside world. Do not fear the word *epilepsy*. Understand epilepsy, and the world will follow your lead.

Knowledge is power: Education about epilepsy is key. Adults with epilepsy, or the parents of children with epilepsy, should understand the types of seizures, the risks and benefits of the various antiepileptic drugs, the factors that can cause seizures or help prevent them, and which activities are safe and which are dangerous. Education about epilepsy can come from pamphlets and books, the Internet, videotapes, support groups, health care workers, conferences, and the Epilepsy Foundation. A new Website—www.epilepsy.com—is devoted to fostering more knowledge about epilepsy through the innovative presentation of information, including editorials about topics such as medications and their side effects, online access to nurses and doctors, access to research studies, presentations about alternative therapies, and other epilepsy-related topics. The site encourages patients and families who are affected by epilepsy to share their views about their experiences. Although most of my own medical information about epilepsy comes from textbooks, scientific articles, and professional lectures, the people I have cared for—my patients and their families—have been my greatest source of knowledge about living with epilepsy.

A little knowledge, however, can be confusing and frightening. For instance, anyone who reads the *Physician's Desk Reference*, which describes all the prescription drugs on the market, may be surprised to learn about the many side effects of antiepileptic drugs. The list seems almost endless. Some of these effects are serious, and even fatal. But the risks must be weighed against the benefits. For a child who is having so many absence seizures that the ability to learn, play, and socialize with other children is affected, the benefits of medication outweigh the risks. An antiepileptic drug may have a 1 in 100,000 chance of causing death, and although the fear of this chance is real, it should not deter someone from using the drug if the potential benefits are substantial.

Adults with epilepsy should become advocates for themselves. Parents of children who have epilepsy should become their advocates. They should speak out if the medical care seems wrong or violates common sense. If they are dissatisfied with the seizure control or the negative side effects of therapy, they should discuss them with the doctor. The current regimen may truly be the best possible one, but sometimes a second opinion is helpful. Parents of a child with epilepsy also must make sure that the child's educational needs are met, as provided for by law. Perhaps even more important, they should nurture the child's independence. Adults with epilepsy must make sure that their rights to employment and their driving privileges are fairly considered. The safeguards against discrimination in the Americans with Disabilities Act and other legal provisions are described in this book.

This book can be read from cover to cover, or certain sections or chapters can be chosen. Because epilepsy presents different problems and challenges at various stages of life, information pertaining to infants, children, adolescents, adults, women of childbearing age considering parenthood, and the elderly are treated separately. The appendixes provide additional information that will help the reader understand the terminology used in talking or writing about epilepsy, become familiar with the different antiepileptic drugs, find helpful resources, and learn more about the disorder from further reading.

I hope people whose lives are touched by epilepsy find this book informative. If it answers their questions about epilepsy, removes their doubts, dispels their fears, and builds their confidence through knowledge, then it will have served its purpose. I welcome any suggestions that could help a third edition better achieve this goal.

Orrin Devinsky, MD
New York, NY
od4@is4.nyu.edu

Contents

PART THREE
EPILEPSY IN CHILDREN 189

PART FOUR
EPILEPSY IN ADULTS 279

PART FIVE
LEGAL AND FINANCIAL ISSUES IN EPILEPSY 337

PART SIX
RESOURCES FOR PEOPLE WITH EPILEPSY 355

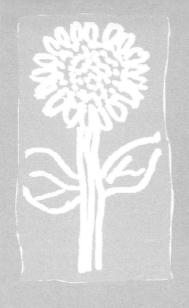

part one

MEDICAL ASPECTS OF EPILEPSY

1

Facts about Epilepsy

Epilepsy has afflicted human beings since the dawn of our species and has been recognized since the earliest medical writings. We now understand that epilepsy is a common disorder resulting from seizures that temporarily impair brain function. Few medical conditions have attracted so much attention and generated so much controversy. Throughout history, people with epilepsy and their families have suffered unfairly because of the ignorance of others. Fortunately, the stigma and fear generated by the words *seizures* and *epilepsy* have progressively diminished during the past century, and most people with epilepsy now lead normal lives.

The Greek physician Hippocrates wrote the first book on epilepsy, titled *On the Sacred Disease*, around 400 B.C. Hippocrates recognized that epilepsy was a brain disorder, and he refuted the ideas that seizures were a curse from the gods and that people with epilepsy held prophetic powers. False ideas die slowly, though, and for centuries epilepsy was considered a curse from the gods or worse. For example, in *Malleus Maleficarum*, a 1494 handbook on witch-hunting written by two Dominican friars under papal authority, one of the characteristics said to identify witches was the presence of seizures. The *Malleus* brought about a wave of persecution and torture and led to more than 200,000 women being put to death. In the early 19th century, people who had severe epilepsy and people with psychiatric disorders were cared for in asylums, but the two groups were separated because seizures were thought to be

3

contagious. In the early 20th century, some U.S. states had laws forbidding people with epilepsy to marry or become parents, and some states permitted sterilizing people with epilepsy.

The modern medical era of epilepsy began in the mid-19th century, under the leadership of three English neurologists: Russell Reynolds, John Hughlings Jackson, and Sir William Richard Gowers. Still standing today is Hughlings Jackson's definition of a seizure as "an occasional, an excessive, and a disorderly discharge of nerve tissue on muscles." Hughlings Jackson also recognized that seizures could alter consciousness, sensation, and behavior.

The past century has brought an explosion of knowledge about the functions of the brain and about epilepsy. Research in epilepsy continues at a vigorous pace, ranging from investigating how microscopic particles in the cell trigger seizures, to developing new antiepileptic drugs, to seeking a better understanding of how epilepsy affects social and intellectual development.

People with Epilepsy Are Not ``Epileptics``

The word *epileptic* should not be used to describe someone who has epilepsy because the term is a "label" that defines a person by one trait. A label is powerful and can create a limiting and negative stereotype. It is better to refer to someone as "a person with epilepsy" or to a group of people as "people with epilepsy."

A Seizure Disorder Is Epilepsy

Because some people fear the word *epilepsy*, they use the term *seizure disorder*, perhaps in an attempt to separate themselves from any association with it. A person who has had two or more seizures has epilepsy, even if the problem first develops in adulthood or is known to be caused by a head injury, a tumor, or other damage to the brain (see Chap. 2).

People with Epilepsy Are Seldom Brain-Damaged

Epilepsy is a disorder of brain *function* that may or may not be associated with damage to brain *structures*. Temporarily disturbed brain function can also occur with extreme fatigue; the use of sleeping pills, sedatives, or general anesthesia; or high fever or serious illness. *Brain damage* implies that something is permanently wrong with the brain's structure. It may occur with head injury, cerebral palsy, or stroke. Injuries to the brain are the cause of seizures in some people with epilepsy, but they are by no means the cause of all of them. Brain injuries range from undetectable to disabling. Although brain cells usually do not regenerate, most people make substantial recoveries after brain injuries. Brain damage, like epilepsy, carries a stigma, and some people may unjustly consider brain-injured patients "incompetent."

People with Epilepsy Usually Are Not Mentally Handicapped

Many people mistakenly believe that people with epilepsy are also mentally handicapped. In most cases, this is not true. Like any other group of people, people with epilepsy have different intellectual abilities. Some are brilliant and some score below average on intelligence tests, but most are somewhere in the middle. They have normal intelligence and lead productive lives. There are some people, however, who have epilepsy associated with brain injuries that cause neurologic impairments, including mental handicap. With only rare exceptions, seizures do not cause mental handicap.

People with Epilepsy Are Not Violent or Crazy

The belief that people with epilepsy are violent is an unfortunate image that is both wrong and destructive. Most people with epilepsy have no greater tendency toward irritability and aggressive behaviors than do other people. Many features of seizures and their immediate aftereffects can be easily misunderstood as "crazy" or "violent." Unfortunately, police officers and even medical personnel may confuse seizure-related actions with these negative behaviors. However, the behavior relating to a seizure merely represents semiconscious or confused actions resulting from the seizure. Some people having a seizure may not respond to questions, speak gibberish, undress, repeat a word or phrase, crumple papers, or appear frightened and scream. Some people are confused immediately after having a seizure, and if they are restrained or prevented from moving about, they can become agitated and combative. Some people may be able to respond to questions and carry on a conversation fairly well after a seizure, but several hours later they will have no recollection of the conversation.

In some people, problems associated with epilepsy, such as injury to specific brain areas or sensitivity to certain medications, can contribute to aggressive or confused behavior. The issue of aggression and epilepsy is discussed in Chapter 28. Anxiety and depression may be slightly more common among people with epilepsy.

Seizures Do Not Cause Brain Damage

Single brief seizures do not cause brain damage. Although tonic-clonic (grand mal) seizures lasting longer than 20 to 60 minutes may injure the brain, there is no evidence that shorter seizures, lasting less than 20 minutes, cause permanent injury to the brain. Prolonged or repetitive complex partial seizures (a type of seizure that occurs in clusters without an intervening return of consciousness) also can potentially cause long-lasting impairment of brain function. Prolonged episodes of other types of seizures are unlikely to injure the brain.

Some people have difficulty with memory and other intellectual functions after a seizure. These problems may be caused by the aftereffects of the seizure on the brain, the effects of antiepileptic drugs, or both. Usually, however, these problems do not mean that the brain has been damaged by the seizure. In some people, there may be a cumulative, negative effect of many tonic-clonic or complex partial seizures on brain function.

Epilepsy Is Not Necessarily Inherited

Most cases of epilepsy are not inherited, although some types are genetically transmitted (that is, passed on through the family). Most of these types are easily controlled with medication.

Epilepsy Is Not a Lifelong Disorder

Most persons with epilepsy have seizures and require medication for only a small portion of their lives. Most childhood forms of epilepsy are outgrown by adulthood. For many forms of epilepsy in children and adults, when the person has been free of seizures for 2 to 4 years medications often can be slowly withdrawn and then discontinued under a doctor's supervision.

Epilepsy Is Not a Curse

Epilepsy has nothing to do with curses, possession, or other supernatural processes, such as punishment for past sins. Like asthma, diabetes, and high blood pressure, epilepsy is a medical problem.

Epilepsy Should Not Be a Barrier to Success

Epilepsy is perfectly compatible with a normal, happy, and full life. The person's quality of life, however, may be affected by the frequency and severity of the seizures, the effects of medications, and associated disorders. Some types of epilepsy are harder to control than others. Living successfully with epilepsy requires a positive outlook, a supportive environment, and good medical care. Coping with the reaction of other people to the disorder can be the most difficult part of living with epilepsy.

Acquiring a positive outlook may be easier said than done, especially for those who have grown up with insecurity and fear. Instilling a sense of self-esteem in children is important. Many children with chronic medical illnesses—such as epilepsy, asthma, or diabetes—have low self-esteem, perhaps caused in part by the reactions of others and in part by parental concern that fosters dependence and insecurity. Children develop strong self-esteem and independence through praise for their accomplishments and emphasis on their potential abilities.

The Brain and Epilepsy

The human brain is an extraordinarily complex organ that controls life-support functions such as breathing and temperature regulation, primitive survival behaviors such as eating and drinking, sleep-wake cycles, emotions, sensations, movements, and intellect. The part of our brain that differs most from the brain of other animals is the *cerebral cortex*, which forms the large outer surface of the upper brain (*cerebrum*). The outer surface contains numerous folds that increase the surface area and allow more cerebral cortex to be packed into the skull. This gives us more "brain power" (Fig. 1).

Anatomy of the Brain

THE CEREBRUM

The cerebrum, or upper brain, is composed of white matter and gray matter (Fig. 2). The gray matter forms the cerebral cortex and consists largely of nerve cells (*neurons*) and supportive cells (*glial cells*). The nerve cells work like computer chips, analyzing and processing information and then sending signals through the nerve fibers. The white matter lies

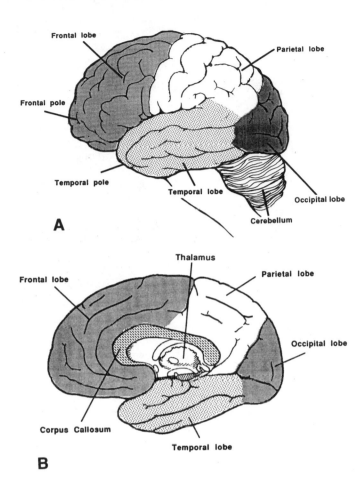

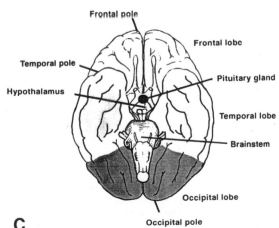

FIGURE 1. Three views of the brain. (*A*) Outer surface (*side view*). (*B*) Inner surface (*cross-sectional view*). (*C*) Lower surface (*bottom view*).

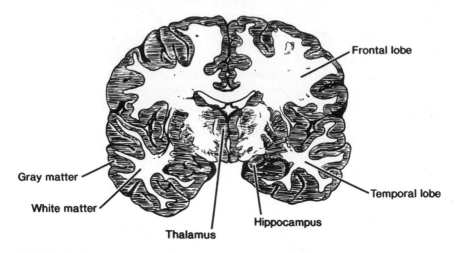

FIGURE 2. Cross-section of the brain showing the gray matter and the white matter.

beneath the cerebral cortex and is composed of nerve fibers. The nerve fibers act like telephone wires, connecting different areas of the brain, spinal cord, muscles, and glands.

The cerebrum is divided into left and right halves, called cerebral hemispheres. These are connected by a large white fiber bundle called the *corpus callosum* (Fig. 1*B*). Each cerebral hemisphere contains four lobes: frontal, parietal, occipital, and temporal. Each lobe contains many different areas that have different functions. For example, in almost all right-handed persons, the area that controls speech lies in the left frontal lobe, and the area that controls understanding of spoken and written language lies in the left temporal lobe. Some brain functions are fairly well confined to specific areas, but most rely on a network of related areas. For functions requiring an integrated network, other areas often can compensate for damage to one area. For example, the ability to focus our attention and concentrate involves both cerebral hemispheres, as well as other areas located in the brain stem (see The Brain Stem and the Spinal Cord). Damage or disruption of function in certain critical areas of this "attention network" can severely disrupt our ability to stay focused. But disruption or damage in other, less critical areas of the network will cause only a mild and temporary disorder of attention.

The right half of the brain controls the left side of the body, and the left half of the brain controls the right side of the body. Therefore, damage to the left cerebral cortex from a head injury or a stroke can cause weakness and loss of sensation on the right side of the body if the motor (movement) or sensory areas of the left cerebral cortex or the fiber bundles that connect these areas with other parts of the brain are damaged.

The cerebral cortex contains areas called the neocortex, including the language areas of the left cerebral hemisphere. The deep, central portions of the frontal and temporal lobes contain the limbic cortex, which controls emotions and memory (Fig. 3C). The limbic cortex is particularly important in epilepsy because in most cases it is the area from which partial seizures arise. The functions of the different parts of the brain are summarized in Figure 3.

Injury or disordered function of the cerebral cortex can cause seizures. If seizures arise from a specific area of the brain, then the initial symptoms of the seizure often reflect the functions of that area. For example, if a seizure starts from the area of the right hemisphere that controls movements in the left thumb, then the seizure may begin with jerking movements of the left thumb or hand. The motor cortex of each hemisphere is organized so that groups of muscles are controlled by specific areas. The lowest part of the motor cortex controls the vocal cords and mouth, the middle part controls the hand and arm, and the upper part controls the leg on the opposite side of the body (Fig. 4).

THE BRAIN STEM AND SPINAL CORD

The lower part of the brain contains the brain stem (Fig. 5), which controls sleep-wake cycles, breathing, and heartbeat. The upper part of the brain stem contains the thalamus and hypothalamus (Figs. 1B and 1C). The spinal cord begins as a continuation of the lower part of the brain stem.

The Thalamus

The *thalamus* processes and filters all sensory information except for the sense of smell. The thalamus serves as a relay station to send important messages about bodily sensations (e.g., the touch of a mosquito landing on the left hand or the sounds and visual impressions of a car) to the cerebral cortex for conscious awareness. At the same time, it helps filter out unimportant messages (e.g., the light pressure of a ring on your finger). The thalamus is also important in pain perception and in regulating the level of consciousness; patients with damage to the thalamus may enter a nearly continuous sleeplike state from which they are difficult to arouse. The thalamus plays an important role in

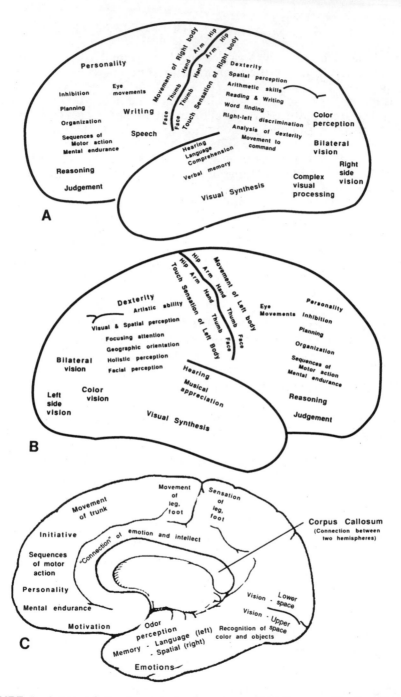

FIGURE 3. Areas of the human brain responsible for specific functions. (*A*) Left hemisphere (*side view*). (*B*) Right hemisphere (*side view*). (*C*) Inner surface (*cross-sectional view*). The areas in the frontal lobe and the side views of the parietal lobe are not so precisely distributed as the drawings indicate, and the areas overlap in their control of some functions.

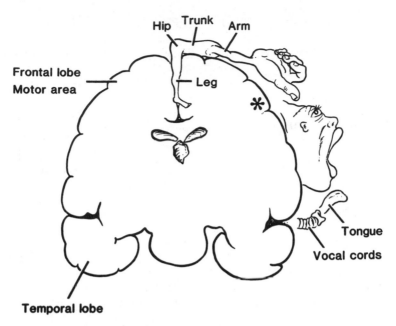

FIGURE 4. A cartoon showing the parts of the body whose movements are controlled by various areas of the motor cortex in the right hemisphere; the asterisk indicates the hand area.

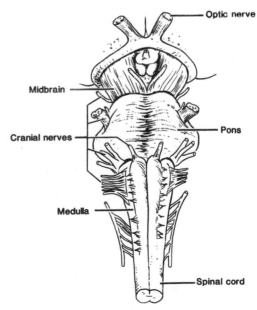

FIGURE 5. The brain stem.

generalized epilepsies and initiates the generalized spike-and-wave patterns seen on the electroencephalogram in these disorders (see Chap. 8).

The Hypothalamus

The *hypothalamus* regulates endocrine (hormone) functions through its control over the pituitary gland. Hormones are proteins released into the bloodstream by an endocrine gland to influence the activity of other parts of the body. The hormones released by the pituitary gland control the activity of other endocrine glands, such as the ovaries, testicles, thyroid, parathyroid, and adrenal glands. The limbic areas of the temporal lobes influence the hypothalamus, which in turn alters pituitary gland functions. This may explain changes in certain hormone functions in people with epilepsy, such as irregular menstrual cycles. Hormones also influence the limbic areas. For example, the stress hormone cortisol and the sex hormones estrogen, progesterone, and testosterone all attach to cells in the limbic areas and affect the functions of these cells. This probably explains why some women are more prone to seizures, migraine attacks, or emotional changes at certain times during their menstrual cycle.

The Lower Brain Stem

The lower part of the brain stem (Fig. 5) controls movement and sensation of the face, eye movements, taste, heartbeat, breathing, and other bodily functions, such as how much acid is produced by the stomach.

The Cerebellum

The *cerebellum*, located behind the brain stem, helps coordinate complex movements and is one of the reasons why we get better when we practice difficult tasks such as playing the piano. The cerebellum also has a role in regulating intellectual and behavioral functions.

The Spinal Cord

The *spinal cord* receives and sends information to the body about senses and movement. For example, cells in the motor area of the left cerebral cortex send fibers ("brain wires") down through the brain stem. In the lower brain stem, these fibers cross over to the opposite (right) side and continue downward into the right side of the spinal cord. This explains why the left cerebral cortex controls movements of the right side of the body. In the spinal cord, these fibers activate other cells, which in turn send fibers into the nerves that pass into the arm and directly activate the muscles to make the hand move.

Similarly, there are touch receptors in the hand. When these receptors are activated by touch, they excite nerve impulses to flow up the same nerves in the arm. The sensory fibers (axons) carrying information toward the spinal cord are bundled with the motor fibers (axons) carrying signals from the spinal cord to the muscles. These bundles of sensory and motor fibers are called the peripheral nerves. This sensory information then passes up the spinal cord to the lower brain stem, where there is a relay station. This is a group of nerve cells that receive the information and pass it on to a new fiber called an axon, which crosses over to the opposite half of the brain stem and goes up to another relay station in the thalamus. This crossing-over explains why touch information from the right hand ends up in the left cerebral cortex.

From the thalamus, the information finally makes its way to the parietal lobe of the brain, the area that brings touch sensation to conscious awareness. The motor and touch sensation areas of each hemisphere communicate with each other. This communication allows us to make precise, complex movements and to know instinctively where the parts of our body are in space. Without it there would be no basketball stars or concert pianists.

THE CENTRAL AND PERIPHERAL NERVOUS SYSTEMS

Together, the brain and spinal cord are called the *central nervous system*. The nerves in the face, arms, and legs make up the *peripheral nervous system*. Epilepsy is a disorder of the central nervous system—specifically the brain. Some chiropractors say that problems in the spinal cord or in the blood vessels associated with the spinal bones of the neck may contribute to epilepsy. There is no evidence to support these claims, except in extremely rare cases in which strokes from blockages of these blood vessels are followed by epilepsy. In such cases, chiropractic manipulation of the neck can be dangerous.

Nerve Cells of the Brain

Nerve cells (neurons) are the building blocks of the brain. Nerve cells are so small that a microscope is needed to see them. There are approximately 14 billion nerve cells in the brain and spinal cord. Nerve cells are usually composed of three parts: the cell body, axon, and dendrites

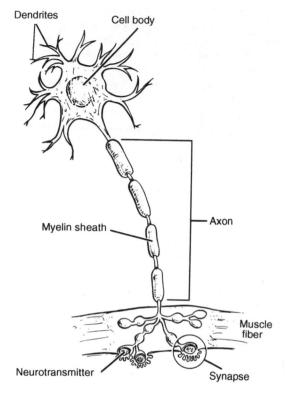

FIGURE 6. A neuron (nerve cell).

(Fig. 6). The cell body (*soma*) contains the enzymes and chemicals that regulate the metabolism of the cell and genetic information to power and direct the cell's activities. The *axon* is the long portion of a nerve cell that resembles a wire. Axons are the critical, "transmitting" parts of the nerve fibers in both the central and peripheral nervous systems. The axons that go from the motor area in the cerebral cortex to the leg area in the spinal cord can be more than 4 feet long. The message to wiggle your toes quite literally goes down the axon. Therefore, axons act like copper wires in a telephone system.

Most axons are surrounded by a fatty covering called *myelin,* which serves the same function that plastic does around telephone wires—to insulate the wires from each other and prevent "cross-talk" between the different wires. The heavier the coating of myelin, the faster an axon transmits its messages. The fastest axons in the nervous system transmit messages at a rate of approximately 350 feet per second.

Axons carry chemical messengers known as *neurotransmitters* from the cell body to the end of the axon, where they are passed to other nerve cells. The space between the end of the axon and either a muscle fiber or the dendrite of another nerve cell is called the *synapse*. *Dendrites* serve as the cell's receiving antennas. The neurotransmitters released from the axon travel across the synapse to interact with receptors on the muscle or dendrite.

Most nerve cells have thousands of synapses on their dendrites, with various kinds of receptors into which neurotransmitters fit the way a key fits into a lock. A specific key is needed for a specific lock—there are no "master keys" in the brain. These chemical neurotransmitters may increase (excite) or decrease (inhibit) the cell's activity and thereby change the electrical activity and chemical composition of the cell. Thus, both electrical and chemical systems are critical for nerve cell functions and for the transmission of information in the nervous system.

Each nerve cell is bombarded by hundreds of impulses every second. One of the wonders of the human brain is how the billions of individual computers (nerve cells) in the brain function in a coordinated fashion to control our movements and breathing and, most importantly, allow us to think and feel.

Neurotransmitters

Neurotransmitters are the chemical messengers of the brain. These substances are produced in the nerve cell body, carried down the inside of the axon, and released at its end. The neurotransmitters then cross the synapse, a tiny space between the walls of the axon and the dendrite, to bind to receptors located on the dendrite.

There are many kinds of neurotransmitters, but each individual nerve cell produces only one major type. Some of the neurotransmitters are carried a long distance within the nervous system. Others have local effects; that is, they are produced by and released onto cells that are close to each other. Neurotransmitters are important in diseases of the nervous system. In Parkinson's disease, for example, there is degeneration of the cells in the brain stem that manufacture dopamine, an important neurotransmitter that regulates movement. Loss of nerve cells may contribute to the development of epilepsy in some cases. For example, prolonged lack of oxygen may cause a selective loss of cells in the hippocampus (see Fig. 2), which may lead to epilepsy.

Some of the major brain neurotransmitters can be classified as *excitatory*. They stimulate or increase brain electrical activity; that is, they cause nerve cells to fire. Others are *inhibitory*. They shut off or decrease brain electrical activity; that is, they cause nerve cells to stop firing. According to one theory, epilepsy is caused by an imbalance between neurotransmitters that cause nerve cells to fire and those that cause them to stop firing. Either a deficiency of inhibitory neurotransmitters such as GABA or an excess of excitatory neurotransmitters such as glutamate increases the likelihood that a seizure will occur. Much research is being conducted in this area. Many of the new drugs being developed to treat epilepsy act by increasing activity in the inhibitory systems, which turn cells off, or by decreasing activity in the excitatory systems, which turn cells on.

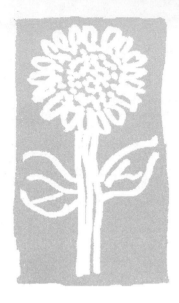

Seizures

A seizure is not a disease. Rather, a seizure is a symptom of many different disorders that can affect the brain. A person with diabetes whose blood sugar becomes extremely low or high can have a seizure. A person who drinks too much alcohol for many years can have seizures, especially during the first several days after drinking is stopped. High fevers, especially in infants and young children, can cause seizures. Head injury, stroke, brain tumors, and brain infections also can cause seizures.

Definition of Seizures and Epilepsy

A *seizure* is a brief, excessive surge of electrical activity in the brain that causes a change in how a person feels, senses things, or behaves. Seizures can cause an incredible range of effects. A sensation of "pins and needles" in the thumb for a few seconds can be a seizure. So can a smell of burnt rubber and a strange feeling in the belly, a ringing sound that keeps increasing in volume, staring with loss of awareness for several minutes, or convulsive movements. Many patients consider only their tonic-clonic convulsive seizures to be "seizures" and regard other seizure symptoms such as jerks and auras to be nothing important or perhaps "minor spells." However, even very minor symptoms are seizures if they are changes in behavior that result from an abnormal brain electrical discharge.

Epilepsy is a disorder in which a person has two or more seizures without a clear cause (such as alcohol withdrawal). In other words, epilepsy is a condition of *recurrent* and *unprovoked seizures.* The seizures may be the result of a hereditary tendency or a brain injury. Often, particularly in people without apparent risk factors who are otherwise healthy, the cause is unknown. It is a common misconception that all seizures, regardless of their cause, can be referred to as epilepsy.

For many persons, the diagnosis of *epilepsy* seems more serious and frightening than *seizure disorder.* However, epilepsy is a seizure disorder. Accepting the condition for what it is, name and all, is often the first step toward leading a normal life. Epilepsy refers to all individuals who have had two or more seizures, regardless of seizure severity, the age at which the seizures began, or their origin, except for clearly identified causes such as heart problems, alcohol withdrawal, or extremely low blood sugar.

Impairment of Consciousness

A simple definition of *consciousness* is the ability to respond and to remember. People with some kinds of seizures do not recall the seizure and don't even know that they have had a seizure. Others are aware that they had a seizure, but are absolutely convinced that they had no loss or impairment of consciousness when, in fact, they did. Therefore, it is helpful to have a family member or friend test the person during a seizure by asking him or her to follow commands such as "show me your left hand" and "remember the word yellow." If the person can follow the command and remember the word, consciousness was preserved, at least during the time tested.

Although neurologists describe consciousness during seizures as either *impaired* or *preserved,* the two categories are not as clearly separate as one might imagine. The degree of impairment or preservation of consciousness varies from seizure to seizure. Consciousness is affected if either responsiveness or memory is impaired during an attack, but these two criteria do not have the same importance for the person's functioning. For example, during a seizure someone may be able to respond to most commands, but later be unable to recall some details of the seizure. In certain cases, individuals may be able to operate dangerous equipment safely or perform complex tasks during a seizure regardless of whether they can later recall what happened. Some seizures, however, may impair a person's ability to move voluntarily. The person is unable to speak or raise his or her hand when asked, but may be able to recall the entire event. This person did not have impaired consciousness, but had impaired motor control. Even in the same individual, the degree of impairment of function can vary dramatically from seizure to seizure.

Classification of Seizures

Seizures can be broadly separated into two groups: (1) primary generalized seizures and (2) partial seizures (Table 1). Primary generalized seizures begin with a widespread, excessive electrical discharge involving both sides of the brain at the same time. In contrast, partial seizures begin with an abnormal electrical discharge restricted to one region of the brain. Distinguishing primary generalized seizures from partial seizures is important because the types of tests needed and the drugs used to treat these disorders differ. A description of what happened before, during, and after the seizure and recordings of electrical activity generated by the brain (*brain waves*) help the doctor determine the type of seizure. In particular, the moments before a seizure or the first few seconds of a seizure are important to the doctor. Brain waves are recorded with an electroencephalograph machine; the test is called an electroencephalogram (EEG). It can detect abnormal electrical impulses in people with epilepsy (see Chap. 8).

TABLE 1
CLASSIFICATION OF EPILEPTIC SEIZURES

PRIMARY GENERALIZED SEIZURES

Absence seizures (typical and atypical)

Myoclonic seizures

Atonic seizures

Clonic seizures

Tonic seizures

Tonic-clonic seizures

PARTIAL SEIZURES (SEIZURES ORIGINATING IN SPECIFIC PARTS OF THE BRAIN)

Simple partial seizures (consciousness not impaired)
   With motor symptoms (jerking, stiffening)
   With somatosensory (touch) or specialized sensory (smell, hearing, taste, sight)
      symptoms
   With autonomic symptoms (heart rate change, internal sensations)
   With psychic symptoms (*déja vu,* dreamy state)

Complex partial seizures (consciousness impaired, automatisms usually present)
   Beginning as simple partial seizures
   Beginning with impairment of consciousness

Partial seizures secondarily generalized to tonic-clonic seizures

In primary generalized seizures, the EEG shows a widespread increase in electrical activity. In partial seizures, the brain waves show a more restricted, or local, increase of electrical activity. The EEG may be normal in people with epilepsy, however, and occasionally it shows "epilepsy waves" in people who have never had a seizure.

Hereditary factors are more important in primary generalized seizures than in partial seizures. In some cases, it can be difficult to distinguish primary generalized seizures from partial seizures because many of their features overlap. For example, a tonic-clonic seizure may begin as a primary generalized seizure or as a partial seizure, and a staring spell can be an absence seizure (a type of primary generalized seizure) or a complex partial seizure. We will describe all of these types of seizures in the next part of the chapter.

PRIMARY GENERALIZED SEIZURES

Primary generalized seizures begin from both sides of the brain at the same time. The principal types of primary generalized seizures are called absence seizures, atypical absence seizures, myoclonic seizures, atonic seizures, clonic seizures, tonic seizures, and tonic-clonic seizures.

Absence Seizures

> Frank, a 7-year-old boy, often "blanks out" for a few seconds and sometimes for 10 to 20 seconds. His teacher calls his name, but he doesn't seem to hear her. He usually blinks repetitively, and his eyes may roll up a bit, but with the short seizures he just stares. Then he is right back where he left off. Some days he has more than 50 of these spells.

Absence (petit mal) seizures are brief episodes of staring with impairment of awareness and responsiveness. The episode usually lasts less than 10 seconds, but may last as long as 20 seconds. The seizure begins and ends suddenly. There is no warning before the seizure, and immediately afterward the person is alert and attentive and usually unaware that a seizure has occurred. These spells usually begin in children between 4 and 14 years of age. In approximately 75% of these children, absence seizures do not continue after age 18. Absence seizures often may be provoked by rapid breathing (hyperventilation). They usually can be reproduced in the doctor's office with rapid breathing if the patient is not taking medication. For some reason, however, absence seizures are uncommon with rapid breathing during exercise. Children with absence seizures have normal development and intelligence, but may have higher rates of behavioral, educational, and social problems than other children.

Simple absence seizures are just "stares." However, most absence seizures are *complex absence seizures,* in which staring is accompanied by some change in muscle activity, especially if the seizure lasts more than 10 seconds. The most common movements are eye blinks, but others include slight tasting movements of the mouth, hand movements such as rubbing the fingers together, and contraction or relaxation of the muscles.

The EEG is extremely helpful in diagnosing absence seizures. In most cases, a characteristic finding is spike-and-wave discharges at a rate of 3 per second or faster, especially during hyperventilation (see Chap. 8, Fig. 13). Because tests that show images of the brain, such as computed tomography (CT, often called a "CAT scan") and magnetic resonance imaging (MRI) (see Chap. 8), are normal in children with absence seizures, in most cases they are not needed. Absence seizures may be confused with complex partial seizures (discussed later). Absence seizures are usually briefer (less than 20 seconds), however, and are not associated with a warning (aura) or postepisode symptoms such as tiredness.

Atypical Absence Seizures

It is hard for me to tell when Kathy is having one of her staring spells. During the spells, she doesn't respond as quickly as at other times. The problem is that even when she is not having an absence seizure she often doesn't respond very quickly, and she often just stares when she is not having an absence seizure.

Like typical absence seizures, the staring spells of *atypical absence seizures* occur predominantly in children. They usually begin before 6 years of age. Unlike typical absence seizures, atypical absence seizures often begin and end gradually (over seconds), often last more than 10 seconds (the usual duration is 5 to 30 seconds), and usually are not provoked by rapid breathing. The child stares, but often has only a partial reduction in responsiveness. Eye blinking or slight jerking movements of the lips may occur. Children who have these seizures are more likely to have lower-than-average intelligence and difficult-to-control seizures (myoclonic, tonic, and tonic-clonic types in addition to the atypical absence seizures). Atypical absence seizures can be hard to distinguish from the child's usual behavior, especially in those with lower intelligence.

Most children with these seizures have an abnormal EEG, with slow spike-and-wave discharges even when they are not having a seizure. The EEG abnormality is usually not provoked by hyperventilation. Unlike typical absence seizures, atypical absence seizures usually do not stop in later childhood.

Myoclonic Seizures

In the morning I get these "jumps." My arms just go flying up for a second. I often spill my coffee or drop the book I am holding. Occasionally my mouth shuts for a split second. Sometimes I get a few of these jumps in a row. After I have been up for a few hours, I don't get any more of these jumps.

Myoclonic seizures occur as brief, shock-like jerks of a muscle or group of muscles. Myoclonus may occur in people who do not have epilepsy. For example, as many people fall asleep, their body suddenly jerks. This is referred to as *sleep jerks* or *benign nocturnal myoclonus*. Among the abnormal forms of myoclonus are both epileptic and nonepileptic types.

Epileptic myoclonus usually causes abnormal movements on both sides of the body at the same time. The neck, shoulders, upper arms, body, and upper legs are usually involved. Myoclonic seizures occur in a variety of disorders that have different sets of characteristics. How well these seizures can be controlled depends on which of these disorders (syndromes) affects the individual. Many of these syndromes are discussed in more detail in Chapter 4.

Myoclonic seizures in the juvenile myoclonic epilepsy syndrome most often involve the neck, shoulders, and upper arms. The seizures tend to occur within 1 hour after awakening. They are usually well controlled with medication, but the person almost always needs to take medication throughout his or her life.

The Lennox-Gastaut syndrome often includes myoclonic seizures, tonic seizures, and other types. During these attacks, the jerking may be so strong that the person will fall. These seizures also involve the neck, shoulders, and upper arms and the muscles of the face. Seizures in patients with this syndrome are often difficult to control.

Progressive myoclonic epilepsy is a group of disorders associated with deterioration of the nervous system. These disorders are rare when compared with the other types of myoclonic seizures.

Atonic Seizures

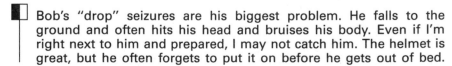

Bob's "drop" seizures are his biggest problem. He falls to the ground and often hits his head and bruises his body. Even if I'm right next to him and prepared, I may not catch him. The helmet is great, but he often forgets to put it on before he gets out of bed.

> Even with carpet in the bedroom and mats in the bathroom, he gets hurt.

In an *atonic seizure,* the person suddenly loses muscle strength. The eyelids may droop, the head may nod, objects may be dropped, or the person may fall to the ground. Atonic seizures usually begin in childhood. Although they last less than 15 seconds, they frequently cause sudden falls, so injury is common. When patients with "drop seizures" are studied carefully, most are found to have *tonic* seizures (associated with muscle contraction) not *atonic* seizures. (See Tonic Seizures.)

Clonic Seizures

Clonic seizures are rare and cause rhythmic jerking movements of the arms and legs. These may be generalized, convulsive seizures with jerking (clonic) movements on both sides of the body, but without the stiffening (tonic) component seen in the more common tonic-clonic seizures. Clonic seizures, unlike tonic-clonic seizures, are not followed by a prolonged period of confusion or tiredness after the seizure has ended.

Some tonic-clonic seizures are preceded by a series of jerking movements. These seizures are referred to as clonic-tonic-clonic seizures and can occur with juvenile myoclonic epilepsy (see Chap. 4).

Tonic Seizures

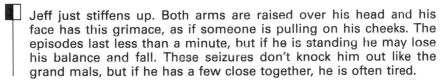

> Jeff just stiffens up. Both arms are raised over his head and his face has this grimace, as if someone is pulling on his cheeks. The episodes last less than a minute, but if he is standing he may lose his balance and fall. These seizures don't knock him out like the grand mals, but if he has a few close together, he is often tired.

Tonic seizures, usually lasting less than 20 seconds, are associated with sudden stiffening movements of the body, arms, or legs and involve both sides of the body. They are more common during sleep. The person often will fall if the seizure occurs while he or she is standing. Tonic seizures are most common in children who have lower-than-average scores on intelligence tests, but they can occur in any child or adult.

Tonic-Clonic Seizures

> These are the seizures that frighten me. They last only a minute or two, but it feels like an eternity. I can often tell they are coming because she is more cranky and out of sorts. When it starts,

> Heather suddenly shrieks with this unnatural cry, then she falls and every muscle in her body seems to be activated. Her teeth clench. I know she can't swallow her tongue, but I still worry that she might. At the very beginning, she is pale, and later, a slight bluish color. Shortly after she falls, her arms and upper body start to jerk while her legs are more or less still stiff. This is the longest part of the seizure. Then it finally stops and she passes into a deep sleep.

Tonic-clonic (grand mal) seizures are convulsive seizures. The person briefly stiffens and loses consciousness, falls, and often utters a cry. It is not a cry from pain, but is caused by air being forced through the contracting vocal cords. The stiffening is followed by jerking of the arms and legs. The seizures usually last 1 to 3 minutes. There may be excessive saliva production, sometimes incorrectly described as "foaming" at the mouth. Biting of the tongue or cheek may cause bleeding. Loss of urine or, rarely, a bowel movement may occur. After the convulsion the person may be tired and confused for minutes or hours and often goes to sleep. He or she also may be agitated or depressed. The time immediately after the seizure is called the *postictal* period. First aid for tonic-clonic seizures is discussed in Chapter 9.

When tonic-clonic seizures last more than 30 minutes or recur in a series of three or more seizures without the person returning to a normal state in between, a dangerous condition called *convulsive status epilepticus* has developed. There is debate about whether convulsive status epilepticus is defined by 5 or 30 minutes of continuous seizure activity, but medical help should be obtained if tonic-clonic seizures last longer than 5 minutes (see Chap. 9). The exact duration of continuous seizure activity that is harmful to the brain is not well defined; children appear to tolerate seizures that last longer than 5 minutes better than adults do.

PARTIAL SEIZURES

Partial seizures begin with an abnormal burst of electrical activity in a restricted area of brain tissue. Most partial seizures arise from the temporal or frontal lobes. Less commonly, partial seizures begin in the visual (occipital lobe) or sensory (parietal lobe) areas of the brain. Head injury, brain infections, stroke, and brain tumors are common causes of partial seizures. In some cases, hereditary factors are important. In most cases, no cause can be identified.

Partial seizures are divided into two main types, depending on whether consciousness is fully preserved. During *simple partial seizures,* the person is alert, is able to respond to questions or commands, and can remember what occurred during the seizure. During *complex partial seizures,* the ability to pay attention or respond to questions or commands is impaired to some degree. Often, there is no memory of what happened during all or part of the seizure. The distinction between simple and complex partial seizures is critical because the ability to drive, operate dangerous equipment, swim alone, and perform other activities usually has to be restricted in people with uncontrolled complex partial seizures.

Simple Partial Seizures

I almost enjoy them. I have the feeling of *déja vu,* like I have lived through this moment, and I even know what is going to be said next. Everything seems brighter and more alive.

It is a pressure that begins in my stomach and then rises up to my chest and throat. When it reaches my chest, I smell the same odor—something burnt, definitely unpleasant. At the same time I feel nervous—not because of the aura, I just get anxious.

Simple partial seizures can cause a remarkably diverse group of symptoms. In some cases, the symptoms are not recognized as a seizure because many symptoms of partial seizures can also be caused by other factors. For example, abdominal discomfort is likely to be the result of a gastrointestinal disorder, but it also can be a symptom of a partial seizure arising in the temporal lobe. Tingling in the little finger that spreads to the forearm may come from a seizure, a migraine, or a peripheral nerve disorder (e.g., "pinched nerve"). There are several types of simple partial seizures: motor seizures, autonomic seizures, and psychic seizures.

Motor seizures involve a change in muscle activity. Most often, the body stiffens or the muscles begin to jerk in one area of the body such as a finger or wrist. The abnormal movements may remain restricted to one body part or may spread to involve other muscles on the same side or both sides of the body. Some partial motor seizures cause weakness of one or more body parts, including the vocal apparatus, which affects the ability to speak. Motor seizures may also include coordinated actions such as laughter or automatic hand movements, with or without consciousness.

Sensory seizures cause changes in sensation. Most often, a person has a hallucination (the sensation of something that is not there), such as a feeling of "pins and needles" in a finger or seeing a red ball. The abnormal sensations may remain restricted to one area of the body or may spread to other areas. There also may be an illusion (the distortion of a true sensation). For example, a car that is standing still may appear to be moving farther away or a person's voice may seem muffled and difficult to understand. Hallucinations and illusions can involve all types of sensations, including touch (e.g., numbness or "pins and needles"), smell (often an unpleasant odor), taste, vision (e.g., a spot of light or a scene with people), hearing (e.g., a click, ringing, or a person's voice), and orientation in space (e.g., a floating or spinning feeling).

Autonomic seizures cause changes in the part of the nervous system that automatically controls bodily functions. The autonomic nervous system is formed by groups of cells and fibers in the hypothalamus, lower brain stem, spinal cord, and peripheral nervous system. However, parts of the cerebral cortex, especially the limbic regions, can strongly influence activity in the autonomic nervous system. This is the reason why strong emotions such as fear are associated with sweating, increases in the heart rate and breathing rate, and a sinking feeling in the chest. The connection between the limbic system and the autonomic nervous system may also be the physiological basis of why we say such things as "In my heart, I feel it's right" or "I just have this feeling in my gut." These visceral sensations are probably linked with the emotions in limbic structures. Partial seizures commonly arise from the limbic system. Therefore, autonomic changes are common during partial seizures. Autonomic partial seizures can cause a strange or unpleasant sensation in the abdomen, chest, or head. There may be changes in heart rate or breathing rate, sweating, or goose bumps that occur for no reason. Autonomic partial seizures are common.

Psychic seizures cause changes in the brain that affect how we think, feel, and experience things. These seizures can cause problems with language function—such as garbled speech, inability to find the right word, and difficulty understanding spoken or written language—and problems with time perception and memory. One type of psychic seizure causes sudden emotions such as fear, anxiety, depression, or happiness. These emotions are spontaneous; they do not result from seeing, hearing, or thinking about something that might trigger the emotion. Other psychic seizures can make a person feel as if:

- He or she has experienced or lived through this moment before (*déja vu*).
- Familiar things are strange and foreign (*jamais vu*).
- They are not themselves (depersonalization).
- The world is not real.
- They are in a dream (derealization) or watching themselves in a movie or from outside their body.

Psychic seizures arise from the limbic areas or more highly advanced areas of the cerebral cortex.

Complex Partial Seizures

Harold's spells begin with a warning; he says he is going to have a seizure and usually sits down. I ask him what he feels, but he either doesn't answer or just says, "I feel it." Then he makes a funny face, like he is both surprised and a bit distressed. He just stares. I call his name, and he may look at me when I call, but he never answers. During this part, he may make these mouth movements, as if he is tasting something. He often grabs the arm of the chair and squeezes it. Other times, he touches his shirt, as if he is picking lint off, even though it's clean. The whole thing lasts a couple of minutes, and then as he comes back he keeps asking questions. He never remembers that he has a warning, and never remembers what he asks or says right after the seizure. He looks tired afterward; if he has two of these spells in the same day he often goes to sleep after the second one.

■ Susan's seizures usually occur during sleep. She makes this grunting sound, like she is clearing her throat. She sits up in bed, opens her eyes, and stares. She sometimes clasps her hands together. I ask her what she is doing, but she doesn't say a word. After a minute or so, she lies back down and goes back to sleep.

With *complex partial seizures* (also known as *psychomotor* or *temporal lobe seizures*), consciousness is impaired, but not lost. In most cases the person stares and is unable to respond to questions or commands or responds incompletely and inaccurately. Automatic movements (*automatisms*) occur in most complex partial seizures. Automatisms can involve the mouth and face (e.g., lip smacking, chewing, tasting, and swallowing movements), the hands and arms (e.g., fumbling, picking, tapping, or clasping movements), vocalizations (e.g., grunts or repetition of words or phrases), or more complex acts (e.g., walking or mixing foods in a bowl). Other, less common automatisms include screaming, crying, running, shouting, bizarre and sometimes "sexual" movements, disrobing, and laughing. Complex partial seizures usually last from 30 seconds to 2 minutes. Auras, or warnings, which are actually simple partial seizures, are common and typically occur seconds before consciousness is altered. After the seizure, lethargy and confusion often occur, but usually last less than 15 minutes. Complex partial seizures occur in persons of all ages.

Some people are unaware that they have had a complex partial seizure. Many of the symptoms are so subtle that others may just think the person is thinking about something, daydreaming, or spacing out. These episodes can cause memory lapses; someone who has a complex partial seizure may perform fairly complex activities and later have no recollection of them. One of the earliest reported medical cases was that of a doctor. One day he found himself walking away from a ward and realized that he was supposed to examine a patient. He found the patient's bed and examined the woman. To his amazement, when he went to write his note, he found that he had been there just before and had written down the correct diagnosis—pneumonia in the bottom of the left lung—but had no recollection of ever having seen the woman. It is likely that he examined her and made his notes either just before or after a complex partial seizure, which "wiped out" his memory for a short period.

Some automatic behaviors pose a danger to persons with complex partial seizures. For example, a child may walk in front of a moving school bus or an adult may cross the street against a red light.

Some unusual automatic behaviors of complex partial seizures can be a source of great embarrassment and concern. For some persons, these unusual automatisms are typical for their seizures. Others may have more common automatisms most of the time, but occasionally have embarrassing behavior, such as disrobing at work. This was a problem, for example, in a person I cared for who worked in an elementary school. As with most other aspects of epilepsy, special precautions can be taken to help minimize the negative effects of such behaviors.

Secondarily Generalized Seizures

They start with a tingling in the right thumb. Then the thumb starts jerking. In a few seconds, the whole right hand is jerking. I learned to start rubbing and scratching my forearm. Sometimes I can stop the seizure this way. Other times the jerking spreads up the arm. When it reaches the shoulder, I pass out and people tell me that my whole body starts to jerk.

I see this colored ball on my right side. The ball seems to grow and fill up my whole view. As the ball grows, everything becomes like a dream and I don't feel real. It is the strangest feeling. The seizure can just stop and my vision is just a little blurry, or it can go all the way, so that I fall to the floor and have a grand mal.

When a burst of excessive electrical activity that starts in a limited area spreads to involve both sides of the brain, the partial seizure may become a *secondarily generalized tonic-clonic seizure*. Secondarily generalized seizures are common, occurring in more than 30% of children and adults with partial epilepsy. Patients may or may not recall an aura, and witnesses may first observe a complex partial seizure that progresses to a tonic-clonic seizure. A secondarily generalized tonic-clonic seizure may be difficult to distinguish from a primary generalized tonic-clonic seizure, especially if it is not witnessed or occurs during sleep. (Most convulsive seizures in sleep begin as partial seizures.) The EEG and MRI are often helpful in distinguishing these seizures.

The Postictal Period

The period immediately after a seizure—called the postictal period—varies depending on the type, duration, and intensity of the seizure, as well as other factors. Absence seizures are not followed by any symptoms—when the seizure ends, the person resumes activity as if nothing had happened. After most complex partial seizures, the person is slightly confused and tired, usually for less than 5 to 15 minutes. Immediately after a tonic-clonic seizure, the person appears frighteningly limp and unresponsive and may be pale or bluish. On awakening, the person often complains of muscle soreness, headache, and pain in the tongue or cheek if those areas were bitten. The person may be confused and tired. Often those who have had a tonic-clonic seizure awaken briefly and then go to sleep.

Other symptoms follow some seizures. Weakness of an arm after a partial motor or tonic-clonic seizure may be symptoms of Todd's paralysis. This condition was first described in the mid-1800s as muscle weakness affecting one side of the body. Seizures may also be followed by impairments in vision, touch sensation, language, and other functions. Often, the nature of the postictal problem can help identify the area where the seizure began. For example, weakness in the right arm and leg may follow a seizure that began in the motor area of the left hemisphere.

For some patients, postictal symptoms can be more troublesome than the seizure itself. In such cases, changes in antiepileptic drugs may not alter the seizures, but may minimize the postictal symptoms. In other cases, treatment of specific symptoms (e.g., using medications for migraine headache to treat postictal headache) can be helpful.

Change in Seizure Patterns

Many people have more than one type of seizure. For example, one person may have both simple and complex partial seizures or simple and complex partial seizures along with secondarily generalized tonic-clonic seizures. Someone else may have both absence and myoclonic seizures or myoclonic and tonic-clonic seizures. In addition, the features of each type of seizure may change from seizure to seizure. More often, the features change over months or years. For instance, a person's simple partial seizures that precede tonic-clonic seizures may change from an unpleasant smell and a strange stomach sensation to simply a sensation of chest discomfort, or there may no longer be any warning at all before the tonic-clonic seizures.

Changes in a person's seizures may result from changes in the patterns of spread of the abnormal electrical discharge. In the case of the person whose aura (simple partial seizure) no longer precedes the tonic-clonic seizure, the area from which the seizure begins and the intensity of the discharge probably have not changed, but the electrical activity may have taken other pathways that allow it to spread more rapidly. In this case, the absence of a warning may prevent the person from avoiding injury even though the seizure is no more severe than before.

Those who have had mild forms of seizures, such as simple partial or absence seizures, later may experience tonic-clonic seizures. In some instances, the change in seizure type may result from factors such as missed medication or lack of sleep. For others, it is just the way their disorder develops; they have always had a small chance of having a tonic-clonic seizure.

We don't know exactly why seizure patterns change over time. There may be some changes in the brain, such as reorganization of connections or an increase or decrease in the concentrations of certain chemicals. If seizures become more frequent or more severe, a medical checkup is advisable.

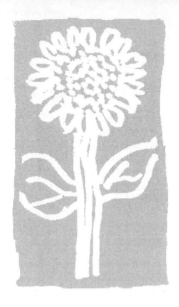

4

Epileptic Syndromes

When a disorder is defined by a characteristic group of features, it is called a *syndrome*. These features may be symptoms or signs of the disorder. *Symptoms* are problems the patient notices or mentions to the doctor. *Signs* are what the doctor observes during the examination or from laboratory studies.

Epileptic syndromes are defined by a cluster of features such as the seizure types, age when seizures begin, electroencephalogram (EEG) findings, and future outlook (prognosis). Classifying an epileptic syndrome often provides information on how long the seizures will persist and what medications are most helpful. Some of the most common or well-defined epileptic syndromes are febrile seizures, benign rolandic epilepsy, juvenile myoclonic epilepsy, infantile spasms, Lennox-Gastaut syndrome, reflex epilepsies, temporal lobe epilepsy, and frontal lobe epilepsy. Rare epilepsy syndromes include progressive myoclonic epilepsies, mitochondrial disorders, Landau-Kleffner syndrome, and Rasmussen's syndrome.

33

Common and Well-Defined Epileptic Syndromes

FEBRILE SEIZURES

Tommy was just 14 months old. He caught a bad cold from one of the children in the playgroup. He had a fever and runny nose. He was taking a nap when I heard this strange banging sound. I ran into his room, and his whole body was stiff and shaking. The whole thing probably lasted less than 10 minutes. They were the longest 10 minutes of my life. He has never had another one and doesn't need any seizure medication. Now when he has a fever I give him Tylenol.

Children aged 3 months to 5 years may have tonic-clonic seizures when they have a high fever. These are called febrile seizures and occur in 2% to 5% of children. There is a slight hereditary tendency toward febrile seizures. Therefore, the chances are slightly increased that a child will have febrile seizures if a parent, brother, sister, or other close relative has had them. The usual situation is a healthy child with normal development, aged 6 months to 2 years, who has a viral illness with high fever. As the child's temperature rapidly rises, he or she has a tonic-clonic seizure. The seizure usually involves muscles on both sides of the body. Unlike tonic-clonic seizures in later childhood and adulthood, febrile seizures often last longer than 5 minutes. In most instances, hospitalization is not necessary, although a prompt medical consultation is essential after the first seizure.

The prognosis for febrile seizures is excellent. There is no reason for a child who has had a single febrile seizure to receive antiepileptic drugs unless the seizure was unusually long or other medical conditions warrant it. Recurrence rates (the chances of having another seizure) vary from 50% if the seizure occurred before age 1 year to 25% if the seizure occurred after that age. In addition, 25% to 50% of recurrent febrile seizures are not preceded by a fever. Instead, the seizure is the first sign of an illness (usually viral) and the fever comes later.

Most children with febrile seizures do not have seizures without fever after age 5. Risk factors for later epilepsy include: (1) abnormal development before the febrile seizure, (2) complex febrile seizures (seizures lasting longer than 15 minutes, more than one seizure in 24 hours, or movements restricted to one side), and (3) a history of seizures without fever in a parent, brother, or sister. If none of these risk factors are present, the chances of later epilepsy are the same or nearly the same as in the general population; if one risk factor is present, the chances of later epilepsy are 2.5%; if two or more risk factors are present, the chances of later epilepsy range from 5% to more than 10%. Rarely, febrile seizures that last more than 30 minutes may cause scar tissue in the temporal lobe and chronic epilepsy that can be effectively treated with medication or a temporal lobectomy (see Chaps. 10, 11, and 12).

Studies have shown that febrile seizures cannot be prevented by baths, applying cool cloths to the child's head or body, or using fever-reducing medications such as acetaminophen (Tylenol) or ibuprofen (Advil). These findings go against the intuition of most parents and pediatricians, but they are proven. Cooling the child's body or head does not regulate the temperature in the brain. Tylenol or Advil can be used to help a feverish child feel better, but it does not prevent febrile seizures. (Aspirin should not be given to young children because of the potential risk of precipitating a serious disorder called Reye's syndrome).

Most children with recurrent febrile seizures do not require daily antiepileptic drug therapy. Children who have had more than three febrile seizures, prolonged febrile seizures, or seizures when they have no fever are usually treated with phenobarbital or valproate. Diazepam (Valium), if given by mouth or rectum at the time of fever, has been used effectively in children with recurrent febrile seizures. The dose that is effective when given by mouth, however, can cause irritability, insomnia, or other troublesome side effects that last for days.

BENIGN ROLANDIC EPILEPSY

> We heard a thud from Timmy's room one night. We rushed in and saw him on the floor, having a whole-body seizure. The next day, the pediatrician asked if Timmy had ever had any tingling or jerking movements in his face or body. We were shocked when Timmy said yes. He said sometimes his tongue would tingle or his cheek would jerk for a little while. The doctor did an EEG and said it was "rolandic epilepsy" and that Timmy didn't have to be treated. That's what we wanted to hear. He had one other, milder seizure a few months later. He ran into our room and woke us up. He couldn't talk because the side of his mouth was twitching, and he was drooling. Fortunately, it was over quickly. It's been 5 years now, and except for a few tingles and twitches, Timmy has been doing great.

Benign rolandic (sylvian) epilepsy (also called BECT, benign epilepsy of childhood with centrotemporal spikes) is a common childhood seizure syndrome, with seizures beginning between 2 and 13 years of age. A hereditary factor is often present. The most characteristic attack is a partial motor seizure (twitching) or a sensory seizure (numbness or tingling sensation) that involves the face or tongue and causes garbled speech. However, tonic-clonic seizures also may occur, especially during sleep. Although the seizures are often infrequent or may occur in clusters

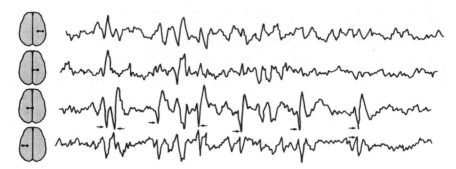

FIGURE 7. An EEG reveals centrotemporal spikes (abnormal epilepsy waves recorded over the central and temporal regions) (*arrows*) from a boy with benign rolandic epilepsy. The brain diagrams on the left indicate the area from which each recording was obtained.

of several a week followed by none for 6 months, some patients need medication. These include children who, in addition to the typical seizure disorder, have daytime seizures, a learning disorder, a mild mental handicap, or multiple seizures at night that leave him or her lethargic in the morning. The seizures are easily controlled with low to moderate doses of carbamazepine, phenytoin, or valproate (or, outside the United States, clobazam). The drug is usually continued until age 15, when the seizures spontaneously stop in almost all patients.

The EEG shows a pattern of spikes over the central and temporal regions of the brain (Fig. 7) and often shows abundant abnormal activity, especially during sleep. This is unusual because the child may have had no seizures or only a single seizure. It shows that an abundance of the kind of brain waves that are markers for increased brain electrical activity and are usually found only in people with epilepsy (*epileptiform activity*) is not related to the severity of the disorder. Siblings or close relatives may have the same EEG pattern during childhood without ever having seizures.

JUVENILE MYOCLONIC EPILEPSY

I have always had these little jerks, ever since I was 12 or 13 years old, but I assumed everybody had them. They never really bothered me until one day I had a big one and fell down. I had a couple of grand mal seizures and was put on medication for a few years, and then the drugs were stopped. During college, whenever I stayed up all night or drank too much, the next day I would get

> lots of those jerks and sometimes a big seizure right after the jerks. I never thought much of those jerks; in fact, my wife, who doesn't have epilepsy, gets them sometimes as she is falling asleep.

Juvenile myoclonic epilepsy (JME) accounts for about 7% of the cases of epilepsy, making it one of the most common epilepsy syndromes. The syndrome is defined by myoclonic seizures (jerks) with or without tonic-clonic or absence seizures. The EEG usually shows a pattern of spikes-and-waves or polyspikes-and-waves. Computed tomography (CT) and magnetic resonance imaging (MRI) scans of the brain are normal and usually are not needed.

Seizures usually begin shortly before or after puberty or sometimes in early adulthood. They usually occur soon after awaking. Persons with JME often have seizures that may be triggered by flickering light, such as strobe lights at dances, TV, video games, or light shining through trees or reflecting off ocean waves or snow. These are called photosensitive seizures. Myoclonic seizures also may be provoked by factors such as decision making or calculations (see Reflex Epilepsy). The intellectual functions of persons with JME are the same as those in the general population.

The disorder is usually lifelong, but the seizures are well controlled with medication. Valproate is the treatment of choice. Myoclonic seizures also may be controlled with acetazolamide, clonazepam, primidone, phenobarbital, lamotrigine, or topiramate. Carbamazepine may actually worsen the myoclonic jerks. Absence and tonic-clonic seizures can be treated with the standard medications (see Table 3).

This syndrome often has a genetic basis. In some families, genes associated with an increased risk of JME are located on chromosomes 6, 8, or 15. Nevertheless, most of children in these families do not develop epilepsy.

INFANTILE SPASMS

> At first I thought Chris was just having the little body jerks when he was moved or startled, like my other children had when they were infants. But then I knew something was wrong. The jerks became more violent, and his tiny body was thrust forward and his arms flew apart. They only lasted a few seconds, but started to occur in groups lasting a few minutes. It was so hard to see such a young baby having these things.

Infantile spasms (West's syndrome), a very uncommon form of epilepsy, begin between 3 and 12 months of age and usually stop by the age of 2 to 4 years. The seizures, or spasms, consist of a sudden jerk followed by stiffening. With some spells, the arms are flung out as the body bends forward ("jackknife seizures"). Other spells have more subtle movements limited to the neck or other body parts. A brain disorder or brain injury, such as birth trauma with oxygen deprivation, precedes the seizures in 60% of these infants, but the others have had no injury and their development is normal. The future course of the disorder and of the child's development is related to the cause of the seizures, the child's intellectual and neurologic development before the seizures begin (the better the condition at that time, the better the outlook), and whether the seizures are controlled quickly. The sooner therapy is begun, the better the results.

Several antiepileptic drugs and hormonal therapy can be used to treat infantile spasms. Some experts recommend a trial of an antiepileptic drug (e.g., vigabatrin, valproate, topiramate) before hormonal therapy, but others use hormonal therapy as the first treatment. Vigabatrin (Sabril) is not available in the United States. It can be obtained in Canada, Mexico and many other countries (see Chap. 11). In countries where it is available, vigabatrin is often used as the initial therapy because it is relatively safe (especially for short-term use) and effective. Vigabatrin is especially effective in children with tuberous sclerosis (a disorder associated with abnormalities involving the brain, skin, heart, and other parts of the body).

If vigabatrin does not control the seizures in 3 or 4 days, adrenocorticotropic hormone (ACTH) is usually used next. ACTH is a hormone made by the pituitary gland. It stimulates the adrenal glands to make and release additional cortisol, which acts much like the steroid hormone prednisone. ACTH has been proven to be slightly more effective than prednisone, but it must be given as an injection once a day for the first several weeks, then every other day. (Steroid hormones, such as prednisone, can be given by mouth.) ACTH stops seizures in more than half of children with infantile spasms.

In the United States, ACTH is often used as the first therapy. In most cases it is given for 3 months. The dosage is highest during the first week and then usually lowered gradually. The adverse effects of ACTH depend on the dose used, the duration of therapy, and the baby's sensitivity to the drug. Although rare allergic reactions may occur, all other adverse effects occur because ACTH stimulates the infant's body to produce cortisol, a steroid hormone. Excessive cortisol can cause severe irritability; increased appetite; high blood pressure; kidney problems; redistribution of body fat that makes the face and trunk fatter and the arms and legs thinner; increased risk of infection or gastrointestinal bleeding; and metabolic changes that alter the concentrations of glucose (sugar), sodium, and potassium in the blood. For most babies with infantile spasms, however, the adverse effects of ACTH can be safely managed. Often the baby will be given another drug after the spasms have stopped and the ACTH therapy has been completed.

When the spasms stop, many children will later develop other seizures. Even without any treatment, infantile spasms will stop in more than 90% of children by the age of 5 years. Untreated children often have frequent spasms for many years, however, and later have partial or generalized seizures or other epileptic syndromes. Approximately one-fifth of the cases of infantile spasms will evolve into the Lennox-Gastaut syndrome.

LENNOX-GASTAUT SYNDROME

The first time I heard Tommy's diagnosis, Lennox-Gastaut syndrome, the words had no meaning. I asked the doctor for information, and he said there wasn't much written for parents. So I went to a medical library and spent the afternoon with a few textbooks and a medical dictionary. Sometimes, I had to ask one of the students to explain the definitions. I was in tears when I left. It sounded totally hopeless; Tommy had no future. Ten years later, Tommy's seizures are under much better control. He loves school (special education classes), has lots of friends, is an incredibly important part of our family, and gives us all great pleasure. He can almost beat me at tennis!

The parent of a child with Lennox-Gastaut syndrome needs lots of patience. Kathy has been on every medication, many of them three or four times. Nothing has ever controlled the seizures well. As the doctors kept going up on the doses, she would undergo terrible personality changes, turn into a zombie, or look drunk. We have finally come to accept the seizures and her mental handicaps. We also have part-time help at home so that we and our other kids could have a more normal life. The more we let go of some our unrealistic hopes and accepted Kathy for who she is, the more our time with Kathy changed from disappointment to joy.

The Lennox-Gastaut syndrome is serious but uncommon. It is defined by three things: (1) difficult-to-control seizures, (2) mental handicap, and (3) a slow spike-and-wave pattern on the EEG. The seizures usually begin between 1 and 6 years of age, but can begin later. The syndrome involves some combination of tonic, atypical absence, myoclonic, and tonic-clonic seizures that are usually resistant to medications. Most children with the Lennox-Gastaut syndrome have intellectual impairment ranging from mild to severe. Behavioral problems are also common and probably relate to a combination of the neurologic injury, seizures, and antiepileptic drugs.

The course of the seizures varies greatly. Some children will later have fairly good seizure control. Others will grow up to have drop attacks and

partial and tonic-clonic seizures. The intellectual and behavioral development of children whose seizures come under fair to good control may be
almost normal, but the development of those who have frequent seizures
and are given high doses of more than one drug may be severely delayed.
This syndrome usually persists into adulthood, and affected persons often
need to live in a residential (adult foster care) group home if their
parents are no longer able to care for them.

Medications that are useful for controlling the seizures of patients with
Lennox-Gastaut syndrome include valproate, carbamazepine, clobazam
(not available in the United States), lamotrigine, and topiramate.
Felbamate also is an effective drug and can often improve behavior and
quality of life. It has a high risk of life-threatening blood or liver
disorders, however, and must be used carefully.

In children or adults with frequent, poorly controlled seizures, it may
be wise to avoid high doses of antiepileptic drugs because they may
intensify the behavioral, social, and intellectual problems, especially
when two or more drugs are used together. It may be better to tolerate
slightly more frequent seizures to have a more alert and attentive child
whose quality of life is much improved.

Vagus nerve stimulation or corpus callosotomy (see Chap. 12) can be
helpful treatments for some patients. Because it has lower risks, we
recommend vagus nerve stimulation before consideration of callosotomy.

REFLEX EPILEPSIES

> It was only later that I realized he was sitting under a fluorescent
> light that was flickering when he had his first seizure. All three of
> his seizures have happened when there have been flashing or
> flickering lights. The last seizure was when they did the EEG with
> the flashing lights. Now we keep Dan away from any light flickers.
> Even driving through shaded areas where the light filters down
> through the leaves and flickers—we just give him a pair of dark
> sunglasses, and he keeps his head down.

Reflex epilepsies are triggered by certain things in the environment.
The most common form of reflex epilepsy is photosensitive epilepsy,
which usually begins in childhood and is often outgrown before
adulthood. In this disorder, flashing lights trigger absence seizures
(staring), myoclonic seizures (jerking of the eyes, head, or arms), or
tonic-clonic seizures. People with reflex epilepsies should try to avoid
flashing lights, but this is not always easy. Even driving past a line of trees
with the sun flickering through can produce the same effect as a strobe
light. For some people, certain rates of blinking or colors are most likely
to provoke seizures. Recently, there has been great interest in the safety

of video games for children or adults with epilepsy. Certain video games can provoke seizures, but this has been reported in only a few people (see Chap. 15).

Other environmental triggers in reflex epilepsy include sounds, such as church bells, a certain type of music or song, or a person's voice; doing arithmetic; reading; certain movements, such as writing; and even thinking about specific topics. Because triggers in the environment may be unavoidable or because seizures may occur without detectable causes, many persons with reflex epilepsy require treatment. Valproate is effective for reflex epilepsies. Other successful medications are carbamaz-epine, clonazepam, clobazam (not available in the United States), phenytoin, lamotrigine, and phenobarbital.

The reflex epilepsies are usually identified as primary generalized epilepsy, which accurately describes photosensitive epilepsy. Other forms of reflex epilepsy are classified as partial epilepsy.

TEMPORAL LOBE EPILEPSY

> I get the strangest feeling; most of it can't be put into words. The whole world suddenly seems more real at first; it's as though everything becomes crystal clear. Then I feel as if I'm here but not here, kind of like being in a dream. It's as if I've lived through this exact moment many times before. I hear what people say, but they don't make sense. I know not to talk during the episode because I just say foolish things. Sometimes I think I'm talking, but later people tell me that I didn't say anything. The whole thing lasts a minute or two.

This description of a partial seizure depicts some of the unusual features of seizures beginning in the temporal lobe. The features of temporal lobe seizures can be extremely varied, but certain patterns are common (see the discussion of simple and complex partial seizures in Chap. 3). The experiences and sensations that accompany these seizures are often impossible to describe, even for the most eloquent adult. Of course, it is even more difficult to obtain an accurate picture of what children are feeling. There may be a mixture of different feelings, emotions, thoughts, and experiences, which may be familiar or com-pletely foreign. In some cases, a series of old memories resurfaces. In other cases, the person may feel as if everything—including his or her home and family—appears strange. Hallucinations of voices, music, people, smells, or tastes may occur.

Experiences during temporal lobe seizures vary in intensity and quality. Sometimes the seizures are so mild that the person barely notices. In other cases, the person may be consumed with fright, intellectual fascination, or even pleasure.

Dostoyevsky, the 19th-century Russian novelist who had epilepsy, gave vivid accounts of apparent temporal lobe seizures in his novel *The Idiot* (see Appendix 4):

> He remembered that during his epileptic fits, or rather immediately preceding them, he had always experienced a moment or two when his whole heart, and mind, and body seemed to wake up with vigour and light; when he became filled with joy and hope, and all his anxieties seemed to be swept away for ever; these moments were but presentiments, as it were, of the one final second . . . in which the fit came upon him. That second, of course, was inexpressible.
>
> Next moment something appeared to burst open before him: a wonderful inner light illuminated his soul. This lasted perhaps half a second, yet he distinctly remembered hearing the beginning of a wail, the strange, dreadful wail, which burst from his lips of its own accord, and which no effort of will on his part could suppress. Next moment he was absolutely unconscious; black darkness blotted out everything. He had fallen in an epileptic fit.

Complex partial seizures, most often with automatic behavior (automatisms) such as lip smacking and rubbing the hands together, are the most common seizure type in temporal lobe epilepsy. Three-quarters of people with this disorder also have simple partial seizures, and about half have tonic-clonic seizures at some time. Some individuals with temporal lobe epilepsy, however, have only simple partial seizures.

Temporal lobe seizures usually begin in the deeper portions of the temporal lobe. This area is part of the limbic system, which controls emotions and memory (see Fig. 3C). Some individuals with temporal lobe epilepsy may have problems with memory, especially if seizures have occurred for more than 5 years, but these memory problems are almost never severe.

In most cases, the seizures can be fully or well controlled with the medications for partial seizures. If drugs are not effective, temporal lobe seizures often can be controlled with surgery. Temporal lobectomy is the most common and successful form of epilepsy surgery (see Chap. 12). Vagus nerve stimulation can be beneficial in cases where temporal lobectomy is not recommended or has failed.

FRONTAL LOBE EPILEPSY

My head starts jerking toward the right side. I try, but I can't stop it. Then my right hand goes up and my head turns toward the hand. I may just stay in that position for half a minute and it's over, or it can become a grand mal seizure.

Usually I don't get any warning—just have tonic-clonic seizures. Occasionally I get a momentary warning before the seizure—a strange feeling in my head.

I spend the night watching Molly sleep sometimes. She will have 5 or 10 seizures in a single night. They are short, usually less than 20 seconds. Her body starts to rock, like she is adjusting her position in the bed, and then she may start to make these kicking movements with her legs, like she is riding a bicycle. She may not have any more seizures for a month or two.

Craig has had the same giggles for more than a decade. Now they occur mainly when he is exercising or stressed. He makes a weird smirk and then giggles for a few seconds. He is usually able to cover it up and the kids don't know. If he misses his medications, he can have a bigger seizure.

After temporal lobe epilepsy, frontal lobe epilepsy is the next most common type of epilepsy featuring partial seizures. The frontal lobes are large (see Fig. 1A, B) and include many areas that do not have a precisely known function. Therefore, when a seizure begins in these areas, there may be no symptoms until it spreads to other areas or to most of the brain, causing a tonic-clonic seizure. When motor areas (areas that control movement) are affected, abnormal movements occur on the opposite side of the body. Seizures beginning in frontal lobe motor areas can result in weakness or the inability to use certain muscles, such as the muscles that allow someone to speak.

Complex partial seizures also may begin in the frontal lobes. In comparison with temporal lobe complex partial seizures, those beginning in the frontal lobe tend to be shorter (usually lasting less than 1 minute), are less likely to be followed by confusion or tiredness, more often occur in a cluster or series, and are more likely to include strange automatisms such as bicycling movements, screaming, or even sexual activity. Sometimes a person remains fully aware during a frontal lobe seizure while having wild movements of the arms and legs. Because of their strange nature, frontal lobe seizures can be misdiagnosed as nonepileptic seizures (see Chap. 8). Although the features of seizures may suggest whether they begin in the frontal or temporal lobes, the only way to definitely determine where they start is to obtain an EEG recording during a seizure.

Partial seizures may also cause laughing (*gelastic seizures*) or crying (*dacrystic seizures*). Crying seizures are rare. Laughing seizures may involve giggling, smirking, or fully developed laughter, with or without the emotion of joy. They can occur as simple or complex partial seizures and are seen in patients with frontal or temporal seizures or seizures arising from the hypothalamus (see Hypothalamic Hamartoma and Epilepsy).

In many cases, frontal lobe seizures can be well controlled with medications for partial seizures. If antiepileptic drugs are not effective, the seizures may be treated surgically or with vagus nerve stimulation (see Chap. 11).

Rare Epilepsy Syndromes

PROGRESSIVE MYOCLONIC EPILEPSIES

At first the doctors just thought Avi had a seizure because he was growing so fast. Then he had more grand mal seizures, and they started him on medication. Each drug seemed to work for a while and then it was as if his body became immune to it. They tried more and more drugs, two or three at a time, and the seizures just became more frequent. The worst part was that Avi was slipping—he was changing. He was not as sharp and quick as he had been. We blamed it on the drugs, but it just got worse and worse. Over a 3-year period, after the seizures began, Avi's mind seemed to get slower and slower. Then came the little seizures that would cause his speech to sputter and hesitate and his mind to turn on and off, like someone was taking a light switch and flicking it up and down.

Progressive myoclonic epilepsies feature a combination of myoclonic and tonic-clonic seizures. Unsteadiness, muscle rigidity, and mental deterioration are often also present. They are rare and frequently result from hereditary metabolic disorders, but sometimes test results are normal and the cause remains unknown.

The medical treatment of progressive myoclonic epilepsy is often successful only for a few months or years. As the disorder progresses, drugs become less effective, and adverse effects may be more severe as more drugs are used at higher doses. In such cases, it is often worthwhile to try lower doses. These patients may require more than one drug. Valproate is most commonly used, but clonazepam, lamotrigine, topiramate, phenobarbital, and carbamazepine are also used. Zonisamide, a new drug, can help control seizures in progressive myoclonic epilepsies (see Chap. 11). Piracetam, which is available in most countries outside the United States, can also be helpful.

MITOCHONDRIAL DISORDERS

Mitochondria, the energy factories of the cell, are inherited through the mother. Abnormalities in mitochondrial genes produce metabolic disorders that affect different parts of the body, including muscle and the brain. Two mitochondrial disorders often are associated with epileptic seizures. One is MELAS: *m*itochondrial *e*ncephalopathy, *l*actic *a*cidosis (meaning too much lactic acid in the blood), and *s*trokelike episodes. MELAS can lead to strokelike episodes at a young age (usually before age 40), seizures, dementia, headaches, vomiting, unsteadiness, and ill effects from exercise. Persons with MELAS can have both generalized (including myoclonic and tonic-clonic) and partial seizures.

The other mitochondrial disorder with epileptic seizures is MERRF (*m*yoclonic *e*pilepsy with *r*agged *r*ed muscle *f*ibers). MERRF is one of the progressive myoclonic epilepsies. It can also be associated with hearing loss, unsteadiness, dementia, and ill effects from exercise. In addition to myoclonic seizures, patients with MERRF often have generalized tonic-clonic seizures that can be controlled with standard medications (see Chap. 11). There are other mitochondrial disorders that do not fit clearly into the MELAS or MERRF syndromes, but which can cause epilepsy and additional neurologic problems.

LANDAU-KLEFFNER SYNDROME

The Landau-Kleffner syndrome (acquired aphasia with seizure disorder in children) is another rare disorder. *Acquired aphasia* means the loss of language abilities that had been present. The EEG shows the presence of epilepsy waves in these children. In the typical case, a child between 3 and 7 years of age experiences language problems, with or without seizures. The language disorder may start suddenly or slowly. It usually affects auditory comprehension (understanding spoken language) the most, but it may affect both understanding speech and speaking ability, or it may affect speaking only. Seizures are usually few and often occur during sleep. Simple partial motor seizures are most common, but tonic-clonic seizures can also occur. Seizure control is rarely a problem.

The EEG is often the key to the diagnosis. A normal EEG, especially one done when the child is awake, does not rule out this disorder. Sleep activates the epilepsy waves; therefore, sleep recordings are extremely important.

The boundaries of the Landau-Kleffner syndrome are imprecise. Some children may first have a delay in language development followed by a loss of speech milestones. Landau-Kleffner syndrome (or a variant of it) may also occur in some children whose language function never develops or in others whose language skills move backward but who very seldom have epilepsy waves on the EEG. The exact relationship between the epilepsy waves on the EEG and the language disorder is imprecise, although in some cases the epilepsy activity may contribute to the language problems.

Standard antiepileptic drugs are ineffective in treating the language disorder. Steroids are effective in some children, improving both the EEG abnormalities and the language problems. A new form of epilepsy surgery—multiple subpial transections (see Chap. 12)—may improve both the EEG abnormalities and the language disorder in a small number of children, but results to confirm this finding are still coming in from various epilepsy centers. Further study is needed to fully define this syndrome and its treatment.

RASMUSSEN'S SYNDROME

Rasmussen's syndrome usually begins between 14 months and 14 years of age and is associated with slowly progressive neurologic deterioration and seizures. Seizures are often the first problem to appear. Simple partial motor seizures are the most common type, but in one-fifth of these children, the first seizure is an episode of partial or tonic-clonic status epilepticus.

Although Rasmussen's syndrome is rarely fatal, its effects are devastating. Progressive weakness on one side (*hemiparesis*) and mental handicap are common. Language disorder (*aphasia*) often occurs if the disorder affects the side of the brain that controls most language functions, which is usually the left side. Mild weakness of an arm or leg is the most common initial symptom besides seizures. The weakness and other neurologic problems often begin 1 to 3 years after the seizures start. CT and MRI scans of the brain show evidence of a slow loss (*atrophy*) of brain substance. Recent studies suggest that the cause of Rasmussen's syndrome is an autoimmune disorder (antibodies are produced against the body's own tissues) directed against receptors on the brain cells. The process may be triggered by a viral infection. A blood test can be helpful in making the diagnosis.

Treatment of this disease with antiepileptic drugs is disappointing. Steroids may be effective, but additional studies are needed. Immunologic therapies (gamma globulin, plasmapheresis) may be helpful in some cases. In children with severe weakness and loss of touch and vision on the side of the body opposite the involved hemisphere of the brain, a surgical procedure called a *functional hemispherectomy* (see Chap. 12) may be successful.

HYPOTHALAMIC HAMARTOMA AND EPILEPSY

Small tumors in the base of the brain that affect the hypothalamus (see Fig. 1C) can cause a syndrome consisting of abnormally early puberty, partial seizures with laughing as a frequent feature, and increased irritability and aggression between the seizures. The partial seizures may be simple or complex, and there may be secondary generalized tonic-clonic seizures. Affected individuals often are short and have mild abnormalities in their physical features (dsymorphisms). MRI is necessary for diagnosis because CT scans are usually normal. If the tumor extends beyond the hypothalamus and below the brain, treatment with surgery may be an option. Antiepileptic drugs and drugs aimed at hormonal and behavioral problems, if needed, can also be beneficial.

An Overview of Epilepsy

Analysis of the number of cases and spread of a disease in a community, known as epidemiological studies, have provided important information on epilepsy. These studies have helped us better define the frequency, causes, and future course of epilepsy.

Epilepsy—More Common than You Think

More than 1.5 million Americans have active epilepsy. *Active epilepsy* is epilepsy that has been treated with antiepileptic drugs during the past 5 years. The total number of active cases of a disorder existing at a certain time is called the *prevalence*. The prevalence of epilepsy is 0.65%; that is, 6.5 out of 1000 people have epilepsy. To put this into perspective, when the stadium for the Rose Bowl is filled with 90,000 fans, nearly 600 of them have epilepsy.

More men than women have epilepsy, and new cases of epilepsy are most common among children, with another peak occurring in the elderly. The highest rate of occurrence of new cases, or the incidence, of epilepsy is during the first year of life. The incidence of epilepsy declines over the first 20 years of life; it then remains stable until age 55 to 60 years, when there may be an increase. This increase is largely related to stroke, brain tumors, and Alzheimer's disease. By age 80 years, the cumulative incidence of epilepsy is between 1.3% and 3.1%. In other words, there is a 1.3% to 3.1% chance that if you live to 80 years of age, you will have active epilepsy at some time during your life. By 40 years of age, there is a 1% to 2% chance of having had epilepsy.

Causes

SEIZURES—A STORM OF BRAIN ELECTRICAL ACTIVITY

The nerve cells of the brain communicate through electrical and chemical messages. The communication processes are interwoven: changes in chemical activity cause changes in electrical activity and vice versa. The brain is organized so that there is a fine balance between excitation and inhibition of electrical activity, and there are systems in the brain that limit the spread of electrical activity.

During an epileptic seizure, the regulatory systems that maintain the normal balance between excitation and inhibition of the brain's electrical activity break down. For example, there may be a loss of inhibitory nerve cells (cells that turn off other cells when they become too active) or overproduction of a neurotransmitter that stimulates cells to discharge electrical signals.

For an electrical discharge in the brain to alter a person's behavior, the function or structure of the brain cells must be abnormal. In most seizures, a small group of abnormal cells cause changes in neighboring cells or in cells with which they have strong connections. Ultimately, groups of cells are activated all at once; that is, the electrical discharges of many cells become linked, creating a storm of activity.

Patients often ask why there may be an interval of many years between an injury to the brain and the first seizure. We now have some insights into the process leading to the development of seizures, called *epileptogenesis*. Research done on animals may provide more information. In this research, an area of an animal's brain is stimulated once a day with a small current of electricity. At first, the stimulations may cause no measurable change in the brain's electrical activity or the animal's behavior. After a week, there may be a small, local storm of electrical activity after the stimulation. The animal's behavior may or may not change. After several weeks, the storm may be followed within seconds by storms in the same area of the opposite hemisphere of the brain or in areas near the original storm of activity. When these electrical storms occur, the animal may show signs of a seizure, such as facial grimacing or blank staring. As the stimulation is repeated, the electrical storms and visible seizure signs become more intense. Eventually the animal experiences a tonic-clonic (grand mal) seizure. Finally, in some animals, tonic-clonic or other seizures may occur spontaneously; that is, seizures occur without the electrical stimulation. Thus, a "fire" has been "kindled" in the brain. In more advanced species, such as baboons and rhesus monkeys, the "kindling" process proceeds more slowly.

Of course, kindling experiments have never been done in humans. But the similarity between the patterns of seizures, the electroencephalogram (EEG) activity, and the changes found in the brains of animals kindled to have seizures and the patterns in humans with epilepsy support the notion that kindling occurs in humans. A brain injury in humans probably somehow triggers abnormal electrical currents, which may progress over several years. This kindling process potentially explains the delay in the development of epilepsy.

THE INFLUENCE OF LIFE EVENTS

Some factors, including brain tumors, abnormal collections of blood vessels in the brain, bleeding into the brain, and lack of oxygen or blood flow to the brain, are clearly associated with an increased risk of seizures and epilepsy. The causes of epilepsy vary with the age at which seizures develop (Fig. 8).

Babies who are small for gestational age (in other words, who have a low birth weight compared with other infants born after the same number of weeks of pregnancy) have an increased risk of epilepsy. Infants with seizures in the first month of life also have an increased risk of developing epilepsy.

Epidemiological studies have identified many other factors that cause epilepsy. The risk of developing epilepsy is increased more than 10-fold in people who have had a head injury involving a concussion with loss of consciousness for more than 30 minutes, some memory impairment after the injury (posttraumatic amnesia), abnormalities such as weakness or impaired coordination on the neurologic examination, or skull fracture. Similarly increased risk follows central nervous system infections such as meningitis, encephalitis, or cerebral abscess; cerebral palsy and mental handicap; Alzheimer's disease; complicated (complex) febrile seizures; stroke resulting from blockage of arteries or veins; and alcohol abuse.

Factors associated with a smaller increase in the risk of developing epilepsy (less than 10-fold) include use of illegal drugs, a family history of epilepsy or febrile seizures, multiple sclerosis, and seizures occurring within days after head injury (early posttraumatic seizures). Mild head injury, such as a concussion with momentary loss of consciousness after a motor-vehicle accident or during sports, is not a cause of epilepsy.

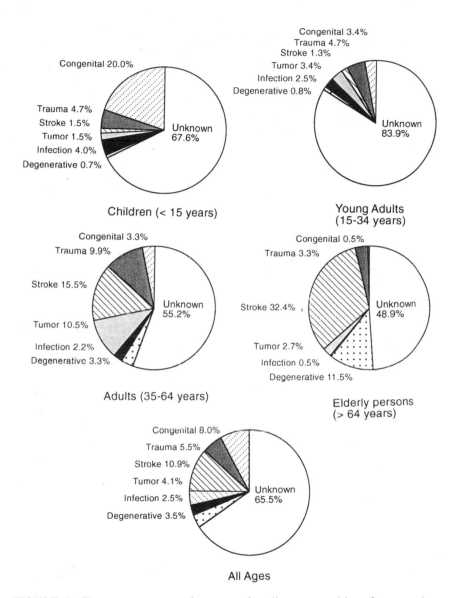

FIGURE 8. The percentage of cases of epilepsy resulting from various causes, shown for persons of all ages and different age groups. (From Hauser, WA: Seizure disorders: The changes with age. Epilepsia (Suppl 4)33:S6–S14, 1992, with permission.)

Epidemiological studies have failed to establish a clear relationship between vaccination and epilepsy. In some cases, however, vaccination may cause a fever associated with a febrile convulsion.

Hereditary Influences

Hereditary (genetic) factors are important in some cases of epilepsy. When epilepsy develops at a young age, there is an increased risk of epilepsy among the affected person's siblings and children. It is more common for genetic factors to be present in primary generalized epilepsy than in partial epilepsy.

Among patients with primary generalized epilepsy and the spike-and-wave abnormality on the EEG, the risk of epilepsy in a brother or sister is approximately 4%. When a child with absence or tonic-clonic seizures has generalized epilepsy waves on the EEG (generalized spike-and-wave pattern) and one of that child's brothers or sisters also has the spike-and-wave abnormality, another child in the family has an 8% risk of developing epilepsy. When a parent and a child have primary generalized epilepsy, there is a 10% risk that the parent's other children will have isolated seizures or epilepsy.

Heredity may influence the likelihood that a person will develop partial epilepsy after experiencing a clear cause of seizures, such as serious head injury with loss of consciousness for longer than an hour. The rate of seizures is higher among the family members of people who develop epilepsy after head trauma than among the relatives of people who do not.

One form of partial epilepsy with a strong genetic component is the syndrome of benign rolandic epilepsy. A brother or sister of a child with benign rolandic epilepsy has as much as a 35% chance of showing the characteristic EEG abnormality, and 15% of those with the abnormality will develop seizures. These represent only 5% of all children in the family, however.

The children of parents with epilepsy also have an increased risk. Overall, the chance that a child of a parent with epilepsy will have unprovoked seizures by age 25 is 6%, compared with 1% to 2% in the general population. Epilepsy is roughly twice as common among the children of women with epilepsy than among the children of men with epilepsy.

In cases where heredity is important, a single gene or several genes may be the determining factor. Recent studies have linked several epilepsy syndromes to specific genes.

Prognosis

RISK OF RECURRENT SEIZURES AFTER A FIRST SEIZURE

After a single, unprovoked seizure, the risk of having more (*recurrence*) is approximately 50%. The next seizure most likely will occur within a year. If someone experiences two seizures, the chances of having a third one are about 80%. The risk of recurrence is roughly twice as high for individuals with a known brain injury or other type of brain abnormality (*symptomatic epilepsy*) than it is for those with no known injury (*idiopathic epilepsy*). It is also higher for those with partial seizures or an abnormal EEG.

People who long ago had a seizure at the time of an injury to the brain, such as head trauma or brain infection, are more likely to develop epilepsy than if they had not had a seizure at the time of the injury. People with abnormalities on a neurologic examination appear to be at slightly greater risk of a second seizure than are those with normal results.

The EEG is another important predictor of recurrence after a single seizure. People with abnormalities characteristic of epilepsy (*epileptiform abnormalities*), such as spike-and-wave discharges, spikes, or sharp waves, have approximately twice the chance of having another seizure than do people with normal EEGs or with other kinds of abnormalities, such as mild slowing (see Chap. 8 and Table 7, p. 216). The presence of epileptiform activity on the EEG is key in predicting recurrent seizures in people with no history of brain injury or abnormality.

We are not sure whether epilepsy in a family member increases the risk of recurrence after a person's first seizure. Most studies have found either no increase or only a slightly increased recurrence rate.

REMISSION AND RISK OF RECURRENCE

After the diagnosis of epilepsy is made and effective therapy is prescribed, approximately two-thirds of people will be seizure-free for 5 years. The longer the interval between seizures, the greater the chances of permanent remission (freedom from seizures). Twenty years after the diagnosis of epilepsy, approximately three-quarters of people will have been seizure-free for 5 years. The longer the time that people continue to have seizures after the diagnosis of epilepsy is made, the lower the chances of a remission. Nevertheless, even people with intractable epilepsy (seizures that cannot be controlled with tolerable medication doses) may become seizure-free.

People with primary generalized seizures, especially tonic-clonic seizures, have a better chance of remission than those with other types. Also, those who are young when the diagnosis of epilepsy is made are more likely to stop having seizures than are people who are older when they first are diagnosed. The remission rate is also higher if the person has no known brain injury or abnormality and if the results of their neurologic examination are normal.

The role of the EEG in predicting whether epilepsy will go into remission remains uncertain. The characteristic EEG pattern of centrotemporal spikes (see Fig. 7) in benign rolandic epilepsy virtually guarantees remission by age 15 years. People with the widespread spike-and-wave EEG pattern that is characteristic of some types of primary generalized epilepsy are less likely to become seizure-free than are those without these abnormal patterns. This difference partly reflects the group of patients with juvenile myoclonic epilepsy who often have such EEG abnormalities and have low remission rates. However, the overall value of other patterns of epilepsy waves on the EEG in predicting remission is uncertain.

People with epilepsy who have been seizure-free for 5 years may later have seizures again. Overall, about 1.5% of people who have been seizure-free for 5 years have another seizure. Such a relapse is more likely in people with complex partial seizures and those who are more than 20 years old.

There is some risk of relapse after antiepileptic drugs are discontinued, but the drugs may also play a role in the remission of epilepsy. More than 100 years ago, the English neurologist Sir William Gowers suggested that "seizures beget seizures." Once you have one seizure, you are more likely to have another simply because your brain "learns" how to have a seizure. This may partly result from the kindling process mentioned at the beginning of this chapter. Although his concept remains unproven, there is informal evidence that he may have been right in some cases. In children, this may be true only after 10 or more tonic-clonic seizures have occurred. The longer someone remains seizure-free while taking antiepileptic drugs, the better chance he or she has of remaining seizure-free when the medication is stopped. Just as the brain learns to have seizures, it may also "forget" to have seizures. Antiepileptic drugs may enhance the forgetting process by controlling seizures. This effect of antiepileptic drugs, however, is unproven.

Many people who are seizure-free for 2 to 4 years can stop taking their medications without having further seizures. About 20% to 35% of children and 30% to 65% of adults will have seizures again after medication is withdrawn, however. Currently, most neurologists in the United States consider withdrawing antiepileptic drugs after someone has been seizure-free for 1 to 2 years. In Europe medication is often withdrawn after 6 months without seizures for children with a good prognosis. Whether the person takes part in activities that may be hazardous if they had a seizure, such as driving or swimming, may influence the doctor's decision of when it is appropriate to consider withdrawing the antiepileptic drugs (see Chap. 10).

Epilepsy and Life Span

People with infrequent seizures have death rates comparable to the general population, and the average person with epilepsy lives a normal life span. Overall, however, epilepsy is associated with a slight reduction in life span. In part, this reduction is because of the effects of conditions such as stroke and brain tumors, which can both provoke seizures and shorten life. The increased risk of death associated with epilepsy is almost entirely limited to the first 10 years after the diagnosis is made.

FATAL SEIZURES

Although fatalities from epilepsy are possible, single seizures that impair consciousness are almost never fatal. However, convulsive (tonic-clonic) status epilepticus (see Chap. 3) is a medical emergency and may cause permanent injury or death if treatment is delayed or ineffective.

Accidents and injuries are increased for people with epilepsy. A tonic-clonic seizure may cause someone to fall in front of a train, for example, or to roll over in bed and suffocate (as may have happened to Florence Griffith Joyner, the Olympic track star). A complex partial seizure may cause a person to cross a busy street without caution. The most dangerous setting for someone with episodes of impaired consciousness is driving a motor vehicle, where a brief lapse can prove deadly. Death from drowning is also more common among people with epilepsy and can even occur in a tub with only a few inches of water.

Although seizures causing a fatal injury are *extremely rare,* prevention is the best medicine. People with seizures that impair consciousness or motor control should try to avoid situations that place them at risk. However, the reality is that ordinary activities of daily living—crossing streets and taking trains or subways—can be dangerous. There must be balance between safety and leading an active, productive, and enjoyable life (see Chap. 24). Nearly all people with epilepsy can achieve this balance.

UNEXPLAINED DEATH IN EPILEPSY

There is a mysterious, rare condition known as SUDEP (sudden unexplained death in epilepsy) in which young or middle-aged persons with epilepsy die without a clearly defined cause. They are often found dead in bed without signs of having had a convulsive seizure, although about a third of them show evidence of a seizure close to the time of death. In most cases they are found lying on their stomach. Although the cause of death is unknown, some researchers suggest that a seizure causes an irregularity in the heart rhythm. More recent studies have suggested that a combination of impaired breathing (apnea), increased fluid in the lungs (which impairs the exchange of oxygen and carbon dioxide), and being face down on the bedding all combine to cause death from impaired respiration. In many cases, death probably occurs after the seizure has ended.

A few safety precautions can minimize the chances of SUDEP:

• Patients should take the medications prescribed for them.
• Adult patients with a high likelihood of tonic-clonic seizures in sleep should be watched if possible. (SUDEP is extremely rare in children with epilepsy.)
• Basic first aid, including rolling the person onto one side, should be provided (see Chap. 9).

It is important to understand that sudden, unexplained death in epilepsy is rare. The risk of SUDEP for a person with epilepsy is about 1 in 3000 per year. The risk for people with intractable epilepsy who have frequent seizures and take large doses of many antiepileptic drugs is about 1 in 300 per year. Among all patients with epilepsy, SUDEP accounts for less than 2% of deaths. The risk is highest in adults ages 15 to 44, accounting for about 8% of deaths in this group.

Acknowledgment

Much of this chapter was derived from the authoritative book, *Epilepsy: Frequency, Causes, and Consequences,* by WA Hauser and DC Hesdorffer. Demos Publications, New York, 1990.

Seizure-Provoking Factors

Many people with epilepsy can identify certain factors that increase their chances of having a seizure. It is well established that some factors, such as missed medication, sleep deprivation, and the premenstrual period, can provoke seizures. Proving or refuting an association between seizures and other factors, such as emotional stress or a full moon, is more complicated than it seems, and the medical world has not thoroughly examined this subject.

Many patients are surprised when missed medication or sleep deprivation leads to a so-called breakthrough seizure because at other times they had missed medication or skimped on sleep without having a seizure. This apparent inconsistency may occur because often more than one factor contributes to the seizure. For example, missing a single dose of medication may provoke a seizure in a person who also has not had enough sleep or in a woman around the time of her menstrual period, but not at other times. The risk of breakthrough seizures is often related to the intensity and number of seizure-provoking factors. An unfortunately common example is binge drinking by college students—they stay out late, drink excessively, and often forget to take their medication. In many other cases, we cannot define all of the variables that provoke (or control) seizures in an individual.

Seizure Calendar

Patients with epilepsy should strongly consider keeping a seizure calendar. It is simple and can often help answer questions about changes in the type or frequency of seizures over time, the effect of different medications on seizure control, adverse effects of medications, and seizure-provoking factors. The most basic seizure calendar includes the type of seizure and the date and time of the seizure. If a precipitating factor is suspected (e.g., lack of sleep, missed medication, stress, or menstrual period), it also should be written down. It is helpful to record the medication, dosage, and levels of the drug in the blood. For women, it may be useful to keep track of the relationship between seizures and the menstrual cycles. This can be done by recording the basal body temperature each day (taking the temperature shortly after awakening), although this rarely provides essential information.

Missed Medication

There are about half a dozen fairly well-defined factors that can provoke seizures, but there likely are many others. Most people do not think that missing their medication will lead to seizures, but it is almost certainly the most common cause of both breakthrough seizures and life-threatening *convulsive status epilepticus* (prolonged seizures that require emergency medical treatment). Convulsive status epilepticus is most likely to occur following the abrupt complete stopping of antiepileptic medications.

The most common and least harmful instance is the occasional missing of a single dose. People are more likely to miss a dose when medications are taken three or four times per day than if they are taken only once or twice daily. When medication is given only once per day, however, missing one dose means missing a full day of medication; therefore, it is more likely to cause seizures than if the medication is taken two to four times a day. Missing several doses in a row increases the likelihood of a breakthrough seizure. This sometimes happens when patients go away for a weekend, forget to pack their medication, and hope they can "get away without it for a few days."

Medications are missed for many reasons, and various strategies can be used to prevent such errors. The patient should never have less than a 1- to 2-week supply of medication. Those who order large quantities of antiepileptic drugs by mail are wise to have a spare 2- to 4-week supply. It is a good idea to keep extra medication at work, in the car, and in one's wallet or purse.

(Remember to "restock" the emergency supply so that it does not go out of date. This is especially important for emergency supplies that are stored in places that may become quite hot and shorten the shelf-life of a medication, such as the glove compartment of a car.) The school nurse or teacher should keep extra medication for children. When going on a trip, it is smart to pack two separate supplies of medication: one in a carry-on bag and one for luggage that is checked. The hand-carried medications are "insurance" in case the checked bag is misplaced or stolen.

Patients can help themselves to remember to take all their medication by establishing some cues. Their daily pattern can be helpful in determining what time of day or activity would be a good point to stop and take the pills. Is there a specific time of day, such as 8 A.M. or 8 P.M.? Can the pills be taken with meals, two or three times daily? Can dosing be linked with brushing the teeth, taking a shower, or some other bathroom activity? The person should make a special effort to remember to take the pills if the routine is interrupted, such as sleeping late or skipping lunch. Pillboxes are available to organize medication by day of the week and time of day. There are even wristwatches and pillboxes that can be easily programmed to provide a reminder.

Some people with epilepsy decide to discontinue their medication without a doctor's advice. This is a dangerous decision. Abruptly stopping some antiepileptic drugs can cause withdrawal symptoms, including prolonged tonic-clonic seizures even if they have never occurred before. Also, changes in one drug can dramatically change the blood levels and effectiveness of other drugs and in some cases cause serious adverse effects. Medications should never be stopped suddenly unless the doctor recommends it. If a doctor feels that it is unsafe to continue taking a medication (e.g., the patient gets a rash), but if suddenly stopping the drug poses a risk of status epilepticus, he or she may prescribe another medication or the person may be hospitalized during the time the drug is withdrawn.

The patient should always be comfortable enough with the doctor or nurse to discuss his or her wants and needs. Stopping an antiepileptic drug—whatever the reason—should always be discussed first with the doctor. If the doctor feels it is too dangerous or unwise to stop the drugs and the patient still feels strongly, it may be necessary to obtain a second opinion—but the medication should not be stopped without a doctor's advice.

REFILLING THE PRESCRIPTION

If the number of pills starts to get low and there are refills on the last prescription, get another supply from the pharmacy well before running out completely. If there are no refills left, the patient can ask the doctor to telephone the pharmacy. Patients must *never* wait until the last minute to call the doctor or pharmacy.

Most doctors and clinics are available to speak with patients 24 hours a day. A patient rarely will need to call a doctor at 3 A.M. for a refill, but it can be done if it is an emergency. If not, the patient should call the doctor in the morning. If it is a weekend, it is best not to wait until Monday to call if waiting means running out of pills. If the doctor is unavailable and no other doctor is taking the calls, the patient might consider calling or visiting a 24-hour doctor service, outpatient clinic, or an emergency room. A patient who has no medication, or only a few pills, can get more medication in almost any location. The patient's doctor can telephone a pharmacy or hospital even if the patient is in a foreign country. If that is impossible, the patient can go to a local doctor or hospital. Where there is a will, there is always a way—patients with epilepsy must not run out of medications.

TRAVELING ACROSS TIME ZONES

When traveling across time zones, it is important that the amount of medication taken over a 24- or 48-hour period remain the same as if the patient were at home, and the interval between doses should be approximately the same. In general, because changes in time zones increase the likelihood of sleep deprivation, it is better to err on the side of taking slightly too much medication or too-frequent doses.

Each drug has a *half-life* (the time required for the concentration of the drug in the blood to decline to half of its original value). Medications with a short half-life, such as carbamazepine (the regular form, not extended-release) and valproate, pose a slightly greater problem than those with a longer half-life, such as phenytoin or phenobarbital. For drugs with a short half-life, it is important to keep the interval between doses as close to the usual routine as possible. Otherwise, the person risks adverse effects from high drug levels in the blood or seizures from low drug levels. It's not necessary to use an alarm clock to take the medications at exactly the same interval. With medications that have a long half-life, the timing is less critical because the drug levels do not fluctuate as much in the intervals between doses.

If the seizures have been difficult to control, if there are problems with dose-related adverse effects, or if time-zone differences are confusing, the patient should ask the doctor about taking medications during travel. In some people, benzodiazepines such as lorazepam (Ativan), clonazepam (Klonopin), or diazepam (Valium) may be used to increase sleep time on the plane, decrease jet lag, and reduce the risk of a seizure while traveling.

Sleep Deprivation

Sleep deprivation, or lack of sleep, can trigger a seizure. Indeed, some people suffer a single seizure for the only time in their entire life after doing an "all-nighter" at college or after a prolonged period of poor sleep associated with a major life stress. For people with epilepsy, lack of proper sleep can increase their chances of having a seizure or even increase the intensity and duration of a seizure. Doctors take advantage of this phenomenon by asking people with suspected epilepsy to stay up all night before having an electroencephalogram (EEG) to "activate the brain" and make it more likely that abnormal brain electrical activity will be revealed. Sleep deprivation also makes it more likely that the patient will fall asleep during the EEG, increasing the chances of recording certain electrical abnormalities. Similarly, when doctors in an epilepsy center are using video-EEG to study seizures, they will often ask the patient to stay up all night to provoke a seizure.

We don't know why sleep deprivation provokes seizures. The sleep-wake cycle (circadian rhythm) is associated with prominent changes in brain electrical activity and hormonal activity, so seizures and the sleep-wake cycle are often clearly related. Some people have all of their seizures while sleeping, some have most of their seizures just before or shortly after they wake up, others have seizures as they are falling asleep or waking up, and still others have seizures randomly spread throughout the day or night.

Most doctors recommend that people with epilepsy get adequate sleep. Defining "adequate sleep" is difficult, but a simple definition is a night's sleep that leaves a person feeling refreshed the next day. Although it is hard to specify a minimum number of hours, in general people with epilepsy should try to sleep at least 7 hours a night. For most individuals, going to bed very late (e.g., 3 A.M. instead of 11 P.M.) can be compensated for by sleeping late (e.g., 10 A.M. instead of 6 A.M.) to avoid sleep deprivation. However, for some patients with epilepsy, the disruption of the sleep-wake cycle may make seizures more likely even if they sleep their usual total time.

For people who have problems with falling asleep and staying asleep, some simple measures may be helpful: make sure the sleeping environment is quiet and dark, go to bed at least half an hour before trying to fall asleep, avoid caffeinated beverages within 6 hours of going to sleep, have no more than one alcoholic beverage a day, exercise daily but do not exercise shortly before going to sleep, and read in bed instead of watching television. Those people who find that reading a good novel keeps them up and TV puts them to sleep, however, should turn on the TV.

Sleeping pills should be used only under a doctor's supervision and almost never for more than 2 or 3 weeks. Even with short-term use, they must be handled carefully because stopping certain types of sleeping pills, especially the benzodiazepines such as triazolam (Halcion), clonazepam (Klonopin), and temazepam (Restoril), can trigger seizures in susceptible people. During periods of tremendous stress, however, such as loss of a job or a relationship, the judicious use of sleeping pills for several nights can help to prevent a seizure caused by sleep deprivation.

People who have come to depend on sleeping pills should consult their doctors about getting off of them. Gradual reduction of the dosage, possible substitution of non–habit-forming medications that promote sleep, and the simple measures described previously can be helpful. Diphenhydramine (Benadryl) is an over-the-counter medication that is not habit-forming and can promote sleep, but its use also can provoke seizures in some people with epilepsy. Melatonin is another over-the-counter drug used to promote sleep; it appears to be safe for most people with epilepsy, but scientific studies are lacking.

Children require more sleep than adults do. The pediatrician can offer guidance on how much sleep the average child requires at different ages and tips on helping to maintain a regular sleep routine. A good book on this subject is *Solve Your Child's Sleep Problems* (see Appendix 4). If a child consistently has more seizures when he or she does not sleep enough, the parents should try to recognize and avoid the things that cause sleep deprivation.

Alcohol Use

A relationship between alcohol use and increased seizure frequency has been recognized for centuries. During the past century, however, the role of alcohol in epilepsy has been more clearly defined. Alcohol in small to moderate amounts actually has properties to counteract seizures; that is, alcohol has antiepileptic effects. It should never be consumed in the hope of controlling seizures, however. Alcohol rarely provokes seizures while the person is drinking, but it may cause "withdrawal" seizures 6 to 72 hours after drinking has stopped.

Withdrawal seizures are most common among people who have abused alcohol for years. When alcohol consumption is stopped suddenly or markedly reduced over a short time, a seizure may occur. This is an example of provoked seizures rather than true epilepsy. In a similar way, the abrupt withdrawal of barbiturates—such as phenobarbital and primidone—or benzodiazepines—such as diazepam, lorazepam, and clonazepam—may cause a seizure after prolonged use.

Alcohol withdrawal can also provoke seizures in a person with epilepsy who does not have a long history of heavy drinking. Many people with epilepsy are at a markedly increased risk of seizures after consuming three or more alcoholic beverages.

Long-standing alcohol abuse can increase a person's risk of developing epilepsy. In such cases, the relative roles of alcohol withdrawal, alcohol intoxication, head injury, and the lack of certain vitamins or minerals such as magnesium remain uncertain. All of these factors probably contribute to some degree to the development of seizures in people who chronically abuse alcohol.

The use of alcohol by people with epilepsy is controversial. In general, they are less likely than others to use or abuse alcohol. This largely reflects patients following their doctors' recommendations and the warnings on their medication bottles. Several studies, however, have shown that adults with epilepsy may have one or two alcoholic beverages a day without any worsening of their seizures or changes in the blood levels of their antiepileptic medications. (Acute consumption of three or more alcoholic beverages can inhibit metabolism of some antiepileptic drugs [e.g., phenytoin] and lead to increased drug levels and an increased risk of side effects. Chronic use of alcohol will cause the liver enzymes that break down antiepileptic drugs to work harder, resulting in lower drug levels and an increased risk of seizures.)

Moderate to heavy alcohol consumption is never recommended for people with epilepsy. Alcohol and some antiepileptic drugs share similar adverse effects, such as tiredness, unsteadiness, slurred speech, and the lessening of respiration. The result is that people who are sensitive to the adverse effects of alcohol or antiepileptic drugs may find the combination especially troublesome and extremely dangerous when driving. Further, the consumption of large amounts of alcohol, as in college drinking contests, can be extremely dangerous when combined with antiepileptic drugs. There is also good evidence that if a people with epilepsy consume three or more alcoholic beverages over a short time, their seizures will worsen 6 to 72 hours after drinking is stopped. Finally, those who consume large amounts of alcohol tend to sleep poorly and forget to take their antiepileptic drugs. If there is a chance that they may wake up away from home, they should make sure that they have a supply of morning medications on hand. People with a history of alcoholism or drug abuse who also have epilepsy should not drink alcohol.

Drug Abuse

Cocaine can cause seizures. All forms of cocaine consumption, including snorting, injecting it into the skin or veins, and smoking crack with a pipe, can cause seizures. Seizures can occur within seconds, minutes, or hours after the cocaine has been consumed. Seizures caused by cocaine are uniquely dangerous and may be associated with heart attacks, interruption of the heart's normal rhythm (cardiac arrhythmia), and death. Seizures caused by cocaine use can occur in someone who has never had a seizure—not just in people with epilepsy. The 1986 death of college basketball star Len Bias resulted from a cocaine-related seizure. Those who have epilepsy definitely should avoid cocaine.

Amphetamines, like cocaine, are brain stimulants. They are often prescribed to treat attention deficit disorder, hyperactivity, and narcolepsy. When used under a doctor's supervision, amphetamines or other stimulants do not appear to increase the likelihood of seizures in people with epilepsy. When amphetamines and related drugs are abused, however, they can lead to sleep deprivation, confusion, and major psychiatric disorders. This can cause people with epilepsy to forget to take their antiepileptic drugs, which increases the risk of seizures. Very high doses of amphetamines can cause severe tonic-clonic seizures, heart attacks, and death.

Marijuana (cannabis or pot) is obtained from the flowering tops of hemp plants. The active ingredient in marijuana is tetrahydrocannabinol (THC). In the 19th century, marijuana was used to treat epilepsy. Studies in animals have suggested that THC and cannibidiol, a substance in marijuana, have some antiepileptic properties but they also may have seizure-provoking effects. Some preliminary studies in humans have suggested that cannibidiol may reduce seizure frequency, but additional studies are needed to define any potential therapeutic role for marijuana or its components. Because it causes a variety of adverse effects, marijuana is not recommended for the treatment of epilepsy. Furthermore, as is the case with alcohol, even if marijuana or one of its components had some antiepileptic effects in humans, abrupt withdrawal of the substance after recreational use may increase the likelihood of seizures.

Heroin and related *narcotics* (drugs derived from opium and manufactured drugs that are chemically similar to opium) are dangerous when abused. Narcotics can be used medically to treat severe pain. These drugs do not directly affect the chances that someone with epilepsy will have a seizure. However, narcotic use often leads to failure to take prescribed antiepileptic medications. Further, when taken in large amounts, narcotics can cause serious oxygen deprivation to the brain. These problems can lead to seizures. Among the narcotics, meperidine (Demerol) may have the greatest potential to cause seizures.

Nicotine (in tobacco) and caffeine (in coffee, tea, chocolate, and other foods) are drugs that are often used and abused in our society. There is no evidence that using nicotine or caffeine in usual amounts affects seizure control, but there are stories of susceptible people in whom seizures were provoked by their abuse. Cigarette smoking also can be dangerous in people who have seizures that impair consciousness or motor control because a dropped cigarette can cause a fire.

Menstrual Cycle

Approximately half of the women of childbearing age who have epilepsy report an increase in seizures around the time of their monthly menstrual period. Seizures occurring predominantly around the time of menstruation are referred to as *catamenial epilepsy*. Seizures may take place shortly before menstruation, during and immediately after it, or at the time of ovulation (midcycle). Studies reveal that the premenstrual and ovulatory phases are associated with the highest seizure frequencies.

The hormonal changes associated with the menstrual cycle are the most likely cause of changes in the seizure frequency. The steroid sex hormones can easily cross the barrier that separates the blood and the brain (the *blood-brain barrier*). The brain contains numerous nerve cells that are directly affected by estrogen and progesterone, the main sex hormones in women. Studies in animals have shown that high doses of estrogen can cause or worsen seizures, whereas high doses of progesterone can act like an antiepileptic drug.

Control of seizures that occur mainly around the time of menstruation remains a difficult problem. For women who have regular menstrual cycles, a slight increase in the dosage of the antiepileptic drugs before the time of increased seizure frequency may be helpful. Some doctors recommend also taking acetazolamide (Diamox), a mild diuretic and antiepileptic drug, but there is no proof of its effectiveness for catamenial epilepsy, particularly when taken every day. It may help to reduce the water retention that occurs in the premenstrual period. Other doctors have prescribed an additional antiepileptic drug such as lorazepam (Ativan) to be taken during the days of the menstrual cycle when seizures are most likely to occur. A few doctors have advocated the use of hormonal agents such as progesterone or birth control pills for women with catamenial epilepsy, but the effectiveness and safety of hormonal therapy for this type of epilepsy remain to be established.

Stress

Stress can affect brain function in many ways. Stress is associated with a variety of unpleasant emotions such as worry, fear, depression, frustration, and anger. It commonly leads to sleep deprivation or disrupted, fragmented sleep. Stress and anxiety can trigger an increase in the breathing rate, known as hyperventilation. Hyperventilation is a well-recognized means of provoking seizures in certain patients, especially those with absence seizures. Stress and preoccupation with problems also may cause some people to miss their medication. Stress can cause hormonal changes such as an increase in the steroid hormone cortisol, which also may influence seizure activity.

Negative emotions, such as worry or fright, may have a direct effect on the brain and may cause seizures. This is a serious result of stress, and the most difficult to prove. The mechanism for this effect of negative emotions could involve the *limbic system* (deep parts of the temporal and frontal lobes). This system, which regulates emotional functions, is one of the most common places for a seizure to arise. It makes sense then that dramatic changes in its activity, such as may occur with intense or prolonged emotional states, could increase the susceptibility to seizures.

If stress appears to provoke seizures, it may be helpful to avoid stressful situations, learn relaxation techniques, or do yoga or tai chi. However, no one can completely avoid stress, and the worst stresses—such as the death of a loved one, serious injury, loss of a job, or financial hardship—are often unpredictable. During stressful times, it is important for people with epilepsy to get enough sleep and not to miss medications.

Parents should try to recognize what is stressful to their child who has epilepsy, particularly if the seizures are difficult to control for unexplained reasons. They should realize that the parent's perspective and the child's perspective are different. What seems trivial to a parent may be stressful to a child. The child can be asked if there are things causing worry or situations that feel uncomfortable. Simply stopping those activities is a bad idea, however. Doing that may signal to such children that they never have to do anything that they do not like to do. It is best to work out some compromise that reduces the stress, but also encourages the child to be active. If the stress is serious, a psychological consultation may be necessary.

Stress is a frequently overlooked cause of seizures in mentally handicapped people. Stress can result from any change in their daily routine, such as a new teacher or new staff member at the residential home. Socializing with others is a wonderful and necessary process for those with or without epilepsy, but the process for those with a mental handicap may be even more stressful than it is for other children because many in the group may have limited social skills, poor impulse control, or increased irritability.

Over-the-Counter Drugs

Some *over-the-counter drugs* (drugs that can be bought without a doctor's prescription) can occasionally cause first-time seizures or increase the frequency of seizures in people with epilepsy (see Appendix 3). Some cold and sleep preparations contain diphenhydramine (e.g., Benadryl) and phenylpropanolamine (PPA). PPA, also present in some diet pills, is currently restricted by the Food and Drug Administration (FDA) because of its association with stroke in young women. Diphenhydramine is also used to treat coughs, itching, and nasal congestion or to induce sleep. These drugs should be avoided by people with epilepsy. (In my experience, this is most important for those with primary generalized epilepsy.) Diphenhydramine ointment applied to the skin for itching appears to be safe for people with epilepsy. Medications for runny and stuffy noses containing pseudoephedrine or phenylephrine appear to be safer than diphenhydramine. However, there are reports of seizures caused by these drugs, too.

For aches and pains, acetaminophen (e.g., Tylenol, Panadol, and Excedrin Aspirin Free) is probably the safest medication. Aspirin also appears safe for most adults, but it should not be given to children. Prolonged high doses of aspirin should be avoided by people taking phenytoin. Drug interactions may cause adverse effects if aspirin is taken by people with high blood levels of valproate or phenytoin. Ibuprofen (e.g., Motrin and Advil) can also interact with phenytoin, leading to increased blood phenytoin levels and possible adverse effects. Propoxyphene (another pain reliever found in over-the-counter preparations), when taken with carbamazepine, can dramatically increase blood carbamazepine levels and possible adverse effects.

Nutritional Deficiencies

Many people are extremely interested in pursuing dietary changes or taking nutritional supplements to improve seizure control. It is reasonable to recommend that people with epilepsy try to eat regularly and eat a balanced diet. It is clear that some foods can alter brain function, but reliable information on which to make recommendations is scarce. For instance, very low levels of sugar in the blood can cause seizures in some people, especially people with diabetes who take too much insulin. There is no proof, however, that mild dips in blood sugar levels that are commonly labeled as hypoglycemia have any relationship to seizures or epilepsy.

People often try to treat seizures with various vitamins, herbs, or amino acids, but there is no evidence that any of these nutritional supplements clearly improve seizure control. Research studies have been unable to confirm the thousands of reports of people who have appeared to respond to these nutritional substances. Promising therapies need not be ignored, even if they are not in the Western tradition of drug therapy, but people with epilepsy would be wise not to embrace a treatment until there is solid proof that it works.

Most nutritional supplements are, in effect, drugs. For example, steroids can be claimed as a natural therapy because steroid hormones are naturally found in the body. There is nothing natural, however, about extremely high doses of steroids, vitamins, amino acids, or other organic compounds. They may even be dangerous, and probably most of them have no real effect on seizure control.

VITAMINS

Vitamins are chemicals that are required in tiny amounts to maintain normal cell function. Some are manufactured by our bodies. Others are made by plants or animals and are contained in the foods we eat. Although our current diet may be unhealthy because of too much fat, sugars, and processed foods, vitamin deficiencies are uncommon in modern Western societies unless the diet is seriously restricted. In rare cases, the body is unable to manufacture or absorb vitamins and the result is a vitamin deficiency, but even then, seizures almost never result.

The only vitamin deficiency known to cause or worsen seizures is a vitamin B_6 (pyridoxine) deficiency. This deficiency occurs mainly in newborns and infants and causes seizures that are difficult to control. To test whether a baby with seizures has a vitamin B_6 deficiency, doctors often prescribe a small dose of the vitamin to see if the seizures stop or decrease in frequency. In some cases, the doctor may administer the vitamin intravenously to a young baby while recording the EEG, which will improve dramatically if there is a vitamin B_6 deficiency. Some doctors may also try vitamin B_6 in older children with difficult-to-control seizures, although there is no solid evidence that it will be helpful.

Antiepileptic drugs may interact with vitamins in the body. Phenytoin and phenobarbital can cause a deficiency of the vitamin folic acid (folate). Folate is important in the production of blood cells and may be important for peripheral nerves. Folate deficiency can cause a predisposition to certain birth defects, especially neural tube defects. The United States Public Health Service recommends that all women of childbearing age should take 0.4 mg of folate per day. Women of childbearing age and people with anemia or other blood cell disorders who are taking antiepileptic drugs should supplement their diet with folate. The recommended dose of folate for women of childbearing age who have epilepsy is between 0.4 and 2.0 mg per day. For women of childbearing age taking more than one antiepileptic drug or those taking moderate to high doses of valproate (i.e., more than 1000 mg per day) or carbamazepine (i.e., more than 700 mg per day) or those who have a family or personal history of a child with a neural tube defect, folate doses of 2.0 to 4.0 mg per day may be recommended. High doses of folate may reduce blood levels of phenytoin, which should be monitored when folate supplementation is used.

Valproate can deplete the liver's stores of carnitine, a substance that functions like a vitamin to help in the metabolism of fats. Some believe that carnitine supplementation can help prevent the rare cases of liver damage caused by valproate, but there is no clear evidence of this effect. Because serious liver damage from valproate is extremely rare, carnitine supplementation should only be considered for individuals at great risk, such as children under 2 years old who are being treated with valproate, especially those who also take other antiepileptic drugs. (This is the group with the highest rate of valproate-associated liver damage.) There have been a few reports that carnitine supplementation has helped older children and adults with other adverse reactions to valproate, such as tremor and tiredness. Formal studies of this effect have not yet been done.

Some unconfirmed reports claim that vitamin E improves seizure control in children, but the response is variable and rarely dramatic. Claims that a therapy is effective based on case reports can be misleading. Vitamin therapies deserve further study in controlled clinical trials.

MINERALS

Minerals are essential nutrients. Low levels of the minerals sodium, calcium, and magnesium can alter the electrical activity of brain cells and cause seizures. Deficiency of these minerals in the diet is rare unless there is severe general malnutrition, but other factors may affect the levels in the body. Low sodium levels may be caused by medications such as diuretics (water pills) or carbamazepine, by excessive water intake, or by hormonal disorders. Low calcium levels most often result from kidney disease or hormonal disorders. Because magnesium levels alter the body's regulation of calcium, low magnesium levels often contribute to or cause low calcium levels. Individuals who chronically abuse alcohol and have poor nutrition often develop low magnesium levels, which can predispose to seizures.

People with epilepsy very seldom need supplementation of sodium, calcium, or magnesium for seizure control. Changes in diet or mineral supplements are reasonable for those who have low levels of these minerals if a medical examination does not find any underlying disorder.

Because many antiepileptic drugs can increase vitamin D metabolism and lead to a deficiency of calcium in the bone (e.g., carbamazepine, phenobarbital, phenytoin, primidone, and valproate), combined calcium and vitamin D supplementation should be taken to help prevent bone loss. For people taking these drugs for more than 5 years, a bone density test can detect this possible complication of antiepileptic drug therapy. If significant thinning of the bone is found, a consultation with a bone metabolism specialist may be helpful.

Certain adverse effects of valproate may be lessened by mineral supplementation. Inflammation of the pancreas (pancreatitis), which is a rare but serious adverse effect of valproate, may be prevented by selenium supplementation. Selenium at a dose of 100 mcg(micrograms) per day has been used to prevent valproate-induced pancreatitis in a child who previously had this problem when taking valproate. Selenium (10–20 mcg per day) and zinc (30–50 mg per day) also may help to counteract the hair loss that some people experience when taking valproate or other drugs. These doses are available in many over-the-counter high-potency multivitamins.

GLYCINE AND HERBS

Glycine, a naturally occurring amino acid, is a neurotransmitter with a possible role in seizure control. Correcting a deficiency of glycine by giving dimethylglycine has been reported to manage some seizures, but controlled studies have not been done.

Herbs have been used for centuries by numerous cultures to treat seizures. So far there is little evidence to support or contradict the use of specific herbs.

Cycles of the Moon

Since the dawn of civilization, people have thought that the moon influences certain behaviors. The moon does affect the magnetic and gravitational activities of the Earth, such as tidal changes. The role of magnetic energy in animal behavior has only recently been recognized.

The moon has been implicated in seizure occurrence for centuries. The moon's role in epilepsy was "proved" and "disproved" on numerous occasions before the modern age of scientific study. Modern neurology rarely even considers the moon's cycles, but some people with epilepsy and parents of children with epilepsy are convinced that seizures are more likely to occur during certain phases of the moon.

The role of the moon in epilepsy is the subject of considerable study in the former Soviet Union, but it has received little attention in modern Western medical studies. The notion of a relationship between the moon's phases and human behavior is worthy of closer study.

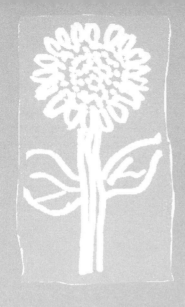

part two

DIAGNOSIS AND TREATMENT OF EPILEPSY

CHAPTER
7

The Health Care Team

Health care is a partnership. The notion that doctors and other health care professionals give orders and patients blindly follow them is out of date. The person with epilepsy—the patient—must become part of the health care team. Other members of the team depend on what the patient tells them. The diagnosis depends largely on the information given in the patient's medical history. Decisions about therapy are influenced by the concerns or fears that the patient expresses. For example, the choice of antiepileptic drugs may depend on the patient's feelings about the drugs' adverse effects and their expense or on the patient's willingness to make lifestyle changes, such as not driving. Under similar circumstances, a variety of choices may be acceptable. Many of the decisions made in medicine depend on such "judgment calls," which should reflect the shared knowledge and wisdom of the patient and members of the health care team.

Doctor and Patient

A good relationship between the doctor and the patient is one of the cornerstones of effective medical care. The doctor and patient are partners in the health care process; they share a common goal, but have different responsibilities in achieving that goal. For some patients, the doctor's visit is a passive event; the doctor checks them over and makes recommendations. A visit should be interactive, however; the doctor needs to know the patient's concerns and wishes. For instance, it is helpful for the doctor to know that a particular patient will do anything—even give up driving—to avoid taking medications and that another patient wants to avoid seizures at almost any cost. These are personal decisions that work best for a specific person in a specific situation. The treatment may need to change if there are changes in the person's situation, such as marriage, a new job that requires a lot of driving, or loss of health insurance.

Communication is central to the doctor-patient relationship. The patient and family members must provide the doctor with the information he or she needs to make a correct diagnosis and prescribe the most effective and best-tolerated treatment. The doctor should use understandable language to discuss with the patient why tests are being obtained, what the tests involve, and perhaps most important, the risks and benefits of therapy. Ideally, the relationship should be comfortable and based on trust. The past several decades have seen a major shift toward greater communication between doctor and patient. Doctors are now much more willing to share information about choices, medical facts, and potential risks.

Time often limits the communication between doctor and patient. In earlier generations, doctors were more available and able to spend more time listening to their patients. Today, patients may feel rushed, and their questions may go unasked or unanswered. The doctor may appear to be more concerned about moving patients in and out of the office, ordering tests, and prescribing drugs than about taking time to listen to the issues bothering the patient. On the other hand, doctors often complain that patients provide too much irrelevant information, which is time consuming. Some patients also like to discuss social, political, and other unrelated topics with their doctors. However enjoyable such conversations may be, patients should limit themselves to issues concerning their health, especially if the doctor's office is busy.

THE FIRST VISIT

There are several ways to help foster a more productive interaction with the doctor. A patient's first consultation with a new doctor often determines the nature of their relationship. The doctor may begin by asking about the main problem that brought the patient to the office. The doctor may then ask the patient to give a fairly detailed account of the symptoms. The doctor may question the patient carefully about events surrounding the seizure:

- Could it have been provoked by sleep deprivation, excessive use of alcohol, or some other factor?
- What was the setting?
- Did the episode occur shortly after standing?
- Was there a warning?
- Exactly what happened during the episode?
- How long did it last?
- Was the patient tired or confused after the episode?
- When did the patient first seek medical attention?
- What tests were done?
- What medication was prescribed?
- What was the response to the medication?
- Have there been more episodes? If so, what were they like?

It is helpful for patients to briefly summarize their medical history in writing. If they were referred by another doctor, the referring doctor may write a letter summarizing the history. Patients should bring with them all important medical records, such as notes from other doctors, seizure calendars (records of seizures), and results of laboratory studies such as blood drug levels and electroencephalogram (EEG) and magnetic resonance imaging (MRI) reports. The actual MRI films and EEG tracings can be borrowed. This information will help the doctor focus his or her questions and will provide important details that might otherwise be forgotten during the visit.

Patients often find it helpful to bring a written list of questions, particularly if the purpose of the visit is to define issues or provide specific answers. Questions are best asked at the end of the visit, after the doctor has had a chance to record the medical history, review previous laboratory studies, and perform a physical examination. It is a good idea to limit the list to five questions; others can be saved for a future visit. In some doctor's offices and clinics, a nurse reviews the doctor's information and recommendations. The nurse can answer many of the patient's questions and may provide materials on epilepsy. This is often helpful, especially if the patient did not understand the doctor's answers to some questions.

When patients leave the doctor's office, they should clearly understand the treatment plan. If things do not make sense or important issues remain unresolved, patients should ask their questions again. They should ask for written instructions, particularly on how to take medications. They should know what to do if another seizure occurs or if they miss taking their medication. If important questions come up after they leave the doctor's office, they should call and ask them. Many questions can be answered by the nurse. Less important questions or bits of information, such as the fact that an uncle has epilepsy, can be communicated by a note or wait until the next visit.

FOLLOW-UP VISITS

Follow-up doctor's appointments usually last 10 to 30 minutes. If the patient is seizure-free and having no adverse effects from the medications, the visit may be brief. If the seizures are worse or the medications have caused new adverse effects, the visit often needs to be longer. Before the patient sees the doctor, a nurse may check blood pressure, review seizure control and dosage of medications, ask about adverse effects of the medications, and discuss any new social or medical problems that have arisen since the last visit. The nurse can answer many questions at this time.

If there is a need to discuss special subjects, such as pregnancy, discontinuing antiepileptic drugs, or epilepsy surgery, a longer appointment may be required. Patients who anticipate such special needs on a visit may want to schedule additional time with the doctor.

The doctor and patient share the same goal: having the person with epilepsy enjoy a good quality of life. There is often a gap between the doctor's perception of how the patient is doing and how the patient feels he or she is doing. Some patients may fear a seizure because of embarrassment or possible injury. If one tonic-clonic seizure a year or one complex partial seizure a month bothers the patient, or if the adverse effects of the medication are a problem, the patient should make sure the doctor knows it. Discussing the patient's concerns helps the doctor understand the disorder and how it affects this patient. The doctor then can tailor treatment strategies and recommendations to his or her specific problems. Often, there must be a balance between seizure control and adverse effects of the medication; that is, giving medication that will make the patient completely seizure-free may produce excessive unwanted effects. Reducing or changing the medication to eliminate these effects may permit some mild seizures to occur but may provide a better overall balance. It may be better to have 2 minutes of mild seizure activity per month and minimal side effects than to have no seizures but feel tired and dizzy most of every day.

It is important that patients communicate their needs to the doctor. For example, some patients may not be able to afford certain drugs and may need to take less expensive ones. (For information on ways to save on the costs of antiepileptic drugs, see Chap. 10). For others, prescription insurance plans make the cost issue irrelevant. Some patients take less than the prescribed amounts of medication to stretch their supply or to avoid bothersome adverse effects. Patients should not adjust their medications without consulting the doctor. If a drug is unaffordable or the medication is causing troublesome adverse effects, the patient should tell the doctor so that adjustments can be considered.

Doctors and patients often fail to talk about sensitive issues such as sexual desire, sexual function, or mood, but they should be discussed if they are a problem. If the doctor does not respond to a sensitive issue, the patient should make sure the doctor understands how seriously the problem affects him or her. The patient also can speak to the nurse. If repeated efforts to make the doctor aware of the problem are unsuccessful, the patient should consider changing doctors.

FINANCIAL ISSUES AND INSURANCE COVERAGE

Most doctors have office or business managers who can answer questions about financial concerns or insurance coverage. In cases of financial hardship, many doctors are willing to accept payment plans or reduced fees. As managed care and health maintenance organizations multiply in our country, the access to doctors both expands and contracts. It expands because people with these health care plans will have access to pediatricians, neurologists, and other physicians. It contracts because the number or choice of doctors available in such plans is usually limited. For example, a specific plan may include only a few neurologists and no *epileptologist* (a neurologist with special training in epilepsy). Furthermore, because specialty care is more expensive, some managed care plans may restrict access to epileptologists. Fortunately, only a minority of people with epilepsy need to see an epileptologist. However, there are potential advantages in a consultation with an epilepsy specialist, including learning new information about new antiepileptic drugs (such as less sedating ones) or getting expertise on issues such as pregnancy or the potential for surgical therapy. Local Epilepsy Foundation (EF) affiliates may be able to provide the names of doctors who accept insurance; doctors who accept Medicaid, Medicare, or worker's compensation; or doctors who are willing to see patients at reduced rates. They may also know of clinics where care is given free of charge.

The types of insurance that cover epilepsy vary tremendously. Many doctors do not accept patients with Medicaid or worker's compensation unless they are willing to pay personally, separate from those forms of coverage. Worker's compensation programs (see Chap. 27) are regulated by the state and have fixed fees for medical services. Doctors who care for people with worker's compensation must accept the allowed fee as full payment.

Patients with Medicaid can often obtain good care at public clinics in teaching hospitals, where the coverage is accepted in full payment. At many teaching hospitals, a patient may be able to attend an epilepsy clinic supervised by an epileptologist. However, the doctors who directly provide the care at teaching-hospital clinics are often residents in training. The residents' fund of knowledge and experience varies tremendously. Most have a limited knowledge of how to diagnose and treat epilepsy. Residents should be supervised by an attending doctor, and the patient should try to speak with both the resident doctor and the attending doctor. Another reason to speak to the attending doctor is that residents' assignments usually rotate from month to month. This means the patient could have a new doctor every month. The attending doctor usually has a more permanent position; consulting with him or her briefly at each visit helps to maintain continuity of care.

Medicare reimburses doctors more fairly than Medicaid does, and many doctors accept Medicare (see Chap. 31). Medicare allows physicians to charge certain maximum rates for services. These rates are often lower than the standard rates charged for a service to a person who does not have Medicare.

SECOND OPINIONS AND CHANGING DOCTORS

A patient with epilepsy usually is first cared for by a primary care doctor (general practitioner, internist, or pediatrician). If the seizures are not controlled within 3 months, the patient should be referred to a neurologist. If the patient is treated by a neurologist for 9 months and the seizures are still uncontrolled, the patient should be referred to an epileptologist.

If the doctor is not meeting a patient's needs, it may be worth obtaining a second opinion or even changing doctors. Before doing this, the patient should consider again the areas in which he or she feels uncertain. In many cases, the patient may begin to feel more comfortable after asking the doctor additional questions or raising certain issues. When a second opinion is obtained, the patient sometimes finds that the first doctor had left no stone unturned and the second doctor agrees with all aspects of the care. On the other hand, the second doctor may have helpful suggestions regarding tests or changes in the treatment regimen.

For a second opinion, it is probably best for the patient to ask the doctor for the name of a neurologist or epileptologist. The patient may also get a list of names from the local affiliate of the EF or from a friend or relative. It is important that care be coordinated. The referring, or primary, doctor and the second doctor should communicate, and the primary doctor should send copies of the patient's records to the second doctor. The patient may wish to continue care with the second doctor, but usually the primary doctor remains in charge of the case.

In some cases, communication and trust between the patient and the doctor may break down. Problems can arise, for example, over time spent during the visit, finances, adverse effects of medication, failure to take medication as prescribed, or language difficulties. Relationships have a "chemistry," and sometimes the chemistry is not right. Changing doctors may be awkward and uncomfortable. It is best for the patient to call the doctor's office and tell the secretary, office manager, nurse, or doctor that he or she is changing doctors. The patient should then ask that the records be forwarded to the new doctor. If questioned about the reason for the change, the patient can simply say, "It is just something I want to do" or can nicely explain why.

The patient will need to write a brief note asking that the records be forwarded to the new doctor or directly to the patient. Patients have a legal right to have a copy of their medical records. The note can be very simple: "Please forward all of my medical records to Dr. —." Be sure to include the doctor's address. It is helpful to call the new doctor's office before the appointment to make sure that the records have arrived. If they have not, the patient should call the first doctor's office and find out if they were sent. Although it is uncommon, there may be a charge for copying the records (there are limits on these charges).

Patients should avoid burning bridges behind them when changing doctors. For example, there may be only two neurologists in a community, and the patient may turn out to like the original one better than the second one or the original neurologist may be on-call when the patient is brought in for an emergency room visit.

Nurses

Nurses are on the front line of medicine. In the emergency room, they are often the first people to obtain information about a problem. In the office and clinic, they often greet patients and review their current medical status. After the doctor orders tests or changes the medication regimen, the nurse more fully explains the test or describes exactly how to take the drugs. The nurse often serves, quite literally, as the translator between the doctor and the patient. In many offices, clinics, and hospitals, nurses provide written instructions and may distribute literature or show videotapes further explaining epilepsy and the doctor's recommendations.

In many medical offices, nurses also answer questions over the telephone and in person. The nurse may spend more time with the patient than the doctor does. Patients should feel comfortable talking with the nurse about problems and should have confidence in the nurse's response. If patients wish to speak with the doctor or want the nurse to check with the doctor, however, they should feel free to ask the nurse to do so.

NURSE-CLINICIANS

In some doctors' offices and in many epilepsy centers, nurse-clinicians play a vital role in patient care. These specially trained nurses help to assess, coordinate, and implement patient education and care. They can answer routine questions over the telephone, such as those about laboratory results, upcoming tests, adverse effects of medications, dosage schedules, interactions between antiepileptic drugs and other medications, and the safety of activities. The nurse-clinician can also be helpful in making referrals to other members of the health care team, such as the social worker or the physical therapist. Because the doctor and nurse-clinician work closely together, their recommendations on specific issues and questions are usually quite similar.

NURSE PRACTITIONERS

Nurse practitioners are nurses with advanced medical education. They are licensed by the state to take a medical history, examine patients, order tests, and prescribe medications, including narcotics and other restricted substances. Nurse practitioners can serve as relatively independent practitioners who diagnose diseases and treat patients.

Nurse practitioners undergo extensive training and licensure examinations. They are supervised by doctors, who review the case histories and treatment plans at intervals specified by the state licensing board.

Physician Assistants

Physician assistants are playing an increasing role in American health care. Their name describes their role: they assist doctors in obtaining the medical history, examining the patient, recommending therapy, drawing blood, ordering tests, speaking with consulting doctors, and performing many other functions.

Social Worker—Counselors

Social workers are valuable members of the treatment team for epilepsy. Unfortunately, social workers with expertise in epilepsy may only be available in comprehensive epilepsy programs, which aren't available in every community. Social workers play many roles. In some centers, the social worker is one of the key providers of patient and family education about epilepsy. In addition, the social worker often provides the community outreach education programs. Often the social worker assists in identifying and obtaining precious resources. These resources include special education programs, respite centers (where a child or adult with special needs can spend some time so that caregivers can rest), home health aides, medical insurance benefits, vocational rehabilitation centers, and referrals to psychologists and other mental health workers. Social workers may also be helpful in referring a person with epilepsy who has experienced discrimination to advocacy groups such as the local Protection and Advocacy Service, Legal Aid Society, or an attorney specializing in this subject. (The Epilepsy Foundation may also be helpful in this regard.)

Social workers sometimes function as counselors or therapists, and their fees can be substantially below those of psychologists and psychiatrists. The counseling sessions provide an important place for people with epilepsy to discuss social and personal issues that the physician may not have time or the expertise to address. Counseling sessions may be especially beneficial for children by helping them to understand issues of independence, maturity, and personal growth. Sometimes social workers help identify parents whose over-protectiveness is adversely affecting a child with epilepsy. Problems of home life—such as a parent or spouse with substance abuse problems or a psychiatric disorder, living in a divorced family, or the death of a loved one—can be discussed, put in perspective, better understood, and coped with after counseling sessions.

Social workers also can inform the doctor about issues that may have a bearing on medical problems, thereby bringing about important changes in medical therapy or referral to a psychologist or psychiatrist. Social workers can also be helpful in crisis situations, when they can help refer patients to the doctors or epilepsy centers that are best able to handle the problem.

EEG Technologists

The EEG is a recording of the electrical activity of the brain. It is discussed in more detail in Chapter 8. The EEG technologist is the person who performs the EEG test. He or she explains the testing procedure to the patient, obtains some background information (age, diagnosis, medications, time of last meal, time of last seizure), applies the electrodes to the patient's scalp, records the EEG, and prepares the EEG record for the doctor's review. The EEG technologist is supervised by the director of the EEG laboratory.

Because the EEG session often takes more than an hour, the technologist spends a good bit of time with the patient and therefore may gather information about the patient's epilepsy that may be helpful to the doctor or other members of the health care team.

Pharmacists

Pharmacists fill prescriptions and dispense drugs. They play an important role in health care. They may have known individuals and families over many years and are often aware of both health and personal issues. Many people feel more comfortable talking to their pharmacist than to their doctor. Pharmacists are knowledgeable and can provide expert information about medications, but they cannot substitute for doctors. Pharmacists can be helpful in discussing the potential adverse effects of medications, costs of drugs, and relative risks and benefits of generic versus brand-name drugs. (See Chap. 10 for a discussion of this issue. Never switch drugs without first checking with the doctor.) For people who are taking several drugs, pharmacists can often provide information on potential drug interactions.

Epilepsy Associations and Support Groups

The Epilepsy Foundation provides important resources at both the local and national levels (see Chap. 32). Local affiliates of the foundation and other epilepsy support groups provide essential services for many people with epilepsy. These groups are sometimes directed by a social worker or may have social workers and counselors on the staff. Depending on the specific group, services include support-group meetings to discuss social and related issues; lectures on health issues; referrals for vocational rehabilitation; lectures to schoolchildren and school nurses about epilepsy; and assistance with referrals to pediatricians, neurologists, epileptologists, and specialized epilepsy centers.

Individual doctors and health care workers at comprehensive epilepsy centers often work together with local epilepsy associations. Patients benefit when the resources of the medical centers and epilepsy associations are pooled.

Specialty Members of the Health Care Team

The health care team is defined by the needs of the patient. In comprehensive epilepsy centers, consultation with a neuropsychologist and psychiatrist is common, especially by patients considered for surgical therapy. Specialists in vocational rehabilitation, physical therapy, occupational therapy, music therapy, speech therapy, or special education may prove important for selected patients.

NEUROPSYCHOLOGISTS

Neuropsychologists assess various aspects of intellectual and behavioral function. The neuropsychologist usually administers a battery of tests that helps to identify relative strengths and weaknesses in areas such as thinking, reasoning, memory, language, perception, motor ability, and behavior. These tests are essential in the assessment for epilepsy surgery, but they are also helpful for showing evidence of improvement or deterioration in certain intellectual functions.

The neuropsychologist also can help to define the effects of the injury to the brain from head trauma, stroke, or tumor. For example, frontal lobe injury from trauma may affect judgment and motivation, making it difficult for the person to understand why it is important to take medications regularly and avoid excessive alcohol use. With a better understanding of the problems and personal dynamics of the patient, the doctor can formulate a more effective treatment plan. Neuropsychologists also perform therapy or other interventions for intellectual or behavioral problems and private psychotherapy for emotional problems related to brain disorders.

For patients considering epilepsy surgery, the neuropsychologist is often directly involved in performing a test called the intracarotid sodium amobarbital test (see Chap. 12). The neuropsychologist also is involved in carrying out electrical stimulation of the brain to map areas of intellectual functions, such as speech and understanding spoken or written language.

PSYCHIATRISTS

People often have negative feelings about psychiatrists, mainly because of stigmas associated with behavioral disorders and misconceptions about the nature of psychiatric care. Psychiatrists do more than simply listen to people. They use a variety of therapies, ranging from counseling and psychotherapy to prescribing medications.

Psychological and psychiatric problems are common in the general population. Some of these problems, such as depression, anxiety, and psychosis, are common among people with epilepsy. Depression may be caused by medications, especially barbiturates. It may also be caused by psychosocial problems, such as loss of a job or a loved one, especially in someone who is dependent on that job or person for support. Depression can also result from biologic factors such as brain lesions (e.g., stroke) and epilepsy. Epilepsy per se does not cause depression, but the biologic processes that underlie epilepsy or result from recurrent abnormal electrical and chemical discharges may predispose toward or cause depression and other behavioral disorders. The psychiatrist can help to identify the problem, determine its cause, and recommend treatment. In some cases, relief from the depression is obtained by adjusting the antiepileptic drugs, adding an antidepressant drug, or counseling the patient about social and medical problems.

If "chemistry" is important in the doctor-patient relationship, it is essential in the psychiatrist-patient relationship. If the patient has a behavioral problem and is not comfortable with a particular psychiatrist, he or she should consider seeing a different one rather than ignoring the problem. Because the psychiatrist may need to prescribe an antidepressant or recommend reducing the dosage of an antiepileptic drug, good communication between the psychiatrist and the primary doctor treating the epilepsy is essential.

PSYCHOLOGISTS

Psychologists can help the patient understand and cope with epilepsy as a neurologic disorder and as a social stigma. They can guide patients and their families in learning to live more positively with epilepsy. Their counseling role is similar to that of social workers, and they can help in treating the patient's mood disorders and problems with self-esteem and independence. As someone to talk to about life stresses and the influences of epilepsy, its treatment, and its consequences, psychologists can be a much-needed resource.

PHYSICAL THERAPISTS

Physical therapists help people who have disorders of movement, coordination, or sensation become more physically able. The movement disorders may be related to problems involving the brain, spinal cord, nerves, or muscles. Mobility and coordination can be enhanced through various programs of stretching, exercise, and skills development. Most individuals with epilepsy do not require physical therapy, but those who do have limited mobility or other physical disorders can get important assistance from a physical therapist.

OCCUPATIONAL THERAPISTS

Some people with epilepsy also have other disorders that affect their ability to perform daily tasks, especially ones requiring fine motor control, such as writing, buttoning clothes, or picking up small objects.

An occupational therapist can offer suggestions for dealing with problems of this kind.

SPEECH-LANGUAGE PATHOLOGISTS

Speech-language pathologists assist people with speech, language, and swallowing disorders. Some problems of this kind may result from disorders of areas of the brain involved in language comprehension, word finding, and the mental formulation of speech. Sometimes speech expression is hampered by motor disorders that do not affect language skills; the disorders impair the coordinated movements required for speech instead. These motor speech disorders can result from abnormalities of the brain, the spinal cord, other nerves, or the muscles of the mouth and throat. Speech therapists assess the nature of the problem and recommend a program of therapy, which varies considerably depending on the problems and the approach of the specific therapist.

VOCATIONAL REHABILITATION COUNSELORS

Vocational rehabilitation counselors help people with disabilities obtain skills needed for employment. Specialized programs, some of which are sponsored by state or community agencies, may be available to facilitate this process (see Chap. 27). Counselors can help by assessing knowledge, skills, and interests and recommending areas that seem worthwhile to pursue. They teach people how to accommodate and overcome aspects of their disability, improve work habits, train for specific job functions, develop more effective interviewing skills, and seek and obtain employment. A person may benefit from several counseling sessions to identify employment agencies or prepare a résumé. In other cases, a vocational rehabilitation program may be helpful. Such programs provide in-depth assessment and training.

The help of vocational rehabilitation counselors can be essential for obtaining a job. One young man who was seizure-free after epilepsy surgery at our center had difficulty obtaining a job in the printing industry, although he had worked in that area for more than 7 years. After a brief vocational rehabilitation program that included training with computers, he found a job in printing and was promoted twice in the year; his training and expertise with computers, added to his background in printing, paid off.

Comprehensive Epilepsy Centers

Epilepsy centers are valuable resources for any person with definite or suspected epilepsy who has unresolved problems related to the disorder. They are discussed in more detail in Chapter 33. Patients may be referred to a comprehensive epilepsy center for a single outpatient visit for an assessment of their current diagnosis and therapy, or they may receive longer-term follow-up and treatment.

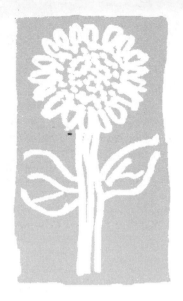

Making the Diagnosis of Epilepsy

Although the diagnosis of epilepsy is usually straightforward, other disorders can cause sudden changes in behavior and may be confused with epilepsy. Moreover, some patients have more than one type of seizure. The correct diagnosis depends on an accurate description of the events occurring before, during, and after the attack. It is essential that the patient—or a witness to the seizure—give the doctor as much information as possible about the episode. If certain details are vague, the doctor should be told. No matter how accurate and complete the information, however, some episodes remain difficult even for experts to diagnose correctly. Every epilepsy specialist has had patients whose attacks were so confusing that the initial diagnosis was incorrect. This is one reason that follow-up care and the additional information it can provide are so important.

Conditions Confused with Epilepsy

Many medical, neurologic, and psychiatric disorders mimic seizures. Before recommending treatment, the doctor wants to be sure that the diagnosis is correct. A detailed discussion of the conditions that can be confused with epilepsy is beyond the scope of this book. Only a few of the disorders that are most often mistaken for an epileptic seizure are presented in this chapter. Chapter 15 discusses some conditions occurring only in children that can be confused with seizures.

FAINTING

Fainting (a brief loss of consciousness, also called syncope) occurs when the brain does not receive enough blood, oxygen, or sugar. Fainting is common and is usually of no consequence in young people. Most often the person is standing and then complains of dizziness, lightheadedness, or abdominal discomfort. He or she then turns pale, begins to sweat, and falls to the ground. The body may stiffen slightly, and the arms or legs may jerk several times. Falling to the floor is a natural remedy for the faint. Many faints result from the heart's inability to pump enough blood up to the brain; when the person is lying down, the heart is at the same level as the brain, and blood flows more easily to the head. An incorrect diagnosis of a seizure may be made when the doctor hears that someone suddenly lost consciousness, fell down, and then had jerking movements. In rare cases of fainting, especially if the person is young and is kept in a standing or sitting position by a well-meaning bystander, a full-blown convulsive seizure can occur after the faint. In most cases of fainting, the loss of consciousness lasts less than 1 minute, and the person is fully alert within 10 to 30 seconds after awakening.

Many disorders can cause fainting. Lowering of the blood pressure related to position, called *orthostatic hypotension,* is a common disorder in which a person faints shortly after arising from a lying or sitting position. Fainting can occur almost immediately upon standing or after several minutes. All people are subject to orthostatic hypotension after prolonged bed rest or after a hot bath. Perhaps the most common instance of orthostatic hypotension is the lightheadedness that occurs when someone gets out of bed quickly after awakening. Other common contributing causes include dehydration from inadequate fluid intake; increased sweating, diarrhea, or vomiting; and prolonged standing in a hot environment. Fainting also may be the result of a disturbance in the rhythm of the heart (e.g., prolonged QT syndrome or ventricular tachycardia or fibrillation), which may require treatment with medication or a pacemaker.

HYPOGLYCEMIA

Hypoglycemia (low blood sugar) is one of the most overdiagnosed disorders in the United States. It does occur as a serious medical problem in some people—most often in people with diabetes who take too much of the hormone insulin. An endocrine tumor of the pancreas is a rare cause of hypoglycemia. Hypoglycemia can cause symptoms of dizziness, lightheadedness, fainting, and even tonic-clonic (grand mal) seizures.

Hypoglycemia is diagnosed without strong supporting evidence in many cases. The diagnosis of hypoglycemia is often based on the results of a glucose tolerance test. For this test, the patient is given a drink with high sugar content and the changes in blood sugar (glucose) are measured at different times over the next several hours. Each time interval has its own expected range of blood sugar levels to reflect the predicted initial rise and later dip in blood sugar after the sugar solution is drunk. After an initial rise in blood sugar, insulin is released from the pancreas into the bloodstream to compensate for the rise and to lower the blood sugar level. In many healthy people, this rebound lowering of the blood sugar level extends beyond the so-called "normal" lower limits, just as the initial rise in blood sugar level extended beyond the "normal" upper limits. According to experts in endocrinology, the results of this test are often interpreted as abnormal although in fact the values for the "normal" resting blood sugar do not apply when the response to a large dose of concentrated sugar solution is assessed. A true diagnosis of hypoglycemia is supported by finding a low blood sugar level when symptoms of hypoglycemia are present and by obtaining relief of the symptoms by consuming foods containing sugar or carbohydrates.

SLEEP ATTACKS

In sleep attacks, a person has an irresistible urge to sleep and suddenly dozes off, usually for only minutes. Upon awakening, he or she feels refreshed. Sleep attacks may be a symptom of narcolepsy, a sleep disorder. These attacks usually occur during boring conditions, but can occur in dangerous settings such as driving. People with narcolepsy may also suffer sudden loss of muscle tone when they experience strong emotions such as vigorous laughing or crying. This may cause them to drop things, nod their head, or fall.

SLEEP APNEA

Sleep apnea is a condition in which breathing is intermittently (often frequently) interrupted during sleep. Most patients with sleep apnea snore loudly. Their sleep is restless with frequent brief awakenings. One effect of the disrupted sleep is excessive daytime sleepiness, often accompanied by irritability and impaired thinking. In a person with epilepsy, sleep apnea can worsen seizure control by impairing restful sleep.

NONEPILEPTIC SEIZURES

Nonepileptic seizures (also known as psychogenic seizures) are attacks that resemble epileptic seizures but result from subconscious mental activity (not abnormal brain electrical activity). Doctors consider most of these episodes psychological in nature, but not purposely produced. The person is usually unaware that the attacks are not "epileptic." Nonepileptic seizures are common, and in many cases, years of therapy for epileptic seizures are spent in vain until the correct diagnosis is made. Approximately 20% of patients with these seizures also have epileptic seizures and require different treatment for each disorder.

Nonepileptic seizures are most common in adolescents and adults, but they also can occur in children and the elderly. They are three times more likely in females. These episodes have been more widely recognized during the past several decades. In comprehensive epilepsy centers, where video-electroencephalogram (video-EEG) monitoring is performed, approximately 20% of referred patients are found to have nonepileptic seizures.

Nonepileptic seizures most often imitate complex partial or tonic-clonic seizures. The degree of resemblance varies considerably. Because doctors rarely witness an attack, the diagnosis is often delayed. Family members report episodes in which the patient stiffens and jerks, and doctors are immediately drawn toward the diagnosis of epilepsy. In studying these attacks, doctors have identified certain features that suggest nonepileptic seizures. These features are wild movements such as thrashing or rolling from side to side; screaming, crying, and moaning during the attack; jerking or stiffening of all extremities with preserved consciousness; stiffening and jerking of the extremities with immediate resumption of normal alertness after the attack (tiredness or confusion typically occurs after a tonic-clonic seizure); altered behavior that waxes and wanes (that is, the jerking or the inability to respond to questions comes and goes); and prolonged episodes (lasting longer than 5 minutes). Any one of these features, however, does not confirm the diagnosis of a nonepileptic attack. Epileptic seizures may occasionally include one or more of these behaviors.

The diagnosis of nonepileptic seizures is most often made with video-EEG monitoring. Doctors often try to have a family member or friend observe the recorded attack to ensure that it is identical or nearly identical to the usual episodes. Certain tests may be safely used to help provoke a seizure of this kind.

The treatment of nonepileptic seizures varies. In some cases, when the doctor tells the person that the attacks are psychological, they stop. Nonepileptic seizures are not necessarily an indication of a serious psychiatric disorder, but the problem needs to be addressed and, in many cases, treated. There may be coexisting depression or anxiety disorders that can be helped with medication. The prognosis for control of these episodes and for the patient's psychological well-being varies. Counseling with a psychologist, psychiatrist, or clinical social worker for a limited time after the diagnosis is often helpful. Accepting the diagnosis (at least as a real possibility) and following through with therapy are important for a successful outcome.

PANIC ATTACKS

Panic attacks are episodes of profound fear and anxiety, often associated with increased heart rate, hyperventilation, shortness of breath, sweating, nausea, chest discomfort, and other bodily (autonomic) symptoms. Certain settings may precipitate panic attacks. Doctors may incorrectly suspect that the person is suffering from partial seizures because simple partial seizures may have both autonomic symptoms and emotional symptoms such as fear or anxiety.

Unlike seizures, which begin suddenly, the panic attacks often build up gradually and last longer than 5 minutes. Many individuals with panic attacks also suffer from depression, and antidepressant medications can treat both the depression and the panic attacks.

Medical History

The medical history is the foundation of the diagnosis of epilepsy. It is essential that the doctor be given all information about the seizure because most doctors never witness a patient's actual attack. The following questions may be asked about the period before the attack:

- Was there lack of sleep or unusual stress?
- Was there any recent illness?

- Had the person taken any medications or drugs, including over-the-counter drugs, alcohol, or illegal drugs?
- What was the person doing immediately before the attack: lying, sitting, standing, getting up from a lying position, heavy exercise?

During the attack:

- What time of day did it occur?
- Did it occur around the transition into or out of sleep?
- How did it begin?
- Was there a warning?
- Were there abnormal movements of the eyes, mouth, face, head, arms, or legs?
- Was the person able to talk and respond appropriately?
- Was there loss of urine or feces?
- Was the tongue or inside of the cheeks bitten?

After the attack:

- Was the person confused or tired?
- Was speech normal?
- Was there a headache?

One of the most valuable pieces of information a doctor has is an accurate description of the typical attack from an eyewitness. It is worthwhile having witnesses accompany the patient to the doctor's office or having the doctor or nurse speak with them about their observations. The witness should write down a detailed description of what they saw soon after the attack because memories fade with time. Save these notes because they may be helpful to another doctor. If the episodes are repeated, it would be very helpful for the doctor if an eyewitness could capture one or more of the attacks on home video.

It is also helpful for patients to review their background with family members. They should ask the following questions:

- Was their birth difficult or traumatic?
- Did they have any seizures with high fevers in infancy or early childhood?
- Did they ever have a head injury? If so, did they lose consciousness after the injury? If consciousness was lost, how long did that last and were they taken to a hospital?
- Did they ever have meningitis (an infection of the membranes around the brain and spinal cord) or encephalitis (a serious viral infection of the brain)?

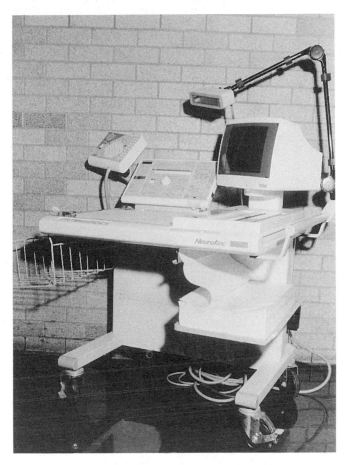

FIGURE 9. An EEG machine.

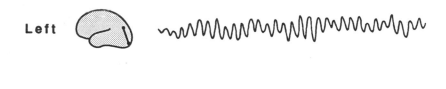

Left

Right

FIGURE 10. EEG traces from a person without epilepsy, at rest. The straight line on each drawing of the brain shows the area from which the EEG recording was made.

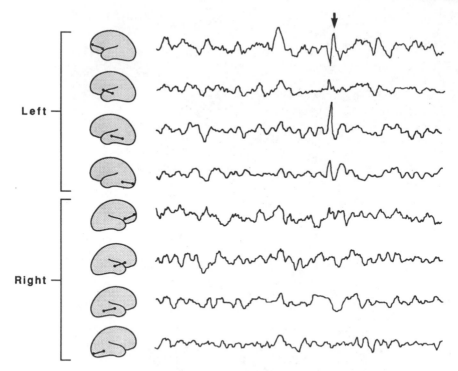

FIGURE 11. EEG traces of spikes and sharp waves (epilepsy waves) from the left temporal lobe of a person with partial epilepsy. The four traces on the bottom, which are from the right frontal and temporal lobes, are normal.

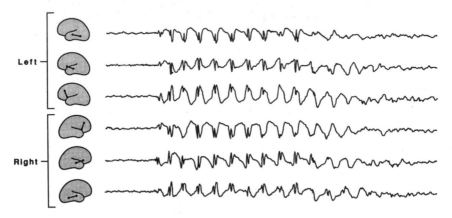

FIGURE 12. EEG traces of spike-and-wave discharges from both the left and right sides of the brain in a person with primary generalized epilepsy. As on Figures 10 and 11, the straight line on each drawing of the brain shows the area from which that EEG recording was made.

Because an EEG usually records the brain activity occurring between seizures, which is called *interictal activity* ("ictal" means seizure), a person with epilepsy may have a normal EEG. The interictal activity will be normal if the brain activity is truly normal during the recording session. Just as people with epilepsy behave normally almost all of the time (e.g., when the duration and frequency of seizures is compared to all the time in a given month), the EEG also is normal most of the time. Also, areas of abnormality may go undetected by the EEG if the abnormality arises deep in the brain (e.g., deep in the temporal lobe), "outside the reach" of the electrodes on the scalp, or if the volume of brain affected is too small to generate abnormal waves of sufficient size. To increase the chances of finding an abnormality on the EEG, it can be recorded in various circumstances:

- During both wakefulness and sleep (sometimes a sleeping pill can be used)
- After sleep deprivation (lack of sleep can cause epilepsy waves on the EEG)
- With 3 to 5 minutes of deep breathing (hyperventilation)
- With flashing lights
- With special electrodes
- For prolonged periods

The actual recording usually lasts 20 to 40 minutes, and the same amount of time is generally needed to prepare for it. Thus, the EEG procedure usually takes 1 to 1 ½ hours. The test is performed by an EEG technologist (see Chap. 7). The patient can help by washing his or her hair the night before or the day of the test, but should not use conditioners, hair creams, sprays, or styling gels.

ROUTINE EEG

The routine EEG is the most common test for epilepsy. The EEG technologist first measures the patient's head so that the electrodes—small, metal, cup-shaped disks attached to wires—can be placed in the correct position. A wax crayon, which can be easily washed off later, is used to mark the points on the scalp. Next, the technologist applies the electrodes, usually using a paste that can hold them in place for several hours. The technologist often scrubs each position on the scalp with a mildly abrasive cream before applying the electrodes. This will help improve the quality of the recording. The electrodes only record the brain waves. They do not stimulate the head with electricity, and they pose no danger to the patient. The EEG machine then records the brain waves as a series of squiggly lines (traces). Today, recordings on paper are often being replaced by computerized, paperless EEGs.

The patient may fall asleep briefly during a routine EEG because the room is quiet and often dimly lit. That is fine and is often helpful because an EEG obtained during both wakefulness and sleep may provide extra information. During the EEG, the technologist may ask patients to open and close their eyes several times, shine flashing lights into their eyes (photic stimulation), or ask them to breathe rapidly or deeply. Patients who have a medical problem that makes it unsafe to hyperventilate, such as asthma or heart disease, should tell the EEG technologist or the doctor. Similarly, pregnant women usually should not undergo hyperventilation or have photic stimulation.

In some cases, the doctor may ask the patient to stay up the entire night before the EEG is performed. This sleep deprivation can increase the likelihood that epilepsy waves will be recorded. If the patient experiences any possible seizure symptoms during the test, he or she should tell the technologist.

Obtaining an EEG in children is usually easy, but it can pose a significant challenge. For babies, it is helpful to perform the EEG around naptime. Electrodes can be applied while the mother holds the child; a bottle may help to calm the baby. Then the baby is allowed to sleep naturally. Sedation is required for some babies and young children to allow the technologist to apply the electrodes and record sleep activity. Children have difficulty lying still during EEG recordings, and the doctors who interpret these studies must separate the waves caused by movement and muscle activity from the brain waves.

After the EEG recording is done, the technologist will remove the electrodes from the patient's scalp. The patient is free to go home and wash the paste out of his or her hair. The paste is lanolin- or water-based, so it can be easily washed off. The doctor usually reads the EEG after the test is completed and the patient has left.

EEG WITH SPECIAL ELECTRODES

Depending on the information the doctor is trying to obtain, special electrodes may be needed. Sphenoidal electrodes (see Chap. 12) are most often used during video-EEG monitoring studies to record electrical activity from deep parts of the temporal and frontal lobes. The patient's cheek is swabbed with an anesthetic. Then a thin needle, which carries a thin wire, is inserted into the cheek. The needle is removed, and the wire is taped to the skin. Patients usually experience little discomfort.

Nasopharyngeal electrodes are used occasionally to record deep brain electrical activity. These electrodes are plastic tubes with a wire inside; the tubes end as a blunt metal tip. The electrodes are inserted through the nose (usually by the EEG technologist), and the metal tip is situated in the upper back part of the nose (the nasopharynx). There may be some discomfort while the electrodes are inserted and slight discomfort while they are left in place for approximately 20 to 30 minutes during the study. Nasopharyngeal electrodes have been used less often during the past few decades because regular electrodes placed in front of and slightly above the ears can often provide the same information with no discomfort to the patient.

AMBULATORY EEG

The brain's electrical activity fluctuates from second to second. The routine EEG provides a 20- to 40-minute sample of brain electrical activity, which is often sufficient. In some patients with epilepsy, however, this recording is normal or shows only minor, nonspecific findings. In such cases, an extended recording that includes long periods of wakefulness and sleep is desired. For example, in some people epilepsy waves may occur only once every 3 or 4 hours or only after an hour of sleep, and a routine EEG will almost always be normal.

The EEG can be recorded for 24 hours with a special recorder that is slightly larger than a portable cassette player. This recorder permits patients to go about their normal routine while the EEG is recorded. Newer recorders have epilepsy wave and seizure detection programs to identify abnormal activity. They also have video recording capacity, which further increases the value of the ambulatory EEG. Patients can wear the recorder on their waist, with the wires running either under or outside of their shirt (Fig. 13). For people with a full head of hair, the electrodes can be fairly well camouflaged. Even so, most people prefer not to go to work or school with the electrodes on their scalp. Because the electrodes must stay on the head for a longer time than for a routine EEG, a special glue called collodion is often used to keep them in place. The technologist can easily remove this glue with acetone or similar solutions.

If the patient scratches his or her head, which may get itchy because of the electrodes, it can appear as abnormal activity on the EEG. Therefore, the patient is usually asked to keep a diary of activities during the day. Most recorders have an "event" button for patients to press if they experience any of the symptoms for which they are being tested, such as episodes of feeling "spacey" or confused. A family member should press the button if the patient is unable to do it.

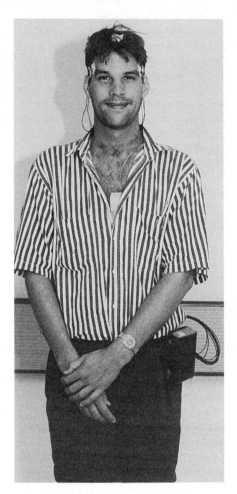

FIGURE 13. Recording the 24-hour ambulatory EEG. The cassette-type recorder, attached to the patient's belt, records the EEG signals from the electrodes on the patient's scalp while he pursues his daily activities.

VIDEO-EEG MONITORING

Our understanding of epilepsy has been greatly advanced by video-EEG monitoring, which allows prolonged simultaneous recording of the patient's behavior and the EEG. The video and EEG images are usually presented on a split screen, permitting precise correlation between seizure activity in the brain and the patient's behavior during seizures (Fig. 14). Video-EEG recordings can be done on hospitalized inpatients or on outpatients. As for ambulatory EEG, the electrodes used for video-EEG recording must be glued to the scalp with collodion.

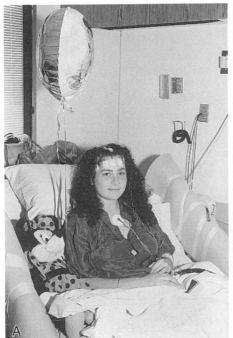
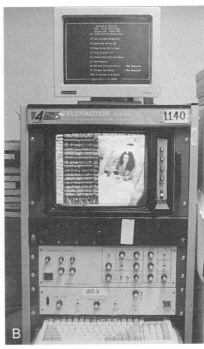

FIGURE 14. Video-EEG monitoring. (*A*) A patient being monitored; a video camera (not shown) records her activities, including any seizures that occur, and the EEG signals from electrodes on her head are transmitted to an adjoining monitor. (*B*) The patient's seizure and EEG are recorded simultaneously and shown as a split-screen display on a television monitor.

Inpatient monitoring with close supervision allows the doctor to reduce and, in some cases, discontinue antiepileptic drugs safely. The medication reduction and possibly sleep deprivation, hyperventilation, exercise, or alcohol intake are used to induce seizures. Video-EEG is most helpful in determining whether seizures with unusual features are actually epileptic, identifying the type of epileptic seizures, and pinpointing the region of the brain from which the seizures begin. This last step is critical in assessing a patient for possible epilepsy surgery.

A patient who is going to have video-EEG monitoring should bring clothing to the hospital that can be buttoned (not pullovers). The patient may also want to bring reading materials or other things to keep busy because a prolonged hospital stay for monitoring can be boring.

MAGNETOENCEPHALOGRAPHY

Magnetoencephalography (MEG) is a recent technological development based on recording magnetic activity that is generated by the brain's electrical activity. Because the physical properties of magnetic waves differ from those of electrical waves, MEG provides different information than the EEG does. Both tests are usually recorded at the same time. MEG recording is achieved using detectors that are placed near the head (Fig. 15A). The test is painless and completely safe. The magnetic waves recorded between seizures can be mapped in three dimensions onto an image of the patient's brain (Fig. 15B) derived from magnetic resonance imaging (MRI, discussed later in this chapter). Unfortunately, the computers needed to analyze the MEG information are complex and costly, making the procedure expensive. Currently, MEG is available at only a few medical centers in the United States, and it is often difficult to get insurance reimbursement for it.

Currently, MEG's main use is to localize the area from which the seizure arises in patients scheduled for epilepsy surgery and to pinpoint the sites of normal sensory function (e.g., touch or vision) so that these vital areas can be spared during the surgery. MEG may be most helpful as part of the presurgical evaluation for patients whose seizures begin outside the temporal lobe and for those with Landau-Kleffner syndrome.

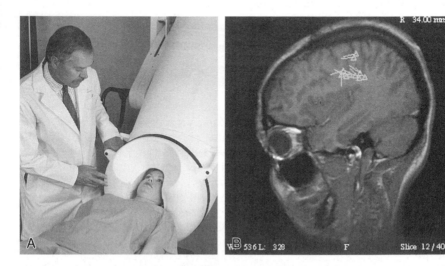

FIGURE 15. (A) A magnetoencephalograph (MEG) machine. (B) MEG area of epilepsy wave mapped onto an MRI image.

Neuroimaging of the Brain

Neuroimaging provides pictures of the brain. The neuroimaging tests most commonly used with epilepsy are computed tomography (CT) and MRI of the head. These tests produce pictures, or scans, of the brain. Like a photograph that shows the surface features of the face, CT or MRI of the head shows the anatomy of the skin, nose, mouth, skull, and brain. Doctors obtain a CT or MRI scan to determine whether an abnormality in the structure of the brain—such as excess spinal fluid (hydrocephalus), scar tissue, or a tangle of blood vessels (vascular malformation)—may be causing the epilepsy. MRI provides much more information than a CT scan does.

In most cases, neuroimaging studies do not need to be done immediately at the time of diagnosis. There are no absolute rules on which people with epilepsy should be studied with a CT or MRI scan. In general, a CT or MRI scan should be obtained when a child or adult has had one or more seizures for which the cause is unknown. There are several important exceptions to this rule, however. First, a CT or MRI scan should be considered if the cause of the seizures is known but has the potential to change (e.g., a benign tumor or a vascular malformation) or if the cause is suspected but indefinite (e.g., a mild head injury). Follow-up scans also may be indicated for someone who has a benign tumor or other brain abnormality. Second, if a person has had epilepsy for more than a decade and has normal results on the neurologic examination, some doctors will recommend a CT or MRI scan because the treatment may depend on the findings. If a patient with partial seizures previously had a normal CT scan but the seizures persist, an MRI scan may provide additional, helpful information. Many doctors will not order a CT or MRI scan for patients with certain well-defined epilepsy syndromes that are often genetic, such as absence seizures, juvenile myoclonic epilepsy, or benign rolandic epilepsy, because the results are almost always normal or unrelated to epilepsy.

CT and MRI show the brain's structure (how it looks). Other neuroimaging methods show its function (how it works). These methods include single-photon emission computed tomography (SPECT), positron emission tomography (PET), and magnetic resonance spectroscopy (MRS). SPECT shows images of how much blood flows through different parts of the brain. PET shows images of how much sugar (glucose) or oxygen is metabolized, or used up, by various areas of the brain. MRS uses technology similar to that of MRI to examine signals generated by elements such as carbon and phosphorous. (MRI studies the hydrogen atoms in water and fat.) MRS data can be used, for example, to learn about metabolic activity in the brain. All these tests are used to evaluate patients before epilepsy surgery or as research tools.

COMPUTED TOMOGRAPHY

CT was introduced in the United States in the early 1970s and revolutionized the practice of neurology and neurosurgery. Like x-rays, CT scans expose the patient to radiation, but the amount is low. The procedure is safe even if it needs to be repeated several times over the years. The scanner is a large machine; the patient's head is in a larger space than with MRI. The CT scan is normal in most people with epilepsy (Fig. 16). Brain abnormalities that might be detected are atrophy (a decrease in brain substance), scar tissue, tumors, or abnormal blood vessels or spinal fluid circulation.

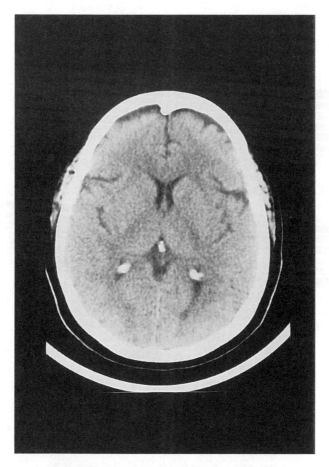

FIGURE 16. CT scan of a normal brain.

MAGNETIC RESONANCE IMAGING

MRI was first introduced in the United States in the early 1980s and further revolutionized the practice of neurology and neurosurgery. MRI is the most important neuroimaging test in epilepsy because it shows even more details of the brain's structure than CT does. The MRI does not use x-rays; it uses a powerful magnet that changes the spin on atomic particles that are normally part of the body, and then measures the changes in the magnetic field as the particles resume their previous course. The patient does not feel anything. The images are a remarkably accurate representation of the brain's structure (Fig. 17). MRI is

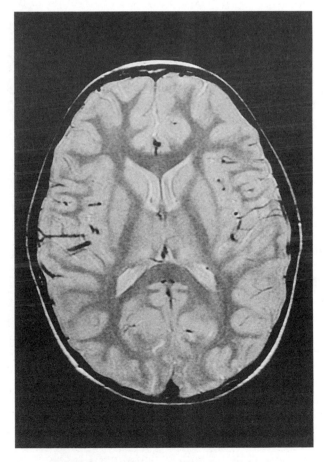

FIGURE 17. MRI scan of a normal brain.

extremely helpful for identifying brain scar tissue, areas of abnormal brain development (dysplasia), small brain tumors, blood vessel abnormalities, and changes in the brain's white matter.

Although the MRI is safe and painless, most MRI machines require that the person's head and upper body be placed in a very confined space. People with claustrophobia (fear of small places), and many people who never knew they were claustrophobic, may become frightened and uncooperative when they see the confinement required for the test. Medications for relaxation can be given (children often require medications to put them to sleep), or a newer type of MRI machine ("open MRI"), which is not so confining, can be used. At present, however, the scans from open MRIs are not as detailed as those of the regular MRIs, and this difference can be important for patients being considered for epilepsy surgery.

SINGLE-PHOTON EMISSION COMPUTED TOMOGRAPHY

SPECT shows the blood flow in the brain. A safe, very-low–strength radioactive compound is injected into the patient's arm, and the particles emitted by the compound are measured. The more blood that flows through a certain area, the more particles are emitted. This test is readily available in most hospitals, but its use as a routine test in epilepsy is unjustified. SPECT scans obtained between seizures may show changes in brain blood flow (decreased flow is sometimes found in the area from which seizures arise), but the findings may be misleading. As illustrated in Figure 18, SPECT scans obtained during or immediately after a seizure may be more helpful than scans obtained between seizures in identifying the brain area from which the seizures arise.

New computer techniques allow doctors to measure the differences between SPECT scans taken during seizures and those taken between seizures and superimpose the resulting "subtraction" SPECT images onto the patient's MRI in an effort to pinpoint the seizure focus. This technique may be most helpful when seizures begin outside the temporal lobe and MRI scans do not reveal a structural abnormality.

POSITRON EMISSION TOMOGRAPHY

PET, which shows the brain's metabolism of oxygen or sugar, requires the injection of a very low dose of a radioactive compound. This test is safe and helpful in identifying the area from which partial seizures arise. It may be performed in the period between seizures. PET scans (Fig. 19) are expensive and very few patients with epilepsy need them. Many insurance carriers are now reimbursing for the use of a PET scan to localize the seizure focus for epilepsy surgery when the scan is medically justified.

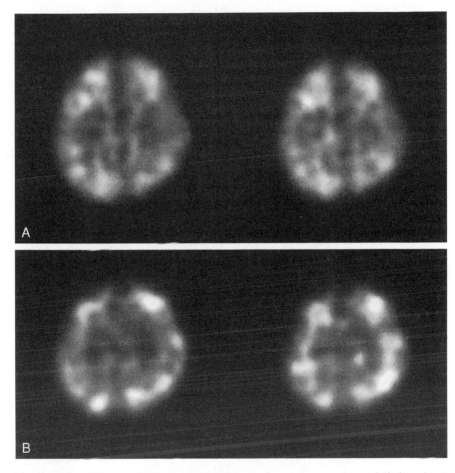

FIGURE 18. Two SPECT scans done on the same patient. (*A*) Interictal images (taken between seizures). (*B*) Ictal images (taken during a seizure). Bright areas on the right side of the ictal images (in the left temporal lobe of the patient's brain) indicate increased blood flow and may mark the area from which the seizure arises, called the seizure focus.

MAGNETIC RESONANCE SPECTROSCOPY

The nuclei of certain atoms have physical qualities (resonance frequencies) that provide chemical information. MRS examines hydrogen and phosphorous atoms to gather information about chemical activity in small areas of the brain. The profiles obtained through MRS provide data about the amounts of specific chemical compounds, such as neurotrans-

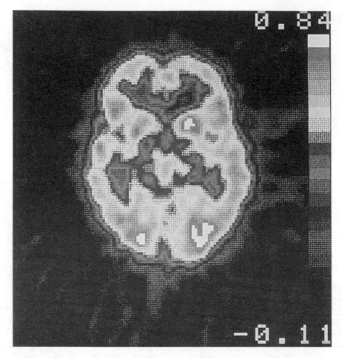

FIGURE 19. PET scan of the brain. PET scans use different colors (not shown) to reveal how well various areas of the brain metabolize oxygen or sugar (glucose). This metabolism is related to brain function. In this scan, for instance, differences are apparent between the functioning of the right and left temporal and parietal lobes. Normally both sides of the brain would be similar.

mitters or energy supplies in areas of the brain. This provides clues to the causes or effects of epilepsy. These data may also help to identify areas of the brain from which seizures arise. MRS is currently an investigational procedure and has no role in making the diagnosis of epilepsy.

ULTRASONOGRAPHY

Most people think of ultrasonography (ultrasound) as a test to observe the development of babies in the womb, but it is also used to diagnose medical and neurologic disorders. Ultrasonography may identify brain abnormalities in babies with neurologic disorders, including seizures. It uses only sound waves, so it is very safe and can be performed easily in either a newborn intensive care unit or an outpatient setting. The sound waves can study the brain through areas of the newborn's skull where the bones have not yet come together, called fontanelles.

Ultrasonography can detect excessive spinal fluid (hydrocephalus) or blood (hemorrhage) in the brain. Sometimes a CT or MRI scan is obtained after ultrasonography to study the abnormality further or to search for abnormalities that may have been missed if the ultrasonography test results are normal.

Lumbar Puncture

Lumbar puncture, or spinal tap, provides a sample of cerebrospinal fluid and measures pressure in the spinal canal (which is usually similar to pressure around the brain). Lumbar puncture, although not a pleasant test, has an undeservedly bad reputation as "very dangerous" and "very painful." For the procedure, a needle is inserted into the sac that contains spinal fluid, several inches below the bottom of the spinal cord. For patients with epilepsy, lumbar puncture is most often used in emergency situations to rule out problems such as bacterial meningitis or viral encephalitis. It may also be used to help diagnose some uncommon disorders in patients with epilepsy, such as Lyme disease, sarcoid (an inflammatory disorder), and lymphoma.

First Aid for Seizures

A person with epilepsy should wear a medical-alert bracelet or necklace that gives the person's diagnosis, medications, telephone numbers of the doctor, and the person to call in case of an emergency. It can help avoid unnecessary actions or costs if a seizure occurs in a public place. Medic-Alert (www.medicalert.org or 888-633-4298) is a nonprofit organization that provides bracelets, necklaces, and cards with important medical information. The organization has a 24-hour emergency response center, which provides information to emergency medical personnel. MedicAlert will also call family contacts to let them know of an emergency.

Although a tonic-clonic seizure is frightening, a single, brief seizure is rarely dangerous to the person having the seizure and never dangerous to anyone else (except perhaps if the person is caring for a baby or driving a car). If the person has a definite history of tonic-clonic seizures, it is rarely necessary to take them to the emergency room or doctor's office after a seizure unless there is evidence or suspicion of an injury or if the seizure was unlike previous ones. If this is the person's first tonic-clonic seizure, however, a prompt consultation with a doctor is essential.

Prolonged, continuous, or repetitive tonic-clonic seizures deserve an urgent call for help. The patient is best transported to a medical facility by ambulance because he or she may need oxygen, and a convulsion in a passenger car can be dangerous for everyone involved.

How long does a seizure have to last to warrant a call for help? There is no absolute answer. This issue is worth discussing with the doctor. In general, if the actual convulsion lasts more than 5 minutes, or if the need for assistance is uncertain, it is best to call for help.

Generalized Tonic-Clonic Seizures

Generalized tonic-clonic (grand mal) seizures are convulsive seizures. They are frightening to watch. The person loses consciousness, falls, stiffens (the tonic portion of the seizure), and jerks (the clonic portion of the seizure). Although a convulsive seizure appears painful, the person is not conscious during the seizure; therefore, he or she is unaware of what is happening. After the seizure there may be discomfort caused by tongue biting, muscle soreness, headache, or bruises from falling. Confusion and tiredness often occur after the attack, in what is called the postictal period. These generalized tonic-clonic seizures usually last less than 3 minutes, but the time can seem like an eternity to family members or friends who are watching it.

Seizures may cause bruises, cuts, sprains, or a bitten tongue, but they rarely cause broken or dislocated bones or other more serious problems. People who spend a good amount of time with someone who is at risk of tonic-clonic seizures should learn first-aid guidelines:

• Try to stay calm. Anxiety and fear are not helpful. Easy to say, hard to do.

• Help the person lie down, and place something soft under the head and neck. Keep the person (especially the head) away from sharp or hard objects, such as the corner of a table.

• Time the duration of convulsive movements, if possible.

• Roll the person onto one side with the head and mouth angled toward the ground so that any excessive saliva or fluids will not accidentally be swallowed or inhaled. This position will also prevent the tongue from falling back and blocking the airway.

• Loosen all tight clothing by unfastening top shirt buttons, belts, and skirt or pant buttons. Remove any eyeglasses or tight neck chains. Do not worry about contact lenses. Trying to remove the small lens during a tonic-clonic seizure can easily scratch the eye.

• Do not hold the person down; you may cause a bone dislocation or get injured yourself.

• Do not put anything in the person's mouth. The tongue cannot be swallowed during a seizure. The muscles for chewing are very strong, so a finger can be bitten or an object can be bitten off and the person can choke on the fragment remaining in the mouth.

- After the seizure is over, do not try to restrain the person. He or she may be confused, and restraint may provoke agitation and a violent reaction.
- Try to keep the person in a safe environment. Walking around is permissible, except near a street, stairs, or any other potentially dangerous place.
- Do not give pills, beverages, or food until the person is fully alert.
- Stay with the person until he or she is fully alert and oriented. Be careful. The person may claim to be fine, but still be quite confused. Ask a series of questions that require more than a yes or no answer. For example, ask "What is your address?" and "What is the date?"
- If this is the person's first tonic-clonic seizure or if the seizure lasts longer than 5 minutes, call an ambulance.
- During and after the seizure, keep onlookers away. One or two people are all that is needed for first aid. Additional people often add confusion. Further, it is embarrassing for the person to awaken to a crowd of people.
- After the seizure is over and calm has been restored, tell the person who had the seizure what actually happened and the duration of the seizure, and, most importantly, provide reassurance and support.

After the seizure, the person may complain of headache, mouth discomfort from tongue- or cheek-biting, or back pain related to the muscular contractions or a fall. Acetaminophen (Tylenol) or ibuprofen (Advil or Motrin) is helpful for minor pains. If back pain is severe, the person should be seen by a doctor because there is the possibility of a fracture (which is usually treated conservatively with rest). Fever may follow a seizure, usually because of the muscle activity and the effects of the seizure. If the fever is unusually high (more than 102°F), lasts more than 6 hours, or develops more than 3 hours after a seizure, it is wise to consult with a doctor. Sometimes secretions pass down the respiratory tract during the seizure and cause pneumonia.

If a person has a history of tonic-clonic seizures that last more than 5 minutes, it often is wise to have drugs on hand that can be given if another such prolonged seizure occurs. This is especially important for patients who live far from a hospital or who are traveling to remote areas (e.g., going camping). Appropriate drugs for this purpose include diazepam given by rectum (Diastat) for all age groups or lorazepam given sublingually (under the tongue) for an older child or a teenager. The doses of these drugs should be carefully reviewed with the physician, including when a second dose of rectal diazepam or sublingual lorazepam may be given if seizure activity persists.

Atonic and Tonic Seizures

Both *atonic seizures*, in which the person has a sudden loss of muscle strength, and *tonic seizures*, in which the person suddenly stiffens, often cause sudden falls with a high potential for injury. Because onset of the seizure and the resulting fall occur in seconds, it is often difficult or impossible to intervene in time. Occasionally, the occurrence or increased frequency of other seizure types (absence or myoclonic seizures) provide a warning that an atonic or tonic seizure is about to happen and the person can sit or lie down. Those who have atonic or tonic seizures without warning need protective headgear and sometimes a face mask to prevent injury. Danmar helmets (see Appendix 4) are made especially for this type of situation; hockey helmets also provide good protection.

Complex Partial Seizures

Complex partial seizures (temporal lobe seizures or psychomotor seizures) are called "complex" because they impair consciousness and "partial" because they begin in a limited area of the brain. Most complex partial seizures are associated with some automatic behaviors, termed *automatisms* (see Chap. 3).

The chance of bodily injury during a complex partial seizure is small. Single and brief complex partial seizures do not damage the brain. Prolonged or repetitive complex partial seizures may cause slight but persistent memory loss. More serious brain injury is rare, however.

During a complex partial seizure, the person usually becomes motionless and stares or makes automatic movements, such as fumbling movements of the hands. When someone has a complex partial seizure, speak quietly and in a reassuring manner because some people have only partial impairment of consciousness and can react to emotional or physical stimulation. Do not yell at the person or restrain him or her (it is rarely necessary). The most important aspect of first aid during a complex partial seizure is to keep the person safe from harm. For example, burns can occur when someone unknowingly touches or falls on a hot object. During and after some complex partial seizures, the person may walk or, in rare cases, run. When this occurs where there is dangerous equipment, on a busy city street, near train tracks, or near high places such as a construction site, there is a potential for serious injury.

Other behaviors during complex partial seizures may cause concern, but are not dangerous to the patient or other people. These include screaming, kicking, ripping up papers, disrobing, making sexual-like movements, and, rarely, masturbating. If someone is known to have unusual automatisms, he or she should be led in a quiet and reassuring manner—not forcibly—out of public places. Specific strategies should be devised to minimize the embarrassing effects for individuals with unusual complex partial seizures.

The greatest danger of an unexpected seizure occurs when the person is driving a car or operating dangerous equipment. Those with seizures that impair consciousness or control of movement should try to avoid these activities. In some cases, potentially dangerous equipment can be used safely if adequate precautions are taken.

If the seizure is prolonged (more than 5 to 10 minutes of impaired consciousness with automatisms) or if there are three or more complex partial seizures, then medical help should be sought. If the patient is known to have a pattern of prolonged or recurrent complex partial seizures, rectal diazepam (Diastat) can be administered at home by family members to stop the seizures. First aid for someone having a complex partial seizure is simple: keep the person away from dangerous situations, use restraint only if it is necessary for his or her safety, and seek medical help for prolonged or recurrent seizures.

Simple Partial Seizures

Simple partial seizures rarely require first aid. Because consciousness is preserved, the person is almost always aware of the seizure and the surroundings. When care or assistance is needed, it should address the specific seizure symptoms. For example, children who experience visual hallucinations that obscure their vision should not play contact sports, such as basketball, during a seizure. If an adult has uncontrolled jerking (clonic movements) of the arm, sharp objects should be removed from the area near the arm. When simple partial seizures are known to progress to complex partial or secondarily generalized tonic-clonic seizures, the person should be quietly and cautiously moved to a safe environment and should stop driving or working with dangerous equipment.

Absence Seizures

Absence seizures usually require no first aid. They are brief and almost never associated with falling or injury. If absence seizures occur in a cluster, it may be wise to remove a child from sports, swimming, or other potentially dangerous activities *during the cluster period.* Very rarely, absence seizures can occur as a continuous state called absence status epilepticus. If this happens, certain medications can be given by mouth or rectum (many patients can take medication by mouth during this type of seizure), or medical attention should be sought.

CHAPTER

10

Principles of Drug Therapy

Antiepileptic drugs are the principal therapy for epilepsy. Choosing the correct drug depends on making an accurate diagnosis of epilepsy. In addition, discussions between the patient and the doctor about the pros and cons of the different drugs can influence drug choice. Relevant issues include how often the medication has to be taken (most patients prefer once or twice a day rather than three or four times), the drug's adverse effects, the drug's cost, and the potential risks for the baby if a woman becomes pregnant while taking the drug. The next chapter will discuss each of the most frequently used antiepileptic drugs and some new and experimental ones.

Although antiepileptic drugs effectively control seizures in most people, they do not *cure* epilepsy. People often remark, "These drugs don't really treat or cure the epilepsy, but just control the condition. They are like Band-Aids." There is a large element of truth in that statement. If scar tissue or an abnormal group of blood vessels in the brain causes seizures, antiepileptic drugs will surely not repair these structural problems. These medications suppress the seizures, but do not "fix" the basic problem. However, the longer someone is seizure-free while taking medications, the better the chances he or she will remain seizure-free when the medications are stopped.

Goals

The goals of antiepileptic drug therapy are very simple: no seizures and no adverse effects. Many people can reach these goals easily, but for many others the balance between seizure control and adverse effects is delicate. This is why communication between the doctor and the patient is critical for the best, individualized management of drug therapy. The patient and the doctor should openly discuss what to expect, what is tolerable, what the patient is experiencing, and the impact of both adverse drug effects and seizures on the patient's quality of life. Although low to moderate doses of antiepileptic drugs work well for most people, some experience unpleasant adverse effects from low doses or their seizures cannot be controlled even with high doses of one or more drugs.

Lack of effective communication between the doctor and patient may cause problems with taking medications. Some patients make the mistake of accepting troublesome adverse effects because they fear that the doctor will reduce the medication and a seizure will occur or because they believe that adverse effects of medication are unavoidable. Some doctors may incorrectly conclude that the complaints are psychological or related to the seizures or other factors if a patient complains of abdominal discomfort and nausea, depression, lack of energy, or feeling "spaced out" while taking low doses of medication. Unfortunately, some people are extremely sensitive to medications and may experience troublesome adverse effects although the level of the drug in their blood is low. Other patients tend to blame every minor problem on a new drug.

Changes in medications should be done systematically, and they should be limited to one drug at a time whenever possible. This strategy enables the doctor to show a relationship between a change and an effect, such as improved seizure control or reduction of an adverse effect.

Time Required for Antiepileptic Drugs to Work

A medication that is taken by mouth has to pass through the stomach and be absorbed in the small intestine. Once absorbed, it passes to the liver, where a fraction of the drug is metabolized, or broken down, and then passed into the bloodstream. In the case of antiepileptic drugs, it eventually reaches the brain. A large portion of some drugs is not metabolized, however; it is eliminated from the body by the kidneys in an unchanged form.

A dose of medication will reach a peak, or maximum, level in the blood 30 minutes to 6 hours after it is taken. The time between taking the medication and reaching the peak level depends on the specific drug, its form (liquid, tablet, capsule, or slow-release), and, in some cases, the food consumed before taking it. The properties of selected antiepileptic drugs when used alone are summarized in Table 5 on pages 142–143.

ABSORPTION AND HALF-LIFE

The goal with antiepileptic drugs is to maintain a relatively constant level in the blood. The time required for the drug's concentration in the blood to be reduced to half the peak level is referred to as the drug's *half-life*. Some drugs, such as carbamazepine, gabapentin, tiagabine, and valproate, have a relatively short half-life; some, such as lamotrigine and phenytoin, have an intermediate half-life; and some, such as phenobarbital, have a long half-life (see Chap. 11). Knowledge of drug half-life is complicated by the different forms in which some drugs are available. For example, carbamazepine is available as a generic tablet, brand-name tablet (Tegretol), chewable brand-name tablet (Tegretol), brand-name sustained-release tablet (Carbatrol and Tegretol XR), and elixir (liquid). Each form has a different half-life. Because of these differences in absorption, switching to a different form of the same drug potentially can cause seizures. For instance, taking a rapidly absorbed form with a shorter half-life may leave a long interval with too little medication in the blood. More rapid absorption may also cause adverse effects. When drugs are used in combination, the half-life of each drug may change.

In general, elixirs are more rapidly absorbed; therefore they have shorter half-lives. Products with delayed absorption have longer half-lives. Drugs in forms that have gradual release and gradual absorption are ideal because they produce the most steady blood drug levels. This allows doses to be taken less often without wide swings in the level of drug in the blood.

Drugs with longer half-lives have more stable blood levels and need to be taken less frequently. Phenobarbital could be given every other day because of its long half-life, but people tend to forget to take their medication if they do not take it every day. Adverse effects also are more likely to occur after taking a single large dose every other day. Drugs with short half-lives, ideally should be taken several times a day to prevent adverse effects during periods of high blood levels and seizures during periods of low levels.

STEADY STATE

Steady state (equilibrium) is the condition in a person who is taking a constant amount of medication and whose blood drug levels are fairly constant. Defined another way, there is a steady state when the amount of drug taken and the amount of drug being metabolized and excreted are equal. In most cases, it takes fives times longer than the half-life of the drug to arrive at equilibrium.

Even when someone has been taking the same drug for a long time and the blood levels are in equilibrium, the levels will fluctuate over the course of the day. Depending on the rate of absorption of the drug and the factors that influence the absorption rate (e.g., taking some drugs after meals slows absorption), there will be peaks in the blood level within hours after the drug is taken and troughs (low points) shortly before or immediately after a dose is taken, especially if there is a long interval between doses. Fluctuations between the peak level and the trough level depend mainly on the half-life of the drug (drugs with short half-lives have greater fluctuations) and the number of times the medication is taken each day (if a drug has a short half-life, taking it frequently will reduce the fluctuations). Dose-related adverse effects are more likely to occur at times of peak levels, and a seizure is more likely to occur at times of trough levels.

Drugs are fully effective when their blood levels have reached a steady state. Some drugs, however, such as carbamazepine, are broken down more rapidly by the liver after someone has been taking it for several weeks. Therefore, a carbamazepine level measured 6 to 8 weeks after the start of therapy is often lower than a level measured 2 weeks after the start of therapy. This effect, in which a drug induces an increase in its own metabolism, is known as *autoinduction*. This process stabilizes by 8 to 12 weeks after the start of therapy.

Adverse Effects of Antiepileptic Drugs

Doctors and patients with epilepsy see medical care from different perspectives. The doctor would like to see the patient regularly, have the patient take medication regularly, and have the patient's seizures well controlled. The patient would like never to see a doctor, never to take a pill, and never have the seizures again. Patients often consider taking pills even worse than seeing a doctor.

In addition to their inconvenience and expense, antiepileptic drugs also may cause adverse effects (see Table 6, pages 144–145). These effects are slight for most people who can be treated with a properly adjusted dosage of just one antiepileptic drug. Before starting to take a medication, the patient should ask the doctor what to expect. Some fatigue, abdominal discomfort, dizziness, or blurred vision may be experienced during the first weeks of taking an antiepileptic drug, but if the medication is started at a low dosage and increased slowly, and if the patient is aware of what to expect, these effects are usually tolerable. They probably will stop after several weeks or months, as tolerance develops.

IDIOSYNCRATIC EFFECTS

The adverse effects may be related or unrelated to the dosage and blood level of the drug. They may be minor or severe, short-lasting and reversible, or long-lasting and potentially irreversible. Unpredictable adverse effects unrelated to the dosage or blood drug level are called *idiosyncratic*. Idiosyncratic adverse effects of antiepileptic drugs include rash, inflammation of the liver or pancreas, and a serious reduction in the number of white blood cells (which are important to the immune system) or platelets (which are important in controlling bleeding). Dangerous but rare idiosyncratic reactions, such as aplastic anemia (severe damage to bone marrow causing a failure in the production of blood cells) and liver failure, are allergic reactions and usually occur within the first 6 months of starting a drug.

If a rash or itchiness develops after a new medication is prescribed, the doctor should be contacted immediately. Drug rashes most commonly begin 5 to 18 days after a medication is started. For some people, allergic reactions start with a fever and the rash only emerges after a few more days. Most rashes are trivial and may even be unrelated to the drug. In people taking more than one drug, the one that was most recently started has probably caused the rash, although rashes may also be caused by viruses, bacteria, allergic reactions, irritation from a laundry detergent, and insect bites. The rash usually resolves shortly after the medication is discontinued. People who have excessive bleeding, abdominal pain and tenderness, hair loss, fever, unusual infections, or other unusual symptoms while taking a drug should promptly inform the doctor.

DOSE-RELATED EFFECTS

Toxicity

Dose-related adverse effects are more common than idiosyncratic effects. When the dosage of an antiepileptic drug is increased, the blood level of the drug may become too high for the person to tolerate and troublesome effects, called *toxicity*, will occur. It is often difficult to predict the exact dosage or blood level of a drug that will cause toxicity in a given person.

The situation can become even more complex because of *active metabolites*—druglike substances derived from the liver's "digestion" of some antiepileptic drugs—that have antiepileptic properties and adverse effects of their own. Most drugs that are metabolized by the liver produce *inactive metabolites,* not active ones. Because active metabolites can contribute to both seizure control and adverse effects, measuring the blood levels of only the original (parent) drug may be misleading. In addition, other drugs may interact with antiepileptic drugs by affecting the level of active metabolites (see Appendix 3).

Adverse effects from medication, including toxicity, are almost never dangerous or permanent. By spreading the total dose more evenly (or frequently) throughout the day; having the patient take medications with meals or at bedtime; lowering the dose; or, when necessary, stopping the medication altogether, the doctor can usually alleviate abdominal discomfort, blurred vision, headache, or fatigue. These are short-term effects related to the amount of medication. Some other adverse effects of medication can be serious, but life-threatening problems are extremely rare. Fewer than 2 people in 150,000 who take antiepileptic drugs will die as a result; the chance of dying in a motor vehicle accident is much greater. Other serious risks include rashes that cause peeling of the skin, infection resulting from a low white-blood-cell count, major bleeding resulting from a low platelet count, and liver damage. In almost every case, when a doctor recommends treatment, the benefits of antiepileptic drugs clearly outweigh the risks.

Most adverse effects of antiepileptic drugs are short-lasting. People often ask, "If I stay on this medication for 5 or 10 years, won't it eventually destroy my liver or kidneys?" The answer is no. Liver function can be easily monitored with blood tests, and if a problem develops, it is reversible in more than 99% of patients when the medication is stopped. That is also true for almost all other kinds of adverse effects. Long-lasting adverse effects, such as nerve damage from phenytoin, are uncommon.

Bone loss from certain antiepileptic drugs may be more common than doctors and patients think it is. Patients taking carbamazepine, phenobarbital, phenytoin, primidone, topiramate, or valproate should consider taking calcium and vitamin D supplements. However, pregnant women should avoid very high doses of vitamin D.

In rare cases, antiepileptic drugs can actually worsen seizures (Table 2). Also, because seizures may be more frequent when a person is sleepy, antiepileptic drugs that cause sedation may occasionally aggravate seizures.

Cognitive Effects

Antiepileptic drugs act by reducing the excitability of nerve cells in the brain. They can also dampen normal activity and impair cognitive function, affecting attention and concentration, energy level, mood, drive ("the will to do things"), and mental and motor speed on tests. As a rule, impairments of this kind are more likely when two or more drugs

TABLE 2
ANTIEPILEPTIC DRUGS THAT MAY AGGRAVATE SEIZURES

Drug	Seizure Type Affected
Carbamazepine	Absence, myoclonic, seizures in benign rolandic epilepsy
Ethosuximide	Myoclonic, tonic-clonic
Gabapentin	Absence, myoclonic
Lamotrigine	Myoclonic or atonic
Oxcarbazepine	Absence, myoclonic, seizures in benign rolandic epilepsy
Phenytoin	Absence, myoclonic, tonic-clonic,* seizures in benign rolandic epilepsy
Tiagabine	Absence, ?myoclonic
Vigabatrin†	Absence, myoclonic

*Tonic-clonic seizures may become worse when the blood phenytoin level exceeds 45 micrograms per milliliter (μg/ml). †Not FDA-approved.

are used (polytherapy) and when levels of drugs in the blood exceed the therapeutic range. Patients often improve when the number of drugs is reduced. Polytherapy can have adverse cognitive effects even when the drug levels are kept within the therapeutic range. Several studies have found an association between higher dosages and increased cognitive impairment. See Chapter 11 for information on the role of specific drugs in such impairment.

Addiction

Many patients fear that once they start taking a medication, they will become "hooked." There is no basis for this fear. The only antiepileptic drugs with addictive potential are benzodiazepines and barbiturates, and addiction with these drugs is rare. The only benzodiazepines that are commonly used as antiepileptic drugs in the United States are clonazepam, clorazepate, and lorazepam. Others, clobazam and nitrazepam, are not available in the United States. Clobazam is used by some patients in the United States who obtain it from other countries. Benzodiazepines can be successfully discontinued, but it must be done gradually to avoid seizures. Some people do experience mild but unpleasant withdrawal symptoms, such as rapid heart rate, sweating, and anxiety, even when the drug is tapered gradually. They also are at higher risk of having more frequent or stronger seizures during benzodiazepine withdrawal.

Barbiturates, which include phenobarbital and mephobarbital, are also used in epilepsy and do have addictive potential, but addiction is extremely rare when they are used for the treatment of epilepsy in adults. Addiction to barbiturates does not occur in children.

Tolerance

Tolerance is the body's response to the repeated administration of a specific drug (or class of drugs) that leads to a decreased medication effect. In other words, the drug becomes less potent over time. Larger doses must be used to obtain the same effect—whether the effect is beneficial (e.g., seizure control) or adverse (e.g., sleepiness). There are two main forms of tolerance: *Metabolic tolerance* is the body's adaptation allowing for more effective elimination of the drug. For example, the liver breaks down the drug more rapidly or more completely. *Pharmacodynamic tolerance* is an adaptive change in the tissue or organ affected by the drug. For example, benzodiazepines such as diazepam and lorazepam act on receptors of the neurotransmitter GABA (see Chap. 2) in the brain. Repeated administration of benzodiazepines reduces the sensitivity of the GABA receptors, so a given dose of the drug is less effective. Regularly using one drug of this type (e.g., clonazepam taken by mouth) will produce tolerance to another type (e.g., rectal diazepam).

A small amount of tolerance can occur for most antiepileptic drugs, but it usually does not affect seizure control. For some patients whose seizures are not well controlled by medications despite numerous attempts, however, tolerance may be part of the problem. Some patients do well with any new drug for a period of weeks or months, but the drug becomes less effective over time. This is an uncommon phenomenon, but it appears to be true in some cases.

Benzodiazepines are the antiepileptic drugs most often associated with the development of tolerance. Although these drugs are among the most powerful in controlling serious and prolonged seizures, they are much less effective in long-term treatment.

Missed Doses

To achieve the goals of antiepileptic drug therapy, patients must take the medication as prescribed. It is common for patients occasionally to forget a dose. For example, the patient may oversleep and, in the rush to get to work or school on time, forget the morning medication, or he or she may simply fall asleep before taking the bedtime dose. The doctor can advise the patient on what to do if a dose of medication is forgotten. If a single dose is missed, it is usually recommended that the missed dose be taken as soon as it is remembered. Patients should not "double up" on the next dose because this may lead to side effects. Instead, the patient should take the missed dose as soon as possible, and then take the next scheduled dose after an interval of at least 2 hours. Spread out the remaining doses for that 24-hour period.

If two doses are missed within the same 24-hour period, it is usually recommended that one dose be taken as soon as it is remembered and the second missed dose be taken 2 to 4 hours later, depending on the medication's half-life and possibility of dose-related adverse effects. Drugs with a half-life longer than 10 hours can be taken about 2 hours later, but patients with a history of adverse effects from high doses should wait about 4 hours. If more than two doses of medication are missed in one 24-hour period, or if medication is missed entirely for more than 24 hours, the patient should call the doctor's office for advice.

Drug Absorption and Food

All antiepileptic drugs can be taken around mealtime. The presence of food in the stomach when medications are taken may delay the absorption of antiepileptic drugs, but it will not reduce it. Occasionally, patients report that they experience fewer adverse effects when they take medication before meals rather than after meals. Some drugs, such as carbamazepine and valproate, often are less likely to cause nausea if they are taken after meals or snacks. For drugs that cause dose-related adverse effects such as tiredness or dizziness, taking the medication with or after meals can help reduce rapid absorption and "peak-level" adverse effects. Although for most patients with epilepsy taking a medication up to 2 hours before or after the regular time will not cause seizures or troublesome side effects, it's a good idea to be consistent about the timing of medication and food—this helps avoid missed doses or adverse effects related to absorption. For example, if the morning dose is usually taken after breakfast and the evening dose is taken on an empty stomach at bedtime, this pattern should be maintained.

First Seizures—to Treat or Not to Treat?

A first seizure can be terrifying. At the time, it may seem to change the person's life permanently. Knowledge and understanding of epilepsy will remove much of the fear about the risk of having another seizure and lessen the anxiety and feelings of vulnerability that arise with the loss of control and unpredictability of a seizure. Other concerns are related to the diagnosis of epilepsy and the real and perceived stigma associated with it, the possibility of physical injury, the possible loss of driving privileges, employment issues, embarrassment, and the effects of antiepileptic drugs on the patient and on the fetus in women of childbearing age. The fact is—most people who have a single seizure do extremely well.

This discussion of first seizures applies only to tonic-clonic (convulsive) seizures. As a rule, when a single absence seizure is reported and confirmed by the typical electroencephalogram (EEG) pattern, the child usually has had many other staring spells that were not reported, and treatment is usually recommended. Similarly, with partial seizures, a person commonly may have had several partial seizures, but one relatively prominent episode (or a convulsion) has finally brought him or her to the doctor. If the diagnosis of a partial seizure is uncertain and the neuroimaging and EEG studies are normal or do not suggest epilepsy, most doctors would not prescribe antiepileptic drugs. If a partial seizure has definitely occurred, however, most doctors recommend treatment because there is a high probability of recurrence. One exception is with benign rolandic epilepsy, in which case many experts do not recommend treatment after a single seizure (see Chap. 4).

There is no simple answer as to whether to treat a single generalized tonic-clonic seizure. The chance of seizure recurrence after a single seizure is approximately 40% to 50% depending on the patient, the seizure type, and the circumstances surrounding the seizure. A person may not require treatment if the results of the neurologic examination and neuroimaging studies are normal, provocative factors such as sleep deprivation or excessive alcohol intake can be eliminated, the EEG is normal, the seizure occurred during sleep, and there is no family history of epilepsy. Table 7 on page 216 shows the risk of a recurrent seizure during the 24 months after an initial seizure in children, based on whether the EEG shows epilepsy waves and whether the neurologic examination found any abnormalities. The risk factors in adults are similar. Some decisions about treatment are more difficult than others. A 10-year-old child with a single seizure during sleep who has normal neurologic examination results and a normal magnetic resonance imaging (MRI) scan and EEG probably should not receive medication. A 30-year-old saleswoman who has a single daytime convulsion and abundant epilepsy activity on the EEG also conforms to most of the guidelines for a decision not to treat, but if she drives hundreds of miles each week in her job and supports two children, treatment may be advisable. Most patients fall between these two extremes. The decision should be based on the chances that another seizure will occur, the patient's lifestyle, the adverse effects of the medications, and the plan for discontinuing medications if seizures do not recur after a certain period.

Selecting a conservative plan for treating the seizures with antiepileptic drugs creates another set of difficult questions. The first antiepileptic drug used will have to be replaced by another drug in about half of people treated, both children and adults, because of more seizures or adverse effects. Questions that arise with treatment include:

• Should the person drive immediately after medications are started, only after the level of the drug in the blood reaches a certain level, or after a set period of time, such as 3 to 12 months?
• If no seizures occur during treatment, how long should treatment last?
• Is it safe to resume driving when the drugs are tapered off and discontinued?

Many of these are legal questions, and the laws and regulations vary in each state.

Primary Antiepileptic Drugs

Each antiepileptic drug is most effective against particular types of seizures. For each type of seizure, one or more drugs may be considered the "best" based on effectiveness and mild side effects. One of these "best" drugs is usually recommended as a first-line, or primary, treatment for the type of seizure that each patient is experiencing (Table 3). Because some medications clearly work best for certain seizure types but can actually worsen other types, correct seizure classification is essential. In prescribing antiepileptic drugs, doctors usually start with just one drug, beginning with a low dose and increasing it slowly unless the patient's condition requires a more rapid buildup. The correct dosage is based on how well the patient is doing (e.g., whether his or her seizures are controlled or whether there are of adverse effects), not on the amount of drug in the patient's blood.

Many patients have seizures of more than one type. For example, a patient may have simple partial seizures consisting of an odd feeling in the stomach and *déjà vu* along with complex partial seizures, in which the stomach feeling progresses to impaired awareness, staring, lip-smacking, and occasional secondary generalized tonic-clonic seizures. For this patient, a medication such as oxcarbazepine or phenytoin (see Chap. 11) is more likely to fully control the tonic-clonic seizures than the complex partial ones. Patients who have only simple and complex partial seizures may find that the complex partial seizures are better controlled than the simple partial seizures.

TABLE 3
PRIMARY AND SECONDARY ANTIEPILEPTIC DRUGS FOR DIFFERENT
SEIZURE TYPES AND EPILEPSY SYNDROMES*

Seizure Type or Epilepsy Syndrome	Primary Drug	Secondary Drug
Generalized		
Absence	Ethosuximide Valproate	Lamotrigine
Myoclonic	Valproate	Acetazolamide Clonazepam Lamotrigine Primidone Topiramate Zonisamide
Tonic-clonic	Valproate Carbamazepine Oxcarbazepine Phenytoin	Lamotrigine Phenobarbital Primidone Topiramate
Childhood-onset absence	Ethosuximide	Valproate Lamotrigine
Adolescent-onset absence	Valproate	Ethosuximide Lamotrigine
Juvenile myoclonic	Valproate	Acetazolamide Clonazepam Primidone Lamotrigine Topiramate
Infantile spasms (West's syndrome)	Adrenocorticotropic hormone (ACTH) Vigabatrin Valproate	Topiramate Benzodiazepine Lamotrigine Tiagabine
Lennox-Gastaut syndrome	Valproate Lamotrigine	Carbamazepine Topiramate Zonisamide Acetazolamide Clonazepam Felbamate
Partial		
Simple partial Complex partial Secondarily generalized tonic-clonic seizures	Carbamazepine Lamotrigine Oxcarbazepine	Gabapentin Levetiracetam Phenobarbital Phenytoin Primidone

*Drugs are listed in order of preferred use.   *(continued)*

TABLE 3
PRIMARY AND SECONDARY ANTIEPILEPTIC DRUGS FOR DIFFERENT
SEIZURE TYPES AND EPILEPSY SYNDROMES* (continued)

Seizure Type or Epilepsy Syndrome	Primary Drug	Secondary Drug
Partial (continued)		
Partial epileptic syndromes		Tiagabine
		Topiramate
		Valproate
		Zonisamide
Benign rolandic epilepsy	Carbamazepine	Phenytoin
	Gabapentin	Topiramate
	Oxcarbazepine	Lamotrigine
	Valproate	

*Drugs are listed in order of preferred use.

Most patients find it easiest to take one small pill once a day. The size and number of the pills may not reflect the drug's effectiveness or adverse effects, however. If 100 mg of drug A has the same beneficial effect as 10 mg (a much smaller pill) of drug B, then drug B is more potent. For example, a patient who had been taking 150 mg of phenobarbital once a day at bedtime may experience better seizure control and fewer adverse effects if he or she gradually changed to taking 500 mg of valproate three times daily, although the amount of drug taken (in milligrams), the size of the pills, and the frequency of dose are all increased. The first goal should be seizure control with minimal or no adverse effects. The number and size of the pills are important, but secondary, issues.

In most patients, a single primary antiepileptic drug provides the best balance between seizure control and adverse effects. Unfortunately, some patients are treated with three or more antiepileptic drugs at moderate doses, and they continue to have both seizures and troublesome adverse effects. This usually is not the best possible therapy. If seizures persist while a patient is taking a single medication that causes no adverse effects, it is usually best to gradually increase the dose until the seizures are controlled or adverse effects develop. A rapid increase in the dose can cause adverse effects and unnecessarily lead the patient and doctor to feel that extreme fatigue, inability to concentrate, feeling like a "zombie," or other problems are inevitable effects of the drug. With many drugs, the key to patient tolerance is a gradual increase in the dosage.

Antiepileptic drugs vary considerably in how they work, how long they remain in the blood (half-life), and how they should be taken.

(More information about specific drugs is found in the next chapter.) It is important that patients not experiment with varying the schedule of their medications without first discussing the proposed changes with the doctor or nurse. Because some medications, such as gabapentin and tiagabine, have relatively short half-lives, they almost always have to be taken more than once a day to improve seizure control and reduce dose-related adverse effects. In an ideal world, medication would be given only once a day and would be released in the body slowly. Unfortunately, steady-release antiepileptic drugs are not always available. We must work with the drugs we have. This means that it is often necessary to take a drug two to four times a day.

The schedule for taking medication should be flexible and adapted to the patient's lifestyle. In most cases, it is easy for the doctor and patient to work out a schedule that is convenient, minimizes adverse effects, and controls seizures.

Secondary Antiepileptic Drugs

The development of a rash, a serious reduction in the number of white blood cells (which fight infection), or other problems may force the doctor to stop a primary antiepileptic drug. In these cases, another primary drug is usually tried alone. Also, if the first primary drug fails to control the seizures, some experts will try another primary or secondary drug alone while others recommend adding a secondary drug to the regimen (see Table 3). When a medication is added to another medication, it is sometimes referred to as *adjunctive therapy*. Although some drugs are called *secondary* because they tend to have fewer good effects and more bad effects than the primary drugs, secondary drugs can be extremely effective in certain instances and do not adversely affect some patients. Many patients are successfully treated using only drugs that are usually considered secondary.

What if the Drug Fails?

The first attempt at antiepileptic drug therapy may be ineffective for several reasons:

- The patient didn't take the medication as prescribed.
- The prescribed doses didn't control the seizures.
- The patient had an allergic reaction (e.g., rash or hives) to the medication.

• The patient experienced adverse medication effects (e.g., tiredness, vision problems, or nausea).

A drug may fail to control seizures for many reasons. First, it may be the wrong medication for the patient's seizure type or epilepsy syndrome. Second, the dose given may be too low. There is no "right" dose that can be determined ahead of time. The amount needed depends on the patient and individual factors such as absorption, metabolism, or severity of epilepsy. If the patient is not having adverse effects, the amount given may be safely increased until the seizures are controlled. Third, the scheduling of the doses may not provide an effective blood drug level at the time when the person is most prone to having a seizure. For example, if seizures tend to occur shortly before or after awakening, the largest dose probably should be given at bedtime to ensure a therapeutic blood drug level when seizures are most likely to occur. For a child with benign rolandic epilepsy who has only had seizures within an hour after falling asleep, a single daily dose given around dinner (several hours before bedtime) may be effective and should minimize daytime side effects. Finally, a drug may simply fail because it is ineffective.

Adverse effects can often be managed by decreasing the dose temporarily until the patient becomes more "used to the drug" (until tolerance develops). In other cases, giving small doses more often, giving the medication after meals, or giving a larger dose at bedtime may reduce or eliminate adverse effects.

If an allergic reaction occurs or if the patient experiences intolerable adverse effects even with low doses, the drug should be discontinued and another drug should be tried alone (monotherapy). If relatively high doses and "therapeutic" blood levels of a drug fail to control seizures, it is reasonable to try another single drug or to consider a trial of two drugs (polytherapy). The decision should be based on a realistic understanding of the potential benefits and adverse effects of one drug versus two drugs. If two drugs are used, it is often helpful to review the change in seizure frequency and severity as well as adverse effects after the dosages have been stabilized. Have the benefits of the second drug outweighed any additional side effects (and financial cost)? For example, a 20% reduction in seizure frequency may not outweigh being bothered by increased tiredness and dizziness for several hours every day. There is an art to selecting and adjusting medication combinations—an art based on full and honest communication between the patient and the doctor.

If a person with epilepsy has been treated unsuccessfully with two different drugs given singly and a combination of two drugs, all at dosages that yield blood levels in the upper therapeutic range, the chances that another drug or combination of drugs will fully control the seizures are less than 10%. Before trying other medications, it may be worthwhile to consult an epilepsy specialist to ensure that the diagnoses of epilepsy, seizure type, and epilepsy syndrome are correct. If the epilepsy diagnoses are correct and the seizures are not easily controllable with medication, then it may be time to consider epilepsy surgery or vagus nerve stimulation.

Blood Testing

Blood tests should be done before any antiepileptic drug is started so the results can be compared with later blood tests. These tests include measurements of electrolyte levels (chemicals in the blood such as sodium and potassium), liver and kidney function tests, blood-cell counts, and monitoring of antiepileptic drug levels. The frequency of testing varies considerably from doctor to doctor and even country to country. For example, in 1989 all 63 child neurologists in Canada issued a consensus statement saying that routine blood testing and laboratory monitoring of antiepileptic drug levels are of doubtful benefit to patients. The Canadian view is that the dosage should be decreased when patients are experiencing bothersome side effects, regardless of the level of drug in the blood. These neurologists suggested that blood drug levels should be monitored only if unexplained seizures occur or if the doctor is not sure that the patient is taking the drug as prescribed. In the United States, however, a blood test is often done routinely several weeks or months after a new drug is started. The timing of later tests depends on the patient's medical history, the drug, and most importantly, the doctor's opinion on the necessity for testing. If a patient has been taking the same drug for more than a year and the results of routine laboratory studies have been normal or unchanged, testing can be done once a year or less often. If new problems arise, such as pain in the upper abdomen, or if seizures increase for no apparent reason, blood tests may need to be rechecked.

Checking the blood level of a drug at consistent times of day and consistent times after the last dose of medication is taken allows the doctor to compare levels at different dosages. Routine blood levels are best measured when the amount of the drug in the bloodstream is at its lowest point (the trough level). This generally corresponds to the time just before the medication is taken. Trough levels fluctuate up to 20% in many patients who take the drug on a consistent schedule. These variations reflect changes in the drug's absorption and metabolism, other medications taken, and handling of the blood specimen at the laboratory.

The so-called therapeutic range of blood levels for antiepileptic drugs is a statistical concept derived from studies of many patients. It is the range of levels at which most patients have good seizure control and few or no adverse effects. The lower and upper limits of this range can vary between different laboratories and doctors. Seizure control without adverse effects, not the blood drug level, is the criterion for judging the efficacy of treatment. For example, if a patient's seizures are well controlled, but the level of drug in the blood is below the expected therapeutic range, the doctor will usually be satisfied and will not increase the dosage to raise the blood drug level. On the other hand, another patient's seizures may have been difficult to control using a single drug, but they have finally responded to a two-drug combination after the dosage of one medication is increased. Blood tests may show that the level of that drug is now slightly above the therapeutic level; that is, the level is in the "toxic range." If the patient is not experiencing adverse effects, the drug dosage should not be decreased.

During the past decade, the trend has been to monitor blood drug levels less frequently. If the patient is feeling well and is seizure-free, the value of monitoring the blood drug level is questionable. In some cases, however, it may be critical to attain a therapeutic blood drug level. For instance, it may be important to ensure that the level is kept in the therapeutic range for a pregnant woman who had seizures when blood drug levels dropped during labor with a previous pregnancy (see Chap. 25).

Drug Interactions

A doctor caring for a person with epilepsy should know about all of the drugs the person is taking. Drug interactions are common and can be dangerous. Antiepileptic drugs interact with each other and with other drugs. The effects of interactions between two drugs vary. Some antiepileptic drugs can lower or raise the blood levels of other types of drugs. Some combinations cause the levels of both drugs to fall, some cause one level to fall and one level to rise, and some cause unpredictable effects. For example, a person taking the antiepileptic drug carbamazepine (Tegretol and Carbatrol) who has an infection for which a doctor prescribes the antibiotic erythromycin (Biaxin) should not take the antibiotic unless the carbamazepine dose is lowered. This is because erythromycin can greatly increase the blood carbamazepine level, causing severe but reversible adverse effects. In another example, the antiepileptic drug phenytoin and the blood thinner or anticoagulant warfarin (Coumadin) can interact and alter the adverse effects and effectiveness of each other.

No list of drug interactions is all-inclusive because doctors and pharmacists continue to learn of interactions between existing drugs and new ones. Therefore, the doctor or dentist who prescribes medication for a person with epilepsy should be aware that he or she is taking an antiepileptic drug. Patients should also tell the pharmacist or doctor about their use of over-the-counter medications because some of them can affect antiepileptic drug levels, cause seizures in someone who has never had a seizure, or increase seizure frequency in a person with epilepsy. The tables in Appendix 3 list drug interactions involving antiepileptic medications.

ANTIEPILEPTIC DRUGS AND BIRTH CONTROL PILLS

Most women with epilepsy can take birth control pills without affecting their seizure control. Usually there is no change when the pills are started, although some women have slightly improved or slightly worsened seizure control. Some antiepileptic drugs (carbamazepine, phenytoin, phenobarbital, primidone, and topiramate) increase the breakdown, or metabolism, of estrogen and progesterone by the liver. These drugs reduce the effectiveness of birth control pills. If a sexually active woman is taking birth control pills and one of these drugs, she should be aware that her chances of getting pregnant are increased.

Breakthrough bleeding between menstrual periods is a clue that the effectiveness of birth control pills is reduced. However, the absence of breakthrough bleeding does not indicate that the woman has adequate contraceptive protection and will not become pregnant. To effectively prevent pregnancy, it is often necessary to use a birth control pill with a higher estrogen content. It also may be wise to add another method of contraception, such as a diaphragm or condom with spermicide. Similarly, birth control pills with a low estrogen content may not be effective when taken for a gynecologic disorder such as endometriosis. Clobazam, gabapentin, lamotrigine, levetiracetam, valproate, and vigabatrin do not interact significantly with birth control pills.

ANTIEPILEPTIC DRUGS AND ALCOHOL

Most people with epilepsy have been warned by doctors and pharmacists not to use alcohol or have been told to limit its use. Alcohol does not seriously alter the effectiveness of antiepileptic drugs, but it can alter the blood levels of some of them. For example, drinking a moderate or large amount of alcohol in a short period can increase blood phenytoin levels. Prolonged use of alcohol can decrease blood levels of phenobarbital and phenytoin (by increasing metabolism) and delay the absorption of carbamazepine (but without altering its blood levels).

People who drink alcoholic beverages while taking antiepileptic drugs may become intoxicated quickly. Many of these drugs have dose-related adverse effects similar to the effects of alcohol, including slurred speech, unsteadiness, dizziness, and tiredness. These effects can be especially dangerous when someone who takes antiepileptic drugs has several drinks; becomes intoxicated; and then has to drive, supervise small children, or operate dangerous equipment. Another danger occurs when someone taking high doses of phenobarbital or primidone drinks a very large amount of alcohol quickly. In this case, the person could lapse into a coma or die.

People with epilepsy should not consume more than two alcoholic beverages per occasion (a "beverage" is 1 oz. of liquor, 6 oz. of wine, or 12 oz. of beer). Drinking more than this can be followed by withdrawal (which is most likely to occur 6 to 48 hours after drinking), during which time seizures are more likely to occur. Drinking more than two alcoholic beverages also is often associated with missing one or more doses of antiepileptic drugs or with sleep deprivation. The combination of multiple risk factors for seizures—missed doses, alcohol withdrawal, and sleep deprivation—can provoke unusually intense or prolonged seizures.

Reducing the Cost of Antiepileptic Drugs

IS IT A GOOD IDEA TO USE GENERIC DRUGS?

Brand-name drugs are manufactured by major pharmaceutical companies and are more expensive than generic drugs. Although generic drugs may be manufactured by large pharmaceutical companies, they are often made by smaller companies and it may be difficult to find out who manufactures the drugs distributed by a specific pharmacy. There is a general trend in medicine toward the use of generic drugs because they are less expensive. For antiepileptic drugs, however, the generics may not be equivalent to the brand-name preparations. The major difference between generic and brand-name medication is not the quality of the drug itself, but the consistency in the amount of medication and the way it is made. The manufacturing process can affect how much of the drug is absorbed and the rate at which it is absorbed. The absorption of brand-name drugs is usually quite consistent. In generic antiepileptic drugs, the absorption may be more variable. For some patients, using generic drugs is associated with fluctuating blood drug levels, leading to a potential increase in seizure frequency when the levels are low and an increase in adverse effects when the blood levels are high.

Although there are some good, reliable generic drug products, it is often difficult to know exactly which manufacturer makes the generic drug that a person receives. Many pharmacies use a distributor, who will buy in large amounts from any company that has a drug available or has the least expensive drug. When the supplier changes, the formulation of the drug may change. Because of these unpredictable situations, most neurologists recommend brand-name epilepsy drugs only.

Most doctors, and also the Epilepsy Foundation (EF), recommend that switching between different manufacturers' products should be avoided because the possible differences in absorption and other factors may affect seizure control or cause adverse effects. These problems are most likely to occur in people who have had trouble achieving seizure control or who have had problems with adverse effects of medication. The change from a brand-name drug to a generic drug should only be made with the doctor's approval. If a generic drug is substituted for a brand-name drug, the pharmacist should tell the patient. The doctor also should be notified so that any additional tests that may be required can be ordered. Once seizure control is established, every effort should be made to keep taking the same manufacturer's product, whether it is a generic or brand-name. If a person is taking a generic drug, it is important that he or she be assured that the manufacturer of the drug will not change. Changing between the products of different manufacturers poses the greatest risk of increased seizures or adverse effects. Patients should always check their antiepileptic drugs before leaving the pharmacy and question the pharmacist if the pills look different.

An interesting aside to the generic issue is that some patients who develop a rash while taking Tegretol (the brand name for carbamazepine) may not be allergic to the drug, but to the red dye used in making it. These patients may wish to use Tegretol extended-release (Tegretol XR) or the Tegretol chewable tablet (white, not red), another brand name (Carbatrol, a sustained-release form of carbamazepine), or a generic preparation.

OTHER WAYS TO CUT COSTS

Antiepileptic drugs are expensive, but there are several ways to cut their costs. When applying for health insurance, if there is a choice between different policies, the subscriber should find out if there is a prescription plan and, if so, how the plan works. It may be useful to compare the possible increased costs of a health care plan that includes partial or complete coverage for medications to the costs of the drugs.

Before purchasing medication, it may be wise to shop around. There may be considerable differences in the price of prescriptions between pharmacies in the same town. It might also pay to shop in some nearby towns. Large pharmacies or chain stores frequently offer lower prices, and some pharmacies offer discounts for the purchase of larger quantities.

Pharmacy services are also available. For example, membership in the EF also includes access to the American Association of Retired Persons pharmacy. There are many other Internet and mail-order pharmacies, some of which are listed in Appendix 4. Local EF affiliates and fellow patients also may have information on obtaining medications at lower prices. Most major manufacturers of brand-name antiepileptic drugs offer a program to make drugs available to patients with limited incomes (see Table 4 and Appendix 4). One such program is administered by

TABLE 4
INFORMATION ON PATIENT ASSISTANCE PROGRAMS

Pharmaceutical Company	Prescription Drugs/ Device	Eligibility	Initial Supply	Renewal Policy
Abbott Laboratories (800) 222-6885	• Depakote (divalproex sodium) tablets • Gabitril (tiagabine) tablets	• U.S. resident • No prescription drug coverage or Medicaid eligibility • Income no more than 200% of poverty level	• 3 months • Sent to physician • No fee	• Three additional 3-month supplies by physician's verbal request • Recertification at end of 12 months, then annually
Athena Rx Home Pharmacy/Elan Pharmaceuticals (800) 537-8899 x7788	• Diastat (rectal diazepam) • Mysoline (primidone) • Zonegran (zonisamide)	• U.S. resident • No third-party coverage including Medicaid, government agencies, or private foundations • Net worth less than $30,000	• 3 months for Mysoline or Zonegran, less than 3 months for Diastat • Sent to patient • No fee	• Recertification at end of 3 months, then every 3 months • 3-month time limit between renewals
Cyberonics (877) 610-1180	• NCP vagal nerve stimulation system	• Inability to pay for NCP system • No insurance coverage	• $5 million of systems provided on a first-come, first-serve basis over 5 years	• N/A
GlaxoSmithKline (800) 722-9294	• Lamictal (lamotrigine)	• U.S. citizen • Uninsured, unable to afford prescription medication, or awaiting approval for other sources of funding	• 30 days • Benefit card given by physician for patient use with prescription at pharmacy • Co-pay fee of $5–$10 per prescription	• Two additional 30-day supplies upon receipt of completed application • Recertification at end of 90 days, then every 90 days

Novartis Pharmaceuticals Corporation (800) 257-3273	• Tegretol (carbamazepine), Tegretol-XR (carbamazepine, extended release) • Trileptal (oxcarbazepine)	• U.S. resident • Special needs because of short-term hardship	• 30 days • Benefit card given by physician for patient use with prescription at pharmacy • Nominal fee based on income	• Five additional 30-day supplies upon receipt of completed application • Recertification at end of 6 months, then every 6 months
Ortho-McNeil Pharmaceutical, Inc. (800) 797-7737	• Topamax (topiramate)	• Unable to pay (income assessed on patient-to-patient basis) • Not covered under private reimbursement plan or government prescription program	• 3 months • Sent to physician • No fee	• Three additional 3-month supplies through physician's written request • Recertification annually
Pfizer Inc. (908) 725-1247	*Parke-Davis Patient Assistance Program:* • Dilantin (phenytoin) • Neurontin (gabapentin) • Zarontin (ethosuximide)	• Not covered under government prescription program or private reimbursement plan • Individual income $16,000 or less, or family income $25,000 or less	• 3 months • Sent to physician • No fee	• Recertification at end of 3 months, then every 3 months

(continued)

[137]

TABLE 4
INFORMATION ON PATIENT ASSISTANCE PROGRAMS *(continued)*

Pharmaceutical Company	Prescription Drugs/ Device	Eligibility	Initial Supply	Renewal Policy
Pfizer Inc. *(continued)*	*Neurontin CAP Program:* (for those whose income exceeds limits above) • Neurontin (gabapentin)	• No prescription drug coverage • More than $138.00 per month spent on Neurontin pre-scription	• 30 days • Benefit card sent to patient for use with prescription at pharmacy • Pays cost of drug in excess of $138.00 per month	• Five additional 30-day supplies • Recertification at end of 6 months, then every 6 months
UCB Pharma, Inc. (800) 477-7877 x2943	• Keppra (levetiracetam)	• U.S. resident • No prescription drug coverage or Medicaid eligibility • Household income not to exceed $15,000 or $25,000 with dependents	• 3 months • Sent to physician • No fee	• Recertification at end of 3 months, then every 3 months

GlaxoSmithKline called the Orange Card Program, which offers discounts on all their outpatient products. Senior citizens age 65 and older are eligible for this program, as well as the disabled who are enrolled in Medicare who have annual incomes at or below 300% of the federal poverty level (annual incomes at or below $26,000 for singles or $35,000 for couples) and who lack public or private insurance programs or other pharmaceutical benefit programs, such as Medicaid. Neurologists, epilepsy centers, and the national and local EF affiliates can provide information on these and other assistance programs.

Discontinuing Antiepileptic Drugs

Getting off antiepileptic drugs is the goal of most people with well-controlled seizures. Chapter 17 discusses the way most children "outgrow" epilepsy and are able to stop their drug therapy. Many of the same principles apply to most adults. Most doctors will consider discontinuing antiepileptic drugs after a seizure-free period of 2 to 4 years. Many doctors will also consider discontinuing the medication of someone who has had only one seizure and has been seizure-free for 6 to 12 months. Patients are unlikely to have future seizures if they had few seizures before taking antiepileptic drugs; if the seizures were easily controlled with a single drug; and if they have normal results on the neurologic examination, MRI, and EEG.

For certain types of seizures, such as benign rolandic epilepsy, it can be predicted with a high degree of certainty that seizures will not recur after age 16 even if medication is discontinued. By contrast, the seizures in juvenile myoclonic epilepsy are often well controlled by the drug valproate, but they are very likely to return if the medication is stopped.

Drugs Used Against Epilepsy

As discussed in Chapter 10, the principal therapy for epilepsy is the use of certain drugs according to a carefully individualized plan. In deciding which drug or drugs to prescribe, the doctor first determines what type of seizures or epilepsy syndrome the patient has. The doctor then chooses the drug most likely to be effective and acceptable for that person. The doctor may discuss with the patient the pros and cons of different drugs, including such factors as cost, how often it must be taken, whether it will interact with other drugs the patient needs to take, and likely adverse effects. This chapter gives some basic facts about each of the most frequently used antiepileptic drugs and provides details about some new and experimental ones. Information on the characteristics and adverse effects of most of the drugs covered is summarized in Tables 5 and 6. Appendix 3 gives information on the ways in which these drugs affect and are affected by other medications.

Drugs Commonly Used Against Epilepsy

The following pages discuss the most commonly used antiepileptic drugs, listed alphabetically. A discussion of the role of benzodiazepines (clonazepam, clobazam, clorazepate, diazepam, lorazepam) follows (see page 153).

ACETAZOLAMIDE

Acetazolamide (Diamox) is used alongside another drug to treat absence and myoclonic seizures. It is also used to treat partial or generalized seizures that occur more often around the time of menstruation (catamenial epilepsy; see Chap. 6). Acetazolamide works by inhibiting an enzyme called carbonic anhydrase. The evidence that it is an effective drug for treating patients with epilepsy is much more limited than for most other drugs. Sometimes it is helpful, however, especially for those with absence or myoclonic seizures.

Some patients develop tolerance to acetazolamide, which means the drug becomes less effective over time. Common adverse effects include dizziness; tingling around the mouth, fingertips, and toes; and increased frequency of urination (because it is a mild diuretic). About 1% to 2% of patients taking it develop kidney stones; patients taking it should drink plenty of fluids, especially in hot environments. Patients on the ketogenic diet (see Chap. 13) or those taking other drugs with similar side effects, such as topiramate or zonisamide, should be especially cautious.

Acetazolamide is available in 125-mg and 250-mg tablets. There is no clearly defined therapeutic range of blood drug levels. Acetazolamide is also used to treat altitude sickness.

CARBAMAZEPINE

Carbamazepine (Tegretol, Tegretol-XR, and Carbatrol) is one of the first-line (primary) drugs for all types of partial seizures and partial epilepsy syndromes (except benign rolandic epilepsy, in which it can increase seizure activity in some children). It is also used to treat bipolar (manic-depressive) disorder and some kinds of pain. It works mainly by reducing abnormal chemical activity in the brain's neurons. Common adverse effects include tiredness, blurred or double vision, nausea, dizziness, or unsteadiness. It also can cause slight reductions in attention, speed of thinking and movement, and response accuracy. Rash occurs in about 5% to 7% of patients. During the first month after starting the medication, it is wise to avoid heavy sunlight exposure because it may increase the risk of rash. Very rare adverse effects include liver or bone marrow failure.

Carbamazepine is available as a generic drug in various strengths (usually 100 and 200 mg). Tegretol is available as a chewable 100-mg tablet (round, white with red speckles, and flavored) and as a 200-mg pink, oblong regular tablet. Tegretol elixir is a liquid that contains 100 mg of the drug in each 5 ml (about 1 teaspoon). Tegretol-XR (extended release) is available in round tablets: 100 mg (yellow), 200 mg (pink), and 400 mg (beige). The shell of the pill, which is not absorbed, has a small hole in it to allow the medication to be slowly released.

Text continued on p. 146

TABLE 5
CHARACTERISTICS OF FREQUENTLY USED ANTIEPILEPTIC DRUGS WHEN USED ALONE

Drug	Daily Dose (mg/lb of patient's weight)	Time to Peak Blood Level[a] (hours)	Therapeutic Blood Levels (μg per ml of blood)	Half-life[b] (hours)
Acetazolamide	4–12	2–4	10–30	10–12
Carbamazepine[c]	4–12	2–12	5–12	8–20
Clonazepam[d]	0.02–0.1[e] 0.04–0.1[f]	1–4	20–80 (ng/ml)	15–40
Clorazepate	0.05–0.2	0.5–2	?	30–60
Ethosuximide[d]	7–25	1–4	50–100	25–70
Felbamate[d]	7–25	1–4	30–100	14–20
Gabapentin[d]	4–15	2–4	4–16	5–7
Lamotrigine[d]	2.5–5	2–4	1–20	7–60[g]
Levetiracetam	7–18	0.75–2.5	?	6–8
Oxcarbazepine	5–18	3–6	? (Only MHD, an active metabolite, is measured)	2 (oxcarbazepine) 9 (MHD metabolite)
Phenobarbital	2–5[e] 0.7–2.5[f]	2–12	12–40	26–140

Phenytoin	2–5	4–8	10–20	14–30[h]
Primidone	5–10	2–5	5–18	12
Tiagabine	0.2–0.5		5–70 ng/ml	4–9
Topiramate	2–5		2–25	20
Valproate[d]	5–25	2–8 1–3[i]	50–140	8–16
Zonisamide	2–5	5–6	10–40	40–60

mg, milligram (one thousandth of a gram); µg, microgram (one millionth of a gram); ng, nanogram (one billionth of a gram).

[a]After blood drug levels reach steady state.

[b]Children metabolize many drugs more rapidly than adults do, so the half-life is often shorter in children.

[c]Active metabolite.

[d]In general, when these drugs are given together with carbamazepine, phenobarbital, phenytoin, or primidone, their blood level is lower and their half-life is shorter.

[e]Dose for young children.

[f]Dose for older children and adults.

[g]Valproate prolongs the half-life of lamotrigine.

[h]The half-life of phenytoin increases as the dose or blood level increase.

[i]After oral dose of valproate.

[143]

TABLE 6
MAJOR ADVERSE EFFECTS OF DRUGS COMMONLY USED TO TREAT EPILEPSY

Drug	Dose-Related Adverse Effects*	Rare Idiosyncratic Adverse Effects	Long-Term Adverse Effects
Acetazolamide	Increased frequency of urination; tingling of face, fingers, toes	Kidney stones	None
Benzodiazepines Clobazam Clonazepam Clorazepate Diazepam Lorazepam	Tiredness, dizziness, unsteadiness, impaired attention and memory, hyperactivity, depression, irritability, aggressivity, drooling (children), nausea, loss of appetite	None	None
Carbamazepine and oxcarbazepine	Nausea, vomiting, blurred or double vision, tiredness, dizziness, unsteadiness, memory problems, slurred speech, low sodium (hyponatremia), rash or fever†	Very low WBC or CBC, liver damage, severe rash, hypersensitivity reaction, heart block (a blockage of electrical impulses in the heart)	Bone loss
Ethosuximide	Nausea and vomiting, loss of appetite, weight loss, behavioral changes, tiredness, dizziness, earache	Very low WBC or CBC	None
Felbamate	Headache, insomnia, irritability, nausea, vomiting, weight loss	Bone marrow or liver failure (combined risk estimated at about 1 in 4500)	None
Gabapentin	Dizziness, tiredness	None	None
Lamotrigine	Insomnia, nausea, unsteadiness	Severe rash	None
Levetiracetam	Tiredness, dizziness, unsteadiness	Unknown	Unknown

Drug	Common/dose-related effects	Serious effects*	Long-term effects
Phenobarbital, mephobarbital, and primidone	Tiredness, depression, hyperactivity, dizziness, memory problems, impotence, slurred speech, nausea, anemia, rash† or fever†, low calcium levels and bone loss	Liver damage, severe rash, hypersensitivity reaction	Bone loss, soft-tissue growths, rheumatologic disorders (e.g., frozen shoulder, stiffening of fingers)
Phenytoin	Tiredness, dizziness, memory problems, rash† or fever, gum overgrowth, growth of facial hair, anemia, acne, slurred speech, low calcium and bone loss	Liver damage, severe rash† and other hypersensitivity reactions, behavioral changes	Bone loss, nerve damage, possible damage to cerebellum (part of brain)
Tiagabine	Dizziness, tiredness, mood changes	None	None
Topiramate	Dizziness, tiredness, decreased appetite, impaired concentration and word finding, memory problems, mood changes	Kidney stones, rash	None
Valproate	Nausea and vomiting, tiredness, weight gain, hair loss, tremor	Liver damage, very low platelet counts, pancreatic inflammation, hearing loss, behavioral changes	Bone loss, hair loss, hair texture change, weight gain
Vigabatrin	Tiredness, weight gain	None	Damage to retina of eye and impairment of peripheral vision
Zonisamide	Drowsiness, dizziness, loss of appetite, GI discomfort	Kidney stones, rash	Possible bone loss

WBC, white blood cell count; CBC, complete blood cell count; GI, gastrointestinal.
*Some of the adverse effects (very low blood-cell or platelet count, liver damage, hypersensitivity reactions, severe rash, pancreatic inflammation) are serious and potentially fatal.
†Rash and fever are common (3% to 6% of patients), but not related to the dosage.

There is no need to worry if the shell is found in the stool—the medicine has been absorbed. However, Tegretol-XR pills pass through some children too rapidly for all of the medication to be absorbed. Carbatrol is another sustained-release form of carbamazepine. It is available in capsule form: 200 mg (gray and turquoise) and 300 mg (black and turquoise).

ETHOSUXIMIDE

Ethosuximide (Zarontin) is used to treat absence seizures only. It has no effect against (or may even worsen) myoclonic, tonic-clonic, or partial seizures. It acts by reducing certain types of chemical activity affecting neurons. Adverse effects include nausea and vomiting, loss of appetite, weight loss, behavioral changes, tiredness, and dizziness. Ethosuximide is available as 250-mg gelatin capsules (amber).

ETHOTOIN

Ethotoin (Peganone), which works against partial seizures, is not used very often. It was introduced as a drug similar to phenytoin (which is discussed later), but with fewer adverse effects. Phenytoin is used much more often, probably because it is more effective in controlling partial seizures. Adverse effects of ethotoin include bitter taste, unsteadiness, dizziness, rash, sleep disturbance, and stomach upset. Ethotoin is available as 250-mg (round, white) and 500-mg (round, white) tablets.

FELBAMATE

Felbamate (Felbatol) is effective in treating partial and secondarily generalized tonic-clonic seizures. It is also effective for Lennox-Gastaut syndrome, and evidence suggests it may help treat various primary generalized seizures. The drug is often given two to three times daily. Common adverse effects are decreased appetite, weight loss, insomnia, headache, and depression. Cognitive and behavioral problems are uncommon and are usually mild. Many patients can tolerate doses of up to 3600 mg per day. Felbamate is available as an elixir for children (600 mg per 5 ml [teaspoon] in fruit punch flavor) and in 400-mg (yellow) and 600-mg (peach) tablets.

After the release of felbamate, a high risk of potentially fatal bone marrow failure or liver failure was identified. These disorders have affected about 1 in 4500 patients taking the drug, and 1 in 9000 has died. As a result, the use of felbamate is now strictly limited to patients in whom the benefits outweigh the risks. Blood-cell counts and liver function tests should be performed often (every 2 weeks is recommended) at least during the first year of therapy, when most of these serious problems occur. These tests can provide an early warning of danger, but are no guarantee against an irreversible and potentially fatal condition.

GABAPENTIN

Gabapentin (Neurontin) is effective for partial and secondarily generalized seizures, but it is not effective for the primary generalized seizures that occur in patients with absence or myoclonic epilepsies. Gabapentin is also helpful for some pain syndromes. It is an amino acid that is chemically related to gamma-aminobutyric acid (GABA), a naturally occurring neurotransmitter (see Chap. 2). Gabapentin probably works by affecting the GABA system. Because it has a short half-life (about 6 hours), it usually needs to be taken three times a day.

Gabapentin seldom causes problems from adverse effects, most of which, such as tiredness and dizziness, improve after several weeks. Tiredness and dizziness are most common when the dose is more than 1200 mg per day, although most adults are able to take doses of 1800 to 3600 mg per day. Other adverse effects include headache, unsteadiness, double vision, tremor, abdominal discomfort, and weight gain. Behavioral problems, such as irritability and hyperactivity, can occur in children. In some individuals, gabapentin has beneficial effects on mood and emotional well-being. Experience with more than 2 million patients suggests that gabapentin does not injure the liver, kidneys, or blood cells.

If the dose of gabapentin is increased beyond 3600 mg per day, a smaller proportion of the medication is absorbed. If a person takes 3600 mg per day, the amount absorbed is about 40% (1440 mg/day) whether the drug is given in three or four doses. However, if a person takes 4800 mg per day, only about 30% is absorbed when given three times a day (1600 mg three times a day; total absorbed = 1440 mg/day) and 35% is absorbed if it is given in four doses (1200 mg four times a day; total absorbed = 1680 mg/day).

One advantage of gabapentin is that it does not interact with any other antiepileptic drugs or oral contraceptives. This is important because it is often used in addition to carbamazepine or phenytoin for partial epilepsy. It is also effective for some patients when used alone.

Gabapentin is available as Neurontin in hard gelatin capsules with doses of 100 mg (white), 300 mg (yellow), and 400 mg (orange). No tablets or liquids are currently available, and there is no generic form.

LAMOTRIGINE

Lamotrigine (Lamictal) is approved for the treatment of partial and secondarily generalized tonic-clonic seizures. It appears to be effective in generalized seizure disorders, including absence and atonic seizures, and in Lennox-Gastaut syndrome and juvenile myoclonic epilepsy. It works in several ways to reduce excessive chemical and electrical activity in the brain. Its half-life, about 30 hours, is changed if other antiepileptic drugs are taken: it is increased by valproate and decreased by phenytoin and carbamazepine. Lamotrigine levels in the blood can be decreased by acetaminophen (Tylenol). It is usually given twice a day, and average adult dosages range from 250 to 500 mg per day.

Patients taking lamotrigine do not often experience adverse effects. Some individuals actually experience beneficial effects on mood and emotional well-being. Adverse effects that may occur include dizziness, unsteadiness, double or blurred vision, headache, nausea and vomiting, diarrhea, impaired coordination, insomnia, tiredness, and rash. The frequency of rash increases if the dosage is rapidly increased, even if the dosage change occurs months after lamotrigine is first given. Rash is especially likely in patients taking valproate. A potentially life-threatening rash (Stevens-Johnson syndrome) can develop. This is more common in children. When patients taking valproate start taking lamotrigine at a very low dosage and increase the dosage slowly, there is seldom a problem. A disadvantage of this approach is that it may take several months to obtain a therapeutic blood level of lamotrigine.

Lamotrigine is available as 2-mg, 5-mg, and 25-mg (chewable); 25-mg (white); 100-mg (peach); 150-mg (cream); and 200-mg (blue) tablets. There are currently no capsules or liquids available, and there is no generic form.

LEVETIRACETAM

Levetiracetam (Keppra) was approved by the U.S. Food and Drug Administration (FDA) in 1999 for use with other antiepileptic drugs in treating adults with partial epilepsy. The way it prevents seizures is unknown, but it seems to work in a different way than other antiepileptic drugs. It can repress abnormal firing of epileptic nerve cells without affecting normal nerve-cell activity. Levetiracetam can be taken with or without food; food will delay absorption by 1 to 2 hours. The half-life is 6 to 8 hours. It undergoes little metabolism in the liver. Instead, most of the drug is excreted unchanged in the urine. It has no known interactions with other antiepileptic drugs or other drugs. The most commonly reported side effect is tiredness. Other adverse effects include weakness, dizziness, unsteadiness, and headache. Behavioral changes occur occasionally, more often with rapid dosage increases, in children, and in patients with developmental disabilities. Rash is rare. The adult dosage is usually 1500 to 3000 mg per day, given in two or three doses.

Levetiracetam is available as Keppra tablets, which are oblong and coated with a film. Doses are 250 mg (blue), 500 mg (yellow), and 750 mg (orange). This drug is not available in any other form or as a generic product.

METHSUXIMIDE

Methsuximide (Celontin) is infrequently used. It can be effective in helping to control absence and partial seizures. Adverse effects include drowsiness, gastrointestinal problems (decreased appetite, nausea, and vomiting), unsteadiness, and rash. It is available as a 300-mg capsule (white with a red stripe).

OXCARBAZEPINE

Oxcarbazepine (Trileptal), as its name suggests, is closely related chemically to carbamazepine. It received FDA approval in 2000 and is now marketed in many other countries as well. Oxcarbazepine appears to be just as effective as carbamazepine for controlling complex partial seizures and primary and secondarily generalized tonic-clonic seizures. It may cause fewer adverse effects in some, but not all, patients. Of patients who had a rash while taking carbamazepine, about 25% will have a rash when later treated with oxcarbazepine. Oxcarbazepine's most common adverse effects are tiredness, dizziness, headache, blurred or double vision, and unsteadiness. It appears to have few cognitive side effects, but it remains unclear whether it causes fewer adverse cognitive effects than carbamazepine. In some patients, the level of sodium in the blood may become low (hyponatremia), which occasionally may increase seizure frequency. Decreased vitamin D levels and bone loss may follow long-term use.

The half-life of the drug itself is about 2 hours, but its antiseizure effect results from the formation of an active byproduct with a half-life of 10 to 15 hours. Oxcarbazepine is available as Trileptal in three sizes of oblong, scored, mustard-yellow tablets: 150 mg, 300 mg, and 600 mg.

PHENYTOIN

Phenytoin (Dilantin), which was approved in the United States in 1938, is a first-line drug for all types of partial seizures. Adults usually take dosages of 200 to 600 mg per day. In emergency settings, it may be given intravenously to achieve therapeutic levels rapidly. Its long half-life (14 to 30 hours) generally allows it to be taken once or twice a day. The half-life may be less than 12 hours in children, patients taking low doses (the higher the dose, the longer the half-life), or those on long-term therapy, however. Once-a-day dosing is not advised for these patients because the trough (lowest) blood levels of the drug may be very low and the risk of seizures may increase.

Adverse effects of phenytoin include tiredness, dizziness, unsteadiness, slurred speech, acne, rash (in about 5% to 7% of patients), and darker or excessive hair on the body (hirsutism). Cognitive and behavioral problems are infrequent and usually mild. After long-term use, patients may experience low calcium levels, bone loss, and soft-tissue growths. Nerve injury also may occur, but it is uncommon. Loss of tissue in the cerebellum of the brain also is uncommon, but may occur. It may be related to periods of very high blood phenytoin levels.

Phenytoin is available as a generic 100-mg capsule. Brand-name Dilantin is available as a 30-mg capsule (white with pink stripe) or a 100-mg capsule (white with a red stripe) or as a 50-mg chewable tablet (Infatab). Dilantin is also available as an elixir (liquid) and as an intravenous preparation, which should only be used in the hospital. A new intravenous preparation, fosphenytoin (Cerebyx), is safer because it does not cause serious skin reactions if it leaks out of the vein. Fosphenytoin is a "prodrug" that is converted into phenytoin by the liver.

TIAGABINE

Tiagabine (Gabitril) is approved for treating partial and secondary generalized tonic-clonic seizures. It prolongs the action of the neurotransmitter GABA by blocking its uptake by cells (see Chap. 2). The half-life of Tiagabine is approximately 6 1/2 hours. Studies have shown that the same total daily dose is just as effective in controlling seizures when given twice a day as when given three times a day. However, tiagabine is often given three times a day. Adults and children older than age 12 years often begin treatment by taking 4 mg per day and increase gradually to a maximum of 32 to 56 mg per day.

Common adverse effects include dizziness, tiredness, nervousness, difficulty concentrating, and tremor. Nausea, vomiting, diarrhea, weakness, irritability, nervousness, or confusion occur less often. For some patients, it has a positive effect on mood.

Tiagabine is available as 4-mg (yellow round), 12-mg (green oval), 16-mg (blue oval), and 20-mg (pink oval) tablets. No capsules or liquids are currently available, and there is no generic form.

TOPIRAMATE

Topiramate (Topamax) is approved to treat partial and secondarily generalized tonic-clonic seizures, and it also appears to be effective in the Lennox-Gastaut syndrome. Some small research studies have suggested that it is also effective for treating infantile spasms and generalized epilepsies, but this is uncertain. Topiramate seems to affect brain cells in more than one way, reducing excessive activity and increasing calming (inhibitory) activity. Its half-life is approximately 21 hours, and it is usually given twice a day. The average daily adult dose ranges from 200 to 500 mg. Topiramate has few significant drug interactions. It can slightly raise blood phenytoin levels, and phenytoin and carbamazepine can lower topiramate levels by 40% to 50%. Because topiramate can cause kidney stones in approximately 1.5% of patients, it should be used cautiously with the ketogenic diet or with other drugs that have similar effects, such as acetazolamide or zonisamide. Patients taking this drug should drink adequate fluids, especially in hot environments.

Adverse effects of topiramate include tiredness, dizziness, unsteadiness, weight loss, constipation, tingling (usually in the fingers and toes or around the mouth), double vision or other vision problems, problems with concentration and attention, slowing of thought processes, speech or memory problems, and mood changes (such as depression, nervousness, or irritability). Most patients tolerate the drug well when it is started at a low dose (25 mg per day) and increased slowly (raising the daily dose by 25 mg every week). The maximum dose for adults is usually 400 to 500 mg per day, although some patients (especially those taking drugs that increase topiramate metabolism, including carbamazepine, phenobarbital, phenytoin, or primidone) tolerate doses of up to 800 mg per day.

Topiramate is available as a 25-mg (white), 100-mg (yellow), and 200-mg (salmon) tablet. The tablets are not scored and should not be broken because the medicine has a bitter taste. Topiramate is also available as a 15-mg sprinkle capsule. Currently no liquid form is available, and there is no generic form.

VALPROATE

Valproate (valproic acid; Depakene and Depakote), which was approved in the United States in 1977, is effective for the treatment of all partial and generalized seizure types and epilepsy syndromes. Valproate is the treatment of choice for several primary generalized epilepsy syndromes (e.g., juvenile myoclonic epilepsy and absence epilepsy with tonic-clonic seizures). It is also an effective preventive therapy when taken every day for migraine headaches and bipolar (manic-depressive) disorder. It acts on receptors for the neurotransmitter GABA and also affects other brain-cell activity.

Adverse effects include tiredness, dizziness, nausea, vomiting, tremor, hair loss, weight gain, and behavioral changes (such as depression in adults and irritability in children). It also can cause slight reductions in attention, speed of thinking and movement, and response accuracy. Long-term use of valproate can cause bone loss, ankle swelling, and changes in the functioning of a woman's ovaries, leading to irregular menstruation and polycystic ovarian syndrome. Rare and dangerous adverse effects include liver damage, very low numbers of platelets (clotting cells) in the blood, inflammation of the pancreas, confusion, and hearing loss. The occurrence of hair loss and pancreatic inflammation may be reduced by taking the minerals selenium (10 to 20 µg per day) and zinc (25 to 50 mg per day); many high-potency multivitamins contain these mineral dosages. The risk of serious adverse effects, such as liver problems, from taking valproate is low. The risk of serious liver problems with valproate use is about 1 in 50,000 adults and children older than 2 years old who are taking the drug. This is lower than the risk of serious injury in a 5-year period as a passenger in a car.

Valproate is available as a generic drug in 125-mg, 250-mg, and 500-mg tablets. Depakene is available as a 250-mg tablet (red). It is also available in liquid form. A delayed-release preparation, divalproex sodium (Depakote), is available as a 125-mg sprinkle capsule and as 125-mg (red), 250-mg (light orange), and 500-mg (pink) tablets. Depakote ER (a gray, 500-mg tablet) is a sustained-release form of divalproex sodium that is approved for once-a-day use to prevent migraine headaches, but its use for once-a-day treatment of epilepsy has not been studied.

VIGABATRIN

Vigabatrin (Sabril) is mainly used to treat complex partial and secondarily generalized tonic-clonic seizures. It is also used to treat infantile spasms and seizures in patients with the Lennox-Gastaut syndrome. It is a derivative of the neurotransmitter GABA and is chemically unrelated to any other existing antiepileptic drug. Vigabatrin was developed in Europe and is now marketed there. Its half-life is 4 to 7 hours, but its main effect continues for at least 6 days after the last dose. Therefore, the effectiveness of vigabatrin does not usually fluctuate when the medication is taken only twice a day.

Vigabatrin typically has few adverse effects. Drowsiness and fatigue are the most common ones. Others include irritability, nervousness, dizziness, headache, depression, and (rarely) psychosis. Unfortunately, as many as 25% of patients taking vigabatrin develop potentially irreversible retinal damage that impairs vision. Because of this safety issue, the FDA has refused to approve vigabatrin for use in the United States. Its use also has been restricted in many other countries, where it is mainly used in treating infantile spasms. Vigabatrin is available as a 500-mg white oval tablet.

ZONISAMIDE

Zonisamide (Zonegran) is used to treat simple and complex partial seizures, primary and secondarily generalized tonic-clonic seizures, tonic seizures, atypical absence seizures, and seizures in progressive myoclonic epilepsy. Preliminary studies suggest that it may also be effective in treating infantile spasms. It was developed in Japan and is now available in the United States. Zonisamide is chemically unrelated to any other antiepileptic drug. It mainly works by reducing excessive stimulation of brain cells.

It is slowly but completely absorbed over 3 to 6 hours, and it is more than 90% metabolized in the liver. The half-life is about 40 to 60 hours.

Adverse effects include drowsiness, dizziness, unsteadiness, loss of appetite, stomach discomfort, headache, rash, and kidney stones. Because zonisamide can cause kidney stones (in about 4% of patients), it should be used cautiously by patients taking other drugs such as acetazolamide and topiramate, which have a similar effect. Patients should drink adequate fluids, especially in hot environments. Zonisamide is available as a 100-mg capsule.

The Role of Benzodiazepines

Benzodiazepines (clonazepam, clobazam, clorazepate, diazepam, lorazepam) are a group of drugs that are often prescribed to treat disorders such as anxiety in people who do not have epilepsy. They also are effective in short-term therapy for all seizure types—both generalized and partial seizures. Tolerance often develops within weeks, however, so the same dose of medication has less effect. Benzodiazepines are often used in the emergency room to stop prolonged seizures. Rectal or sublingual (under the tongue) benzodiazepines can be used outside the hospital to stop prolonged seizures or a series of seizures. Benzodiazepines are sometimes prescribed to stop a cluster of seizures. (An example of a cluster might involve a person who, once a month, has one complex partial seizure in the morning and may have three or four more seizures over the course of the day.) A person who typically has a prolonged warning before seizures (a particular symptom, an unusually long aura, or a series of small seizures) may be able to prevent the larger seizure by taking a benzodiazepine when the warning begins. The use of benzodiazepines in long-term therapy for epilepsy remains controversial, although certain benzodiazepines are effective for certain seizure types (see the following discussion).

Benzodiazepines can cause tiredness, dizziness, unsteadiness, irritability, depression (usually only in adults), nausea, and loss of appetite. Benzodiazepines also can cause hyperactivity and drooling in children. They cause greater cognitive problems than do drugs such as carbamazepine, phenytoin, and valproate. One of the great dangers in using benzodiazepines is the tendency to increase the dose as tolerance develops. To a certain extent this is necessary; however, this practice may increase adverse effects without improving seizure control. Moreover, because these increases are often made gradually over months or years, the subtle changes in personality (e.g., irritability, depression, or decreased motivation) or in cognitive function (e.g., impaired memory) may go unnoticed or may be attributed to the person's "constitution." High doses of benzodiazepines are commonly prescribed for children and adults with developmental disabilities, which may lead to cognitive and behavioral problems.

An important concern with benzodiazepine use for epilepsy patients is the potential that seizures will become more frequent or more severe if they reduce the dosage or stop taking it. The longer the person has been taking the drug and the higher the dosage, the greater the tolerance and therefore the higher the risk of worsening seizure control. Even small, gradual dose reductions can temporarily increase seizure activity, but reducing these sedating medications will often bring long-term rewards in the form of fewer adverse effects.

Although there are arguments against the widespread use of benzodiazepines to treat epilepsy, these medications can be used safely and effectively for some patients. For example, a recent study of clobazam in children with partial epilepsy found it comparable in adverse effects and seizure control to other commonly used drugs such as carbamazepine. In addition, for seizures that mainly occur during sleep or shortly after awakening, benzodiazepines given at bedtime can be very effective in controlling the seizures and improving sleep. Also, rectal diazepam can be extremely helpful to treat seizure clusters and prolonged seizures.

CLOBAZAM

Clobazam (Frisium) has a slightly different chemical ring structure than the other benzodiazepines, which may help reduce the development of tolerance associated with long-term use. Clobazam is approved for use in almost all countries except the United States. This has to do with the costs of the FDA approval process, not because of issues of safety or effectiveness. Clobazam is effective in treating partial and generalized seizures. It is most often used to treat simple, complex, and secondary generalized tonic-clonic seizures. It is used mainly as an add-on (adjunctive) drug in partial epilepsy. Its half-life is 18 hours, although a metabolite with antiepileptic activity has a half-life of 40 hours.

Adverse effects include tiredness, unsteadiness, and irritability. It has been found to be similar to carbamazepine and phenytoin in cognitive and mood effects. The drug should not be stopped abruptly because of the risk of withdrawal seizures.

Besides the brand-name Frisium, clobazam is also available in generic forms. It is produced as either a 10-mg tablet or capsule, depending on the country of origin.

CLONAZEPAM

The benzodiazepine clonazepam (Klonopin) is used to treat absence and myoclonic seizures and can help stop seizure clusters. Clonazepam is available as a generic drug and as the brand-name Klonopin in a 0.5-mg (orange), 1.0-mg (blue), and 2.0-mg (white) round tablet.

CLORAZEPATE

Clorazepate (Tranxene) is used in the treatment of partial seizures as an add-on (adjunctive) therapy. Clorazepate is available as a generic drug and as the brand-name Tranxene in scored triangular tablets in 3.75-mg (gray), 7.5-mg (yellow), and 15 mg (pink) forms; and as Tranxene-SD round (nonscored) tablets in 11.25-mg (purple) and 22.5-mg (tan/peach) forms.

DIAZEPAM

The benzodiazepine diazepam (Valium or Diastat) is used to treat status epilepticus and seizure clusters. Diazepam has been given by mouth to prevent seizure clusters, but this is not the best method because it is absorbed slowly when given that way. It has most often been given intravenously, but during the past 15 years, giving it by rectum has become more common as a way for patients' families and caregivers to treat prolonged or serial seizures. When given rectally, Diazepam is absorbed rapidly. Because it can impair breathing, however, it should only be given rectally using the dose recommended by a doctor. If seizures do not diminish after the first rectal dose, a second one should be given only with a doctor's approval.

Diastat is available as a preloaded syringe for rectal administration of diazepam in the following doses: 2.5 mg, 5 mg, 10 mg, 15 mg, and 20 mg. Other liquid forms of diazepam may also be given rectally (with a very small syringe).

LORAZEPAM

The benzodiazepine lorazepam (Ativan) is used to treat seizure clusters and occasionally chronic epilepsy. Lorazepam can be given orally, sublingually, or intramuscularly and intravenously with injections. It has a half-life of 8 to 20 hours. Like diazepam, it can cause serious breathing impairment, especially when given intravenously at higher doses. Lorazepam should only be used as recommended by a physician. It is available in three sizes (0.5-mg, 1-mg, and 2-mg) of white, pentagon-shaped tablets.

Recently Approved Drugs

Since 1993, after a 15-year gap, the FDA has approved several new antiepileptic drugs for general use. These include felbamate, gabapentin, lamotrigine, levetiracetam, oxcarbazepine, tiagabine, topiramate, and zonisamide. These drugs are chemically unrelated to any other antiepileptic drugs. Their characteristics are summarized in Table 5. New preparations of older drugs have also been approved. These include sustained-release forms of carbamazepine (Tegretol-XR and Carbatrol), a safer form of intravenous phenytoin (fosphenytoin), an intravenous form of valproate (Depakon), and a rectal form of diazepam (Diastat). In addition, several other drugs will be considered during the next few years. The exact position of these new drugs in the treatment of epilepsy will require further study. The recently approved drugs, as well as other drugs that may soon be approved, appear to be effective, safe, and well tolerated by most patients. Whether they will become primary or secondary drugs depends on how they compare with other drugs in carefully designed studies. So far, not enough studies have directly compared these drugs with more commonly used drugs.

The new antiepileptic drugs have undergone extensive testing in animals, healthy volunteers, and people with epilepsy. Their effectiveness does not appear to diminish over time for most patients, and some patients have better seizure control and fewer adverse effects while taking the new drugs than they have had with the older drugs. These are not miracle drugs, however. Only a few people whose seizures could not be fully controlled by the older drugs have achieved full control of their seizures while taking the new drugs. And the newer drugs, like all drugs, do have some adverse effects. Their safety in pregnant and nursing women remains uncertain. Both their effectiveness in controlling seizures and their tendency to cause adverse effects vary considerably from one person to another. Just as epilepsy affects individuals in different ways, the treatment of epilepsy also affects individuals in different ways.

A concern that many patients voice regarding new antiepileptic drugs is "How do you know if they are safe to take for a long time?" It is a good question. Doctors have much more long-term safety information about drugs such as carbamazepine, phenytoin, and valproate than about the recently approved medications. However, it is now more likely that safety concerns will be addressed much earlier than they were in the past. For instance, the relatively high and very serious risk of liver or bone marrow failure associated with felbamate was identified only a year after FDA approval, whereas the effects of valproate on the ovaries were first reported nearly 20 years after FDA approval and remain controversial. Doctors cannot state with certainty that no new adverse effects will be identified after long-term use of new antiepileptic drugs, but the safety profile of the new drugs suggests that some will have fewer long-term side effects than some of the older drugs. For example, gabapentin, lamotrigine, and levetiracetam do not appear to cause bone loss, and none of the new drugs causes the peripheral nerve damage or soft-tissue changes associated with phenytoin or phenobarbital. Overall, doctors know enough to recommend the use of these newer drugs (except felbamate) for routine use in most epilepsy patients. Many doctors use lamotrigine with great caution in children—especially those who are under 12 and are also taking valproate—because of the potential for life-threatening rashes. Increasing the lamotrigine dosage very gradually significantly reduces the risk. Nonetheless, the risks and benefits of any new therapy must always be balanced. The patient and doctor should clearly define the goals when considering a new antiepileptic drug. For example, they should discuss whether a reduction in seizure frequency averaging 35% is worth the possible additional adverse effects, inconvenience, and cost of a second drug.

Investigational Antiepileptic Drugs

Some people do not enjoy a good quality of life when taking antiepileptic drugs. Their seizures are not fully controlled, they suffer from troublesome adverse effects, or both. More than a dozen antiepileptic drugs are now in various stages of development or testing in the United States. Many of them have already been approved for use in Europe, Canada, and other places. The patients enrolled in the tests of the new drugs have seizures that are uncontrolled by the existing medications. This procedure creates a problem, though: if the proven drugs now used by most patients were tested in these patients with uncontrolled seizures, then their well-established effectiveness might not be found because, by definition, these patients have failed to respond to the best available drugs. Newer designs in drug studies are helping to solve this problem.

People with difficult-to-control seizures or troublesome adverse effects from the currently available antiepileptic drugs may want to consider trying one of the investigational or experimental drugs. Almost all studies of these drugs are being performed at comprehensive epilepsy centers. The best way to find out about new drug studies is to call or write nearby comprehensive epilepsy centers. A list of these specialized centers can be obtained from the national Epilepsy Foundation (EF) or local EF affiliates (see Appendix 4).

All drug studies must be approved by an institutional review board or ethics committee at each hospital or medical center. This review process helps to guarantee that the study carefully considers the relative risks and benefits to the patients enrolled and that the risks and benefits are clearly explained in a consent form. The study must be fully explained to the patient, who must understand the consent form before signing it. For children, a parent or legal guardian must sign the consent form. The doctor in charge of the study, called the principal investigator, and the hospital's patient advocate should be available to answer any questions that arise once the study has begun. A patient who considers entering a drug study but then decides not to participate should have no fears that the doctor will be upset or withhold other therapies that he or she would otherwise recommend.

Some of the following drugs are being considered by the FDA for marketing in the United States, and others will be considered in the near future. Consult the resources listed in Appendix 4 for the most up-to-date information.

LOSIGAMONE

Losigamone is chemically unrelated to other antiepileptic drugs. Initial clinical studies suggest that it may be effective in treating partial seizures and that it does not have severe adverse effects. Losigamone may decrease blood levels of valproate. Carbamazepine and phenytoin decrease losigamone levels. The most commonly reported adverse effects are dizziness, headache, and tiredness, but they tend to diminish after several weeks.

PREGABALIN

Pregabalin (isobutyl GABA) is under investigation as therapy for partial seizures and pain disorders. How it works is not known, but it appears to work in close to the same way as gabapentin. Pregabalin was well tolerated in therapeutic doses of 75 to 300 mg per day. Doses of up to 600 mg per day are now being studied. The most commonly reported adverse effects are headache, dizziness, nausea, and tiredness.

REMACEMIDE

Remacemide is chemically unrelated to other antiepileptic drugs. Studies suggest that it could be effective for partial seizures. It may work by inhibiting certain neurotransmitter activity (see Chap. 2) or causing other effects on brain cells. The most common adverse effects are dizziness and gastrointestinal problems, such as nausea.

RUFINAMIDE

In several studies of animals, rufinamide was found to be a powerful and long-acting antiepileptic drug. These studies suggest that it may be effective in treating partial and generalized tonic-clonic seizures and possibly absence seizures. Rufinamide helps to control high-frequency firing of certain nerve-cell activity. Initial studies in humans suggest that it is safe and well tolerated. The most commonly reported adverse effects are dizziness, tiredness, nausea, headache, difficulty concentrating, and double vision. These adverse effects tend to diminish after weeks or months.

INTRAVENOUS GAMMA GLOBULIN

Gamma globulin is composed of antibodies derived from human blood. Antibodies are chemicals that help to fight bacteria, viruses, and other foreign "invaders." Although gamma globulin has been used for decades to bolster the immune system (the body's defense against infection and foreign substances), its use has recently been expanded to children with difficult-to-control forms of epilepsy. Only a limited number of studies have been completed, and the results are preliminary. The use of gamma globulin for epilepsy remains investigational. Although some children may improve with this therapy, many others have no significant reduction in seizures. The effectiveness of gamma globulin for epilepsy remains to be proven.

The gamma globulin is given as an intravenous infusion, usually in the hospital or at home under the supervision of a nurse trained in the procedure. This means that a solution containing the gamma globulin is injected into a vein (usually in the arm) at a prescribed rate. During the infusion—especially the first one—the child must be watched closely for any type of allergic or other reaction and treated promptly if such a reaction occurs. The chances of a serious allergic reaction are small. The child then returns every 2 to 6 weeks for an additional infusion, which may be done as an outpatient or inpatient procedure. The length of therapy varies, but in most cases in which there is a beneficial response, the improvement can be seen within the first few months of treatment.

Many parents ask whether a child can get the human immunodeficiency virus (HIV), which causes the acquired immunodeficiency syndrome (AIDS), from gamma globulin. Because the HIV would be destroyed during the process of preparing gamma globulin, there have been no documented cases of HIV infection from gamma globulin, even before the blood pool was routinely screened for this virus.

Intravenous gamma globulin is expensive and often in short supply. (There are disorders for which it has been proven to be beneficial.) The issues of insurance coverage and expense should be addressed ahead of time.

Getting Drugs Outside the United States

Some investigational and other drugs (e.g., clobazam, vigabatrin) are approved in other countries for the treatment of epilepsy. The legal issues related to importing these drugs under the orders and supervision of a doctor in the United States are not entirely clear. These medications can be obtained from foreign pharmacies by direct purchase (with a doctor's prescription in most countries) or by mail (faxed or mailed prescriptions). When the medications pass through customs (whether you carry them or they are sent by mail or a delivery service such as FedEx), it is helpful to have a note from the doctor documenting the medical disorder for which the patient is being treated, the approval of this medication in another country for that disorder, and the need for its use in the specific person (such as the failure of drugs available in the United States to control seizures).

12

Surgical Therapy

When seizures cannot be controlled by medications or control can be achieved only at the cost of severe or unacceptable adverse effects, surgery is an alternative. Surgical therapy for epilepsy has been used for more than a century, but the past two decades have seen a dramatic increase in its use, reflecting in part an increased awareness by both doctors and patients that it is an effective alternative to medical therapy. As with other surgical procedures, however, the benefits must be carefully weighed against the risks. Also, as with drug therapy, there is no guarantee that the surgery will be successful in controlling the seizures.

Patients with partial epilepsy who are considered for surgical therapy have difficult-to-control seizures that have not responded to aggressive treatment with antiepileptic drugs. As epilepsy surgery has become more widely established, the definition of difficult-to-control seizures has been adjusted. Surgery is now being performed on patients whose seizures have been uncontrolled for only 1 or 2 years. For example, a patient with magnetic resonance imaging (MRI) evidence of a structural abnormality on the temporal lobe from which the seizures arise is an excellent candidate for surgery. In general, a patient should be treated with at least two single drugs and with a combination of two or more drugs before surgery is considered. Medication trials must be adequate; that is, the drugs should be gradually increased to the maximally tolerated dose. In many epilepsy centers, other standard or investigational drugs are tried before surgery is considered.

Traditionally, surgery to control epileptic seizures was performed only after seizures had been occurring for more than a decade. There is some

161

evidence, however, that the earlier the surgery is performed, the better the outcome. A person who has failed to respond to several adequate medication trials is unlikely to achieve complete seizure control by medical therapy. In such cases, the risks and benefits of surgery should be carefully weighed against the costs that continued seizures and high doses of medication impose on all aspects of life, including intellectual, psychological, social, educational, and employment aspects. If the epilepsy is unresponsive to medications and has very troublesome consequences, surgery should be considered sooner rather than later.

Epilepsy surgery can be especially beneficial to people who have seizures associated with benign brain tumors, malformations of blood vessels (arteriovenous malformations, venous angiomas, and cavernous angiomas), and strokes. The surgery may be done either to control the seizures or to remove the abnormality in the brain. For example, in a child who has a stroke shortly after birth and has seizures that cannot be controlled, the goal of surgery would be to control the seizures. In contrast, in a woman with a benign brain tumor and seizures, the primary goal would be to remove the tumor, with control of seizures remaining a secondary issue.

In the case of benign tumors and vascular malformations, simple removal of the abnormal tissue may successfully control the seizures. In many cases, however, especially if the seizures have occurred for more than a year, the area adjacent to the abnormal tissue may be "irritated" and serves as the origin of the seizures. Removing the abnormal tissue may or may not lead to improvement or complete control of the seizures. Occasionally, the structural abnormality may have little to do with uncontrollable seizures. For example, arachnoid cysts of the brain rarely cause seizures that cannot be controlled with medications. Removing the cyst is unlikely to control such seizures unless the cyst is large and exerts pressure on the brain.

Types of Surgery

There are two main types of brain surgery for epilepsy. The first, and by far the most common, removes the area of the brain that causes seizures; this is called resective surgery. It is performed in cases of partial epilepsy, with or without secondarily generalized tonic-clonic seizures. Patients often imagine that the area that causes seizures is tiny (about the size of a pea). In almost all cases, however, the area is much larger (about 1 1/2 to 3 inches long and 1 to 1 1/2 inches wide). Temporal and frontal lobectomy are types of resective surgery.

The second, less common type of epilepsy surgery is the interruption of nerve pathways along which seizure impulses spread. An example is corpus callosotomy, in which no brain tissue is removed, but the large fiber bundle connecting the hemispheres of the brain is severed. Another example is functional hemispherectomy, where one of the hemispheres of the brain is disconnected from the rest of the brain. Candidates for this type of surgery are patients with partial and generalized seizures.

Another type of epilepsy surgery, called multiple subpial transections, is currently under investigation. This procedure may be helpful when the seizures begin in areas of the brain that are vital to functions such as language, movement, or sensation. It can also be helpful in Landau-Kleffner syndrome, an acquired language disorder in children in which frequent epilepsy waves arise in or near language areas of the brain. Stimulation of the vagus nerve is another form of surgery for epilepsy that does not directly affect the brain.

Expectations and Consequences

Patients may have many fears and questions about their epilepsy surgery. Doctors, nurses, psychologists, and social workers can answer questions about the risks, complications, recovery period, and other medical details. In addition, it is often helpful and reassuring to speak with someone who has had a similar surgical procedure.

Epilepsy surgery is major neurosurgery, and some risk is associated with it. The recovery period is rather long. Epilepsy surgery requires a hospital stay of 6 to 8 days or longer after the surgery; in some cases, the stay lasts 2 weeks or longer. There is some mild or moderate temporary discomfort afterward. After being discharged from the hospital, the patient returns home to rest for several weeks and can usually resume normal activities 4 to 8 weeks after the operation.

The actual procedures vary according to the type of operation. The patient is usually under general anesthesia. Sometimes patients are kept awake while the vital areas of the brain, such as those that control language and movement, are mapped with mild electrical stimulation. In such cases, a local anesthetic is used, and the surgery can be performed painlessly because the brain is not sensitive to pain. New short-acting anesthetics allow the patient to sleep during the initial and final portions of the surgery and to be awake only during the mapping procedure.

It is critical to establish realistic expectations before the surgery. Some people are completely free of seizures after surgery, and many others have a marked reduction in the frequency or intensity of seizures. Some patients continue to have auras or occasional complex partial seizures. In some cases, there is no improvement in seizure control. Most people who do become seizure-free after surgery must continue to take antiepileptic drugs; the surgery is not a complete cure for epilepsy. Patients often continue to take the same medication for 6 to 12 months or longer after surgery. Then, some are able to reduce their medication use, depending on the presence or absence of postoperative seizures, the amount of affected tissue removed, and electroencephalogram (EEG) findings. A common question asked by patients considering surgery is, "If epilepsy can be caused by scar tissue and surgery causes scarring, can the surgery cause epilepsy?" It is a good question. Surgery will create a scar, but it is typically much milder than the scars that cause epilepsy. We know that if all or nearly all of the epilepsy-causing tissue is successfully removed, patients usually become seizure-free.

Strange as it may seem, becoming seizure-free after epilepsy surgery can be stressful and may require a major adjustment. Seizure control may create greater pressure to work and to assume new responsibilities, and it may change relationships and other people's expectations. In addition, the surgery may cause memory lapses or other disorders although the seizures are fully controlled. Such problems usually improve with time. Some people feel depressed by all these changes and may need a great deal of encouragement during this period.

Perhaps the greatest setback after epilepsy surgery is the occurrence of a seizure after a period of freedom from them. It can seem as though just when epilepsy is moving further into the background of one's life, it reappears. Emotionally, the recurrence of seizures can be devastating, but it does not mean that seizure control cannot be restored. In many cases, the seizures are caused by missed medications, low blood levels of antiepileptic medication caused by diarrhea or vomiting, a serious infection, childbirth, excessive alcohol ingestion, or other problems. Some patients reduce their medications after surgery, falsely assuming that all of the "epilepsy area" has been removed. If side effects of medication are bothersome, a dose reduction or change in the medication schedule can often help, but it should be done under a doctor's supervision. Seizure control returns after the cause of the new seizures is eliminated. In some patients, a single breakthrough seizure occurs for no identifiable reason. In most others, intermittent seizures occur, but less frequently than before the surgery. In general, the longer the interval of seizure freedom after surgery, the greater the chances are of never having another seizure.

Preoperative Assessment

The first step in deciding whether someone should have epilepsy surgery is to make sure that the seizures are medically refractory (uncontrollable with antiepileptic drugs). A patient may have been treated with numerous medications, but not with high dosages of a single drug, which may be more effective than two or more drugs used at low dosages. Other people may never have been treated with particular drugs or combinations of drugs that might be effective. Most patients with difficult-to-control seizures have been treated with two or more drugs in separate trials and in various combinations and have been treated unsuccessfully for at least 2 years. If the seizures are frequent, relatively short trials of medications can reveal the failure of medical therapy. If the seizures are infrequent, a longer trial of medication is needed to determine that the therapy is ineffective. Therefore, it is important for epilepsy surgery candidates to have a complete record of the antiepileptic drugs that have been tried, including the maximal dosages, blood drug levels, and adverse effects. When the seizures are associated with a blood vessel malformation, benign tumor, or other structural lesion, the proof that the seizures cannot be controlled by drugs is less important in considering epilepsy surgery than it is for other patients.

After a patient's seizures are confirmed to be medically refractory, studies are performed before epilepsy surgery to identify the area of the brain from which the seizures arise and the areas that control vital functions such as language, memory, movement, and sensation. Doctors hope to find that the seizures arise from an area that is not vital for intellectual or other important functions. Some areas of the brain can be removed without any observable or measurable changes in intellect, personality, or mood. The removal of other areas may be associated with slight deterioration or, in some cases, actual improvement in memory or other vital functions.

NONINVASIVE STUDIES

The preoperative assessment begins with a series of consultations and noninvasive tests. Noninvasive tests are ones that do not invade the body or require a surgical procedure and, in general, involve little or no risk. The assessment includes EEG recording and video-EEG monitoring to record epilepsy waves between and during seizures; neuropsychological studies to assess cognitive (intellectual) strengths and weaknesses, which can help to predict the area from which the seizures arise as well as possible complications of the surgery; consultations with psychologists, nurses, and social workers to assess the patient's emotional well-being and social supports and to identify problems that should be addressed before the surgery; and neuroimaging by computed tomography (CT), MRI, single-photon emission computed tomography, or positron emission tomography (PET) (see Chap. 8) to identify abnormalities in the area from which the seizures arise. In some cases, additional tests such as functional MRI, magnetic resonance spectroscopy, or magnetoencephalography (see Chap. 8) may be used.

INVASIVE STUDIES

The preoperative tests may also include invasive procedures. Invasive studies are ones that invade the body. Technically, the insertion of a needle into a vein to draw blood is an invasive procedure, but it is so common and safe that it is not considered invasive. In general, invasive studies are associated with some risk, but the risk varies dramatically with the different types of tests and procedures.

Sphenoidal Electrodes

Many epilepsy centers routinely record the EEG with sphenoidal electrodes. The electrodes are inserted into the cheeks with a needle to record brain electrical activity from regions deep within the temporal and frontal lobes. Many doctors apply an anesthetic to the skin before inserting the electrodes. The needle is immediately withdrawn after insertion, leaving in place a thin wire that is bare at the tip. The patient feels some discomfort during the insertion and for several hours afterward, particularly when yawning or chewing.

The risks of using sphenoidal electrodes are rare and almost always minor. A small amount of bleeding may occur during the needle insertion, but it is rarely a problem. Other risks include infection or a tiny piece of the bare wire remaining in the cheek.

Subdural and Depth Electrodes

Subdural and depth electrodes are used to record electrical activity directly from the brain, and they are often used to map precisely the area from which seizures arise. Whether subdural or depth electrodes must be used depends on the findings from the noninvasive studies and another test called the intracarotid sodium amobarbital test, which will be described later. For example, if the routine scalp-recorded EEG, video-EEG recording, neuropsychological testing, PET scan, and amobarbital test all point to the same area of the brain as the focus of the seizures, most epilepsy centers will proceed without using invasive electrodes. If the information is inconsistent or indefinite, however, subdural or depth electrodes, which are invasive, are often used. For example, the MRI may appear normal, neuropsychological tests and the PET scan may suggest an abnormality in the left temporal lobe, but the video-EEG may suggest that seizures begin in the right temporal area.

With the use of subdural electrodes, the brain can be stimulated electrically for mapping of brain areas involved in language, movement, and other important functions. Seizures can occur with the electrodes in place, and care must be used to protect the patient (and the electrodes) during and after the seizures. In many centers, invasive electrodes are used in an intensive care unit or similar setting. The electrodes may be left in place for several days to weeks, depending on the specific case and how quickly seizures occur after they are placed.

Subdural electrodes (Fig. 20) consist of a series of metal electrodes embedded in plastic and arranged as a strip or a large grid. They cover a large area and record directly from the brain, without interference from the scalp and skull. An operation is required for placement of these electrodes. The *dura mater* is one of the layers of tissue covering the brain. *Subdural* means that the electrodes are placed on the brain underneath the dura mater, but they do not penetrate the brain. In some cases, several strips of electrodes can be inserted through a small hole drilled in the skull, called a burr hole. In other cases, a section of the skull is removed, the electrodes are put in place, and the skull is replaced. If the skull section is not immediately replaced, it is kept sterile and frozen, and the electrodes are covered with the dura mater, the scalp, and a surgical dressing. After the testing is completed, the piece of the skull that was removed is then replaced. There is a moderate amount of discomfort for several days after the subdural electrodes are placed on the brain. In general, the greater the number of electrodes that are used (especially

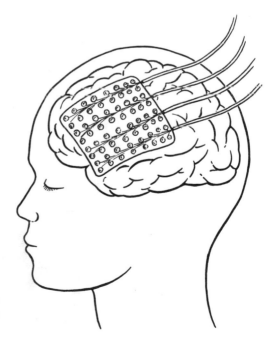

FIGURE 20. Subdural electrodes implanted in the brain.

the grids), the greater the headache. Medicine can be given for pain relief.

The mapping procedures performed with subdural electrodes involve stimulation of the brain with mild electrical currents to temporarily activate or shut down certain brain areas. For example, activating the left motor cortex controlling movement in the right thumb can cause a series of jerks in that finger, or stimulating language areas in the temporal or frontal lobes can cause a person who is counting to suddenly stop speaking. The mapping procedure is almost always painless. If pain occurs, it is momentary and caused by the electrical stimulation, which can be stopped immediately. The major risks of subdural electrodes are infection (which increases during prolonged use, especially after 6 to 8 days), bleeding, and brain swelling.

Depth electrodes (Fig. 21) are thin, wirelike plastic tubes with metal contact points spread out along their length. Unlike subdural and other invasive electrodes, depth electrodes are placed directly into the brain. They do not require a large opening to be made in the skull, as is needed to place a grid of subdural electrodes. Depth electrodes are inserted through burr holes drilled in the skull. The patient is usually, but not always, awake while the electrodes are being placed.

The placement of depth electrodes can be painful, depending on the exact procedure that is used. In some centers, the electrodes are placed

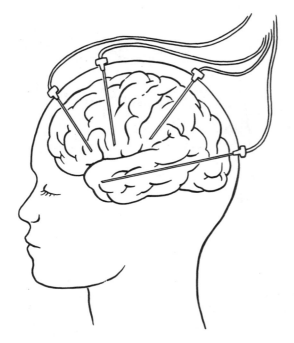

FIGURE 21. Depth electrodes implanted in the brain.

using a frame that attaches to the skull and allows a computer to assist in calculating the exact course of the electrodes in the brain. Attaching the frame can be painful. The pain associated with placing depth electrodes is usually mild or moderate, however, and lasts hours, or occasionally, several days. Medication can reduce the discomfort.

Depth electrodes provide the best recordings of seizures arising in areas deep in the brain, but they also carry some additional risks, especially bleeding within the brain. They are less likely than subdural electrodes to cause infection or brain swelling.

Foramen Ovale Electrodes

The *foramen ovale* is an opening in the skull near the temporal lobe. Electrodes can be inserted into this opening to provide recordings of electrical activity of the lower and middle portions of the temporal lobe, an area from which seizures often arise. These electrodes are intermediate between sphenoidal and subdural or depth electrodes in the information they provide, their invasiveness, and their risk of complications. Overall, foramen ovale electrodes are well tolerated, and in selected cases they can provide important information about the origin of the seizures. One of the problems with them is that they record information from a very limited area of the brain. Therefore, the actual area from which the seizures arise may be missed.

INTRACAROTID SODIUM AMOBARBITAL TEST

In the intracarotid sodium amobarbital test, also called the Wada test, memory and language functions are tested by putting one cerebral hemisphere to sleep with a short-acting anesthetic called amobarbital and studying what functions are still working in the other hemisphere. The test begins with an *angiogram*, a test that examines the flow of a dye through the blood vessels. A thin plastic tube (catheter) is introduced through an artery in the inner portion of the upper thigh. A local anesthetic is given to numb the area, and a needle is then inserted into the artery. The tube is threaded through the needle, and the needle is removed. There is some mild discomfort during the local anesthesia, but the rest of the test is painless. The tube is guided up to the carotid artery in the neck. A small amount of contrast dye is injected through the tube into the artery, and x-rays are taken to study the flow of blood in the brain. The patient may feel some warmth or see flashing lights with the injection of the dye. Next, the radiologist injects the amobarbital, which puts almost half of the cerebral hemisphere to sleep for several minutes.

Immediately after the amobarbital injection, tests are given to see how well language and memory are working with half of the brain sleeping.

This provides information on the functions of the cerebral hemisphere that is sleeping and the hemisphere that is awake. The same procedure is usually repeated on the opposite side to ensure that the patient's level of alertness has returned to normal. Before repeating the procedure, most centers wait 30 to 60 minutes, and some wait a day.

Like any other test involving a cerebral angiogram, this test has the possibility of causing a stroke. The risk is extremely low. The risk is greatest, but still quite low, in older people with atherosclerosis (a disease in which arteries are partially or completely clogged).

Surgical Procedures

TEMPORAL LOBECTOMY

Removal of a portion of the temporal lobe (temporal lobectomy) is the most common and most successful type of epilepsy surgery. In most cases, a modest portion of the brain, measuring approximately 2 1/2 inches long, is removed, (Fig. 22). The temporal lobes are important in memory and emotion. In addition, the upper and back part of one temporal lobe is vital for language comprehension. This "language-dominant" temporal lobe is on the left in nearly all right-handed people and most left-handed people. The preoperative assessment ensures that removal of the area causing seizures will not disrupt memory or language functions. When surgery is performed on the language-dominant side of the brain (usually the left side), however, after the operation there is often a slight reduction in memory and the ability to retrieve infrequently used words. In contrast, after right-sided (nondominant) temporal lobectomy, memory functions often improve slightly. People with frequent seizures who achieve complete or nearly complete seizure control after surgery often have a mild improvement in memory functions. This is especially true for those who have troublesome memory problems after individual seizures or clusters of seizures.

The success rate for seizure control in temporal lobectomy varies:

- 60% to 70% of patients are free of seizures that impair consciousness or cause abnormal movements, but some still experience auras.
- 20% to 25% of patients have some seizures but are significantly improved (greater than 85% reduction of complex partial and tonic-clonic seizures).
- 10% to 15% of patients have no worthwhile improvement.

Therefore, more than 85% of patients enjoy a marked improvement in seizure control. Most of them need less medication after surgery.

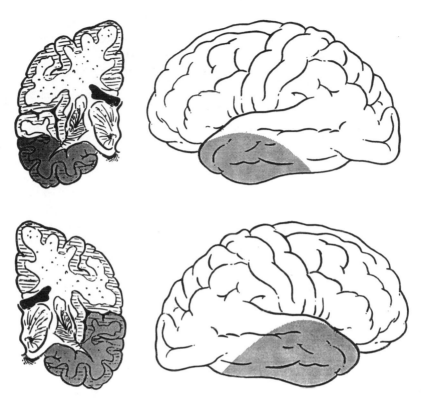

FIGURE 22. Brain tissue removed *(shaded areas)* in a standard temporal lobectomy of the left *(top)* or right *(bottom)* hemisphere. (Cross-sectional views, looking from the front, are on the left side of the figure, and side views are on the right.) A smaller amount of tissue is removed from the left hemisphere than from the right hemisphere because the left temporal lobe contains the area that is vital for language comprehension in most people.

Approximately 25% of those who are seizure-free eventually can discontinue antiepileptic drugs.

The risk of a major complication, such as a stroke with weakness on the opposite side of the body, is about 1% to 2% in temporal lobectomy. The risk can vary between surgeons. If the surgery extends to the back part of the temporal lobe, there is also a risk of loss of vision in the upper quarter of space on the side opposite that of the surgery (superior quadrantanopsia) (Fig. 23). For example, if the surgeon needs to extend the area of removal toward the back part of the right temporal lobe, a defect in vision in the left upper quarter of space is possible. However, this impairment has no real effect on everyday living; affected people are

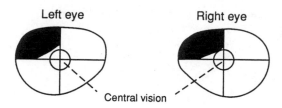

FIGURE 23. Superior quandrantanopsia. The patient's central vision is preserved; only the peripheral vision (to the sides) is affected, and most people are unaware of the problem. In most cases, only a portion of this area is affected.

usually unaware of it. If their vision was excellent before surgery, they still are able to read, drive, and perform tasks requiring extremely precise visual accuracy. In rare cases (fewer than 1 in 200 patients who have temporal lobectomy), the visual loss is more severe and includes an entire half of the visual world on the side opposite the one that was operated on. This impairment, called homonymous hemianopsia, causes functional problems and interferes with reading and driving. Mild memory impairment is common after left temporal lobectomy, and mild memory improvement is common after right temporal lobectomy. Behavioral changes, such as anxiety or depression, occur occasionally (possibly more frequently after right temporal lobectomy). Very rarely, psychosis can develop after surgery. The risk of death from temporal lobectomy is less than 1 in 500 patients.

A common-sense question often asked by patients is, "If you are taking out a piece of my brain, won't I be a different person?" The answer is no. Personality, mood, and overall behavior are hardly ever disrupted or changed by temporal lobectomy. Part of the explanation is that many areas of the brain are redundant; that is, other parts can perform similar functions. Also, some parts of the brain, such as the front (anterior) portions of the temporal lobe and most of the right temporal lobe, are referred to as "silent areas." This means that if these areas are removed or damaged (e.g., in a stroke), changes are minimal or undetectable. In addition, areas that are removed in epilepsy surgery are areas that are not functioning properly, and in some cases, do not function at all. One of the pioneers of epilepsy surgery, Wilder Penfield, suggested that the area of the brain from which seizures arise is "nociferous," which means harmful. Therefore, the area from which seizures arise is associated with problems in the functions normally served by that area, and it can also impair functions of other normal brain areas. In contrast, the problems from a stroke result from the injury to the affected area. The concept of nociferous areas may explain the improvement in memory and other cognitive functions in some patients after epilepsy surgery. In most cases, the area of brain that is removed is abnormal; it usually functions poorly, and when examined under the microscope, it shows evidence of scarring.

FRONTAL LOBECTOMY

The frontal lobes comprise approximately one-third of the cerebral hemisphere (see Fig. 1). This large area is often injured in head trauma and is involved in other brain disorders, such as a stroke or tumor. Partial seizures often arise in the frontal lobes. After a temporal lobe, a frontal lobe is the second most common brain area from which a portion is removed to treat epilepsy.

The back part of the frontal lobes (primary motor cortex) controls movement and cannot be removed without causing severe weakness in muscles on the opposite side. The area just in front of the primary motor cortex is called the motor association cortex. This area also controls movement and communicates between the primary motor cortex and other areas of the brain. The motor association cortex can be removed without causing any weakness. The top part of the motor association cortex, which extends to the most middle part of the frontal lobes (between the eyes), is called the supplementary motor area. This area is a relatively common place for seizures to arise.

The other parts of the frontal lobes are important in personality and behavior. The dramatic personality changes that occur after the destruction or removal of large portions of both frontal lobes (frontal lobotomy) very rarely occur in frontal lobectomy because the operation is always confined to one side and the area removed is usually much smaller than the areas removed in frontal lobotomy. It is possible, however, that mild behavioral changes will develop after frontal lobectomy (and less often, after temporal lobectomy).

The frontal lobes pose a greater challenge in determining the area from which seizures arise. The large size of the frontal lobes makes it difficult to record electrical activity from numerous regions. If depth electrodes are used, only a tiny fraction of the area is sampled. Subdural electrodes are able to sample a greater area, but they require a large grid, which means that only one side can be studied in detail. Regardless of the technique used, it can be difficult to record activity from certain frontal areas.

The success rates for frontal lobectomy are not as good as those for temporal lobectomy:

- 30% to 50% of patients are free of seizures that impair consciousness or cause abnormal movements.

- 20% to 40% of patients are markedly improved (more than 90% reduction of complex partial and tonic-clonic seizures).
- 20% to 30% of patients have no worthwhile improvement.

The risk of major complications, such as a stroke, is about 2%. The risk of behavioral changes is higher than with temporal lobectomy. Behavioral changes associated with frontal lobe impairment are often difficult to measure and define. Personality, motivation, ability to plan and to follow up on a multistep process, ability to organize actions over time, social graces, and demeanor are among the behaviors that the frontal lobes help to serve. Some people with seizures beginning in the frontal lobes may have some mild changes in these behaviors before the surgery.

PARIETAL AND OCCIPITAL LOBECTOMIES

Surgery to remove part of the parietal or occipital lobes, which are located in the back of the brain (see Fig. 1), is most often done when a structural abnormality is identified on the CT or MRI scan. The success rate in controlling seizures is higher when a structural abnormality is present. Other studies, such as invasive electrode recordings, may reveal that seizures come from one of these areas.

The successes and risks of parietal and occipital lobectomies are similar to those of frontal lobectomy. Since neither of these lobes controls movement, however, the risk of weakness is lower and the risk of losing touch sensation or vision is greater. On the dominant (usually left) side, the parietal lobe is important in language functions and conceptualizing skilled motor actions. On the nondominant (usually right) side, the parietal lobe is important for spatial perception and ability to focus attention toward the left side of space. The occipital lobes are essential for vision. The left occipital lobe receives information about vision in the right half of space and vice versa.

CORPUS CALLOSOTOMY

Corpus callosotomy cuts the large fiber bundle (corpus callosum; see Fig. 1B) that connects the two hemispheres of the brain. In contrast with lobectomy, corpus callosotomy does not involve removal of brain tissue. The operation usually involves cutting the front two-thirds of the callosum in the hope that the operation will markedly reduce the seizure frequency. In some cases, a second operation is performed to cut the remaining back third. Corpus callosotomy is most effective for atonic, tonic-clonic, and tonic seizures. Seizure frequency is reduced by an average of 70% to 80% after partial callosotomy and 80% to 90% after complete callosotomy. Partial seizures are often unchanged, but they may be improved or worsened. In many cases, especially after partial callosotomy, seizures are less frequent, but they do persist.

Complications of corpus callosotomy are greater than with frontal or temporal lobe surgery. Behavioral, language, and other problems may affect function and the quality of life, but serious problems are temporary or uncommon. The potential risks of callosotomy must be weighed against its possible benefits, such as a reduction in the frequency of seizures that cause injury and other problems. The people most susceptible to behavioral problems after callosotomy are those in whom language and motor dominance are controlled by different hemispheres; in left-handed people, for example, the left side of the brain controls language, but the right side of the brain controls movement. Some of the problems resulting from callosotomy are caused by injury to the frontal lobes during the operation. Since the corpus callosum is buried deep between the frontal lobes, the middle portions of these lobes must be separated, which poses some risk. Surgical advances may help to minimize this risk.

HEMISPHERECTOMY

The dramatic procedure of hemispherectomy originally involved the removal of one whole side of the brain. Now, it usually involves disconnecting one cerebral hemisphere from the rest of the brain, with removal of only a limited area (Fig. 24). It is only considered in patients, usually children, with severe epilepsy in whom seizures arise from only one side of the brain and in which that hemisphere functions poorly. Before surgery, these patients typically have severe weakness (paralysis) and loss of touch sensation and vision on the opposite side of the body. Therefore, the side of the brain that is to be disconnected is already functioning very poorly and often impairs the functions of the other side of the brain.

If the operation is performed on young children, the opposite hemisphere may make up for the loss. They will never have movement or normal sensation in the hand, forearm, foot, and leg on the side opposite the operation. However, controlled movements are possible in the upper arm and thigh, thus permitting the person to walk. Physical therapy is often needed after hemispherectomy.

The results of hemispherectomy are quite good. More than 75% of the patients experience complete or nearly complete seizure control. If the patient has a progressive disorder, such as Rasmussen's syndrome, the prognosis for seizure control is not as good.

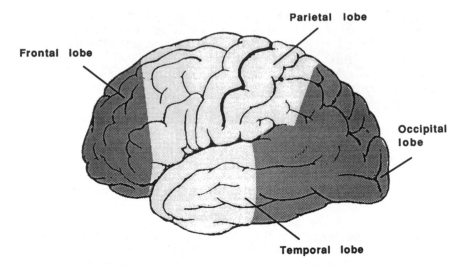

FIGURE 24. Outer surface *(side view)* of the left hemisphere, showing the area of brain removed *(light shading)* and the areas of brain disconnected from the opposite hemisphere *(dark shading)* in a hemispherectomy.

MULTIPLE SUBPIAL TRANSECTIONS

The procedure called multiple subpial transections was pioneered as an alternative to removal of brain tissue. It is used to control partial seizures originating in areas that cannot be safely removed. For example, if the seizure focus involves the dominant temporal-lobe language area (Wernicke's area), which is critical for comprehension, the removal of this area to control seizures would cause a devastating complication: the inability to understand spoken or written language. Similarly, if the primary motor area is part of the seizure focus, its removal would cause permanent weakness on the opposite side of the body.

The operation involves a series of shallow cuts (transections) into the cerebral cortex (Fig. 25). The transections are made only as deep as the gray matter (approximately a quarter of an inch deep). Because of the complex way in which the brain is organized, these cuts are thought to interrupt some fibers that connect neighboring parts of the brain, but they do not appear to cause long-lasting impairment in the critical functions served by these areas. Examination of brain tissue after multiple subpial transections reveals that some nerve cells are destroyed.

Multiple subpial transections can help reduce or eliminate seizures arising from vital functional cortical areas. Transections have been used successfully in Landau-Kleffner syndrome, a disorder in which language problems appear in a child whose language skills were previously

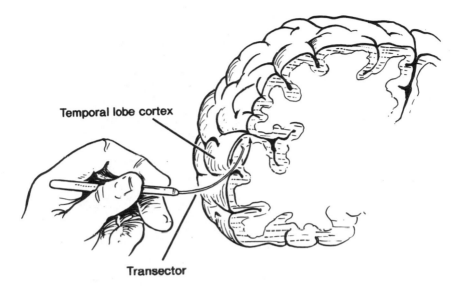

Temporal lobe cortex

Transector

FIGURE 25. Multiple subpial transections of the brain.

developing normally (see Chap. 4, p. 45). One concern is that the epileptic activity may recur after 2 to 20 months. It is uncertain whether this procedure can achieve long-term seizure control.

The procedure is generally well tolerated, but there may be bleeding at the site of the transection. Major complications appear to be rare. Transections in language areas may cause mild impairments in the language function served by that area. The risks and benefits of multiple subpial transections need to be better defined.

STIMULATION OF THE VAGUS NERVE

Electrical stimulation of the vagus nerve is a new technique for controlling seizures. The vagus nerve is part of the autonomic nervous system, which controls bodily functions that are not under voluntary control, such as heart rate. The vagus nerve passes from the brainstem (see Fig. 5) through the neck and into the chest and abdomen. Numerous studies and growing clinical experience confirm that stimulation of this nerve can, in many cases, help control seizures.

The stimulating device (Fig. 26) must be surgically implanted; it has a battery that lasts approximately 5 years. An incision is made along the outer side of the chest on the left side, and the device is implanted under the skin. A second incision is made horizontally in the lower neck, along

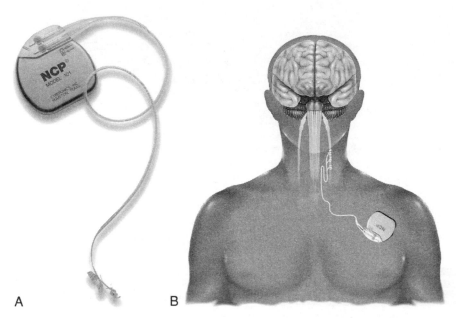

A   B

FIGURE 26. Vagus nerve stimulator. (*A*) Stimulator device and wire. (*B*) Placement of the stimulator, attachment to the vagus nerve, and relationship of the vagus nerve to the brain.

a crease of skin, and the wire from the stimulator is connected to the vagus nerve. The procedure ordinarily requires about 50 to 90 minutes with the patient under general anesthesia and a hospital stay of one night. However, with greater experience, the procedure has been done under local anesthesia with the patient discharged the same day.

The risks of the implantation procedure are low. Approximately 1% of implants cause some damage to the nerve supplying muscles in the voice box, which can result in permanent hoarseness or a change in voice quality. In addition, when the vagus nerve is stimulated, about one-third of patients have some change in their voice quality, which is reversible by reducing the amount of stimulation or adjusting other stimulation features. Even without any change in the level of stimulation, the hoarseness and changes in voice quality tend to diminish and resolve over several weeks or months.

The vagus nerve stimulator was approved by the Food and Drug Administration for use in patients with partial epilepsy who are 12 years of age or older. Many centers have successfully used the device in younger children (as young as 1 year of age) and in patients with primary generalized epilepsy, Lennox-Gastaut syndrome, Landau-Kleffner syndrome, and other convulsive disorders.

The stimulator can be easily activated by holding a special magnet near the implanted device. The strength of the magnet can be adjusted. For people with warnings (auras) before their seizures, activating the stimulator with the magnet when the warning occurs may help to stop the seizure. However, many patients without auras also have improvement in seizure control with the vagus nerve stimulator.

For all patients, the device is programmed to go on for a certain period (e.g., 7 seconds or 30 seconds) and then go off for another period (e.g., 14 seconds or 5 minutes). It continuously cycles, providing intermittent stimulation to the vagus nerve throughout the day and night.

Initial studies revealed that one-third of patients experienced fewer than half as many seizures, another one-third had their seizures reduced by 20% to 50%, and one-third did not have worthwhile improvement. More recent results have been even better:

- 5% to 8% of patients have become seizure-free.
- About 50% of patients have had the number of their seizures cut at least in half. This number includes those who became seizure-free.
- 30% have shown benefit but have had their seizure frequency reduced by less than half.
- About 20% have had no worthwhile benefit.

Epilepsy Surgery During the First 3 Years of Life

Infants and young children who have seizures that cannot be controlled with medications may be candidates for surgery. These children usually have MRI evidence of abnormalities that are restricted (or nearly so) to one area of the brain. In some cases, the abnormality is widespread in one entire hemisphere (e.g., Sturge-Weber syndrome or hemimegalencephaly) and the child's epilepsy is best treated with a hemispherectomy. In other cases, the area of abnormal brain tissue is much more limited, and the removal of less tissue can improve or fully control the seizures.

Many children under 3 years of age who are candidates for epilepsy surgery have had infantile spasms. Infantile spasms are classified as primary generalized seizures and are almost always associated with electrical abnormalities over both sides of the brain both during and between seizures. The spasms also involve muscles on both sides of the body in roughly equal fashion. These features suggest that infantile spasms could never be treated by any form of surgery that removes a limited portion of the brain. However, on the PET scan, some patients with infantile spasms have a restricted area of decreased brain metabolism. When this area overlaps with the area of abnormality shown on the MRI or EEG and the infantile spasms do not respond to medications, the patients may be candidates for removal of the abnormal portions of the brain. Under microscopic examination, the abnormal brain areas that are removed often show an abnormality in the pattern of brain-cell development (cortical dysplasia). Preliminary reports suggest that the operation can improve the child's development and seizure control.

Cost of Epilepsy Surgery

Epilepsy surgery is expensive. Because of the complexities involved in the presurgical planning, it must be performed at a comprehensive epilepsy center that has a team experienced in epilepsy surgery. Strategies, philosophies, and costs differ among epilepsy centers, depending on the part of the country and the extent of the presurgical assessment. At some centers, for example, patients are monitored with video-EEG for prolonged periods; at others, the monitoring periods are shorter. In addition, if invasive electrodes are used, the cost is much greater than if only a routine video-EEG is done. Overall, the cost of epilepsy surgery varies from $35,000 to more than $100,000. Patients should feel free to ask different centers about their average costs, outcomes, rates of complications, and other factors related to the surgery.

   Health insurance plans usually cover epilepsy surgery. If the insurance company denies coverage, it is often worthwhile to have both the patient and the doctor write to the company. The doctor should provide documentation showing that epilepsy surgery is an established procedure for treating people with epilepsy in whom antiepileptic drugs do not control the seizures.

Other Therapies

For centuries, starvation and dehydration have been reported to improve seizure control. In addition, substances as diverse as mistletoe, turpentine, and marijuana have all been claimed to be highly effective in treating epilepsy. In 1858, Sir Edward Henry Sieveking wrote, "There is scarcely a substance in the world, capable of passing through the gullet of man, that has not at one time or other enjoyed a reputation of being an anti-epileptic."[1] Aside from medicinal and dietary therapies, other therapies proposed for controlling epilepsy include the ancient practice of acupuncture and relatively modern relaxation techniques.

Researchers all over the world are continuing to work on developing new therapies, which are still years away from being ready for use with patients. Some of the more promising ideas that may be applied in the future are discussed briefly in Chapter 34.

Dietary Therapy

THE KETOGENIC DIET

Research in the 1930s showed that a ketogenic diet, consisting mostly of fats with little or no carbohydrate and a minimal amount of protein, reduced the frequency of seizures in more than half of the children who followed it. The diet is named the ketogenic diet because a diet rich in fat

[1]Sieveking, EH: On Epilepsy and Epileptiform Seizures: Their Causes, Pathology, and Treatment. J Churchill, London, 1858, p 226.

causes a metabolic change in the body called ketosis. The body metabolizes its own fat and protein, producing chemical substances called ketone bodies.

After the introduction of the antiepileptic drug phenytoin in 1938, the ketogenic diet fell out of use, but new studies during the past several decades have confirmed its therapeutic value in epilepsy. In recent years, a story on a television news program and a television movie informed the public and health professionals about children who were successfully treated with the ketogenic diet. Several new books about the diet have been published also (see Appendix 4). Consequently, the diet is now more widely used.

Many doctors are uncomfortable with prescribing the ketogenic diet because they are unfamiliar with it, unsure of its risks and benefits, or unimpressed with its results. Therefore, it is most often used in epilepsy centers, which usually reserve it for children with seizures that are very difficult to control.

The ketogenic diet is often difficult to enforce, especially for older children and adults, because eating even small amounts of carbohydrates can render it ineffective. Even the tiny amount of carbohydrate in some antibiotic preparations, chewing gum, or toothpaste can be a problem.

The diet is most often used for children between 18 months and 9 years of age whose seizures cannot be controlled by antiepileptic drugs. The best results have been obtained in children with atonic, tonic, and myoclonic seizures, but virtually all types of seizures have been improved or controlled by this diet. Children younger than 1 year of age cannot maintain adequate ketosis to obtain the beneficial effects of the diet. Its successful use by children older than 1 year depends on the child's previous diet, adaptability, and motivation. After the age of 3 to 5 years, children in our society usually have been exposed to foods that they are unwilling to part with. Therefore it can be very difficult for older children or adolescents to use the ketogenic diet unless they are well motivated. School-age children can be remarkably cooperative once the benefits are explained, however, especially if an excellent outcome is achieved. The ketogenic diet also can be used successfully in adults.

Starting and Stopping the Diet

The ketogenic diet should be used only under a doctor's supervision, usually with the help of a dietitian. In most cases, the diet is started while the child is in the hospital. For the first 24 to 48 hours, the child is not allowed to eat anything and is permitted to drink only a certain amount of water or other fluids. The child's blood sugar level often falls during this period of starvation. If the fall in blood sugar is too great, the child may become pale, sweaty, tremorous, irritable, confused, and unresponsive—or the child may even have seizures. If this occurs, he or she will need some sugar or other carbohydrate supplementation. The blood sugar level can be safely monitored in the hospital. Dehydration can also occur. Fluid status requires careful attention when the diet is started.

After several days of starvation, the ketones in the blood and urine rise, and the food allowed on the diet is gradually introduced. The urinary ketones can be easily measured at home by the parents by using an indicator strip. The presence of urinary ketones indicates that the diet has achieved its metabolic goal of ketosis, but they are not an accurate gauge of the concentration of ketones in the blood.

The diet consists primarily of foods high in fat, with the remaining calories made up of protein foods. With the commonly used 4:1 ratio of fats to carbohydrates and protein, 80% to 90% of the foods are fats and 10% to 20% are carbohydrates and protein. Examples of high-fat foods include mayonnaise, butter, and heavy cream. The child is allowed only small portions of cheese, meat, fish, or poultry each day. Fruit is allowed in modest amounts. There is an alternative source of fat, known as MCT (medium-chain triglyceride), which is an oil. The use of MCT allows a slightly greater expansion of nonfat foods in the diet. However, MCT may not be as beneficial in controlling seizures as other fat sources, such as butter and cream.

Because sugar is prohibited in the diet, the parents must be careful about all types of children's medications, cough syrups, vitamins, toothpaste, and any other nonfoods or foods that may contain sugar. Even small amounts of sugar can reverse the effects of the diet and cause a seizure. Therefore, teachers, babysitters, grandparents, siblings, and others who may be with the child in the parents' absence must be knowledgeable about the dietary restrictions.

There are no absolute rules about the length of time someone should stay on the ketogenic diet. If the diet is well tolerated and effective, the doctor will usually recommend continuing the diet for 1 to 3 years, after which the percentage of carbohydrate is gradually increased. Suddenly stopping the diet may cause a temporary increase in seizures, which is similar to the rebound effect that may occur after the abrupt discontinuation of antiepileptic drugs. Therefore, it is usually recommended that the ratio of fats to protein and carbohydrates be gradually reduced.

After the diet is discontinued, some children remain seizure-free without medications. Sometimes, however, the seizures will start to occur again, in which case they may be well controlled with medications that were ineffective before the diet. A patient who was seizure-free on a lower ratio of fats to protein and carbohydrates (e.g., 3:1 or 2:1), but who has seizures when the diet is discontinued, may be helped by continuing the diet at a reduced ratio. This change allows a modest increase in carbohydrates and calories.

Using Antiepileptic Drugs with the Diet

If a child is taking high dosages of several antiepileptic drugs, tapering of one drug is often started during the period of starvation. Barbiturates are often discontinued first because they are the most sedative of the antiepileptic drugs. Also, their blood levels can rise when the diet is started even though the dosage is unchanged. If adequate ketosis is maintained and seizure control improves, a further reduction in medications is often possible. In some cases, all medications can be tapered and stopped.

Potential Risks of the Diet

The long-term effects of a high-fat diet, even if it is used for only several years, are unknown. Many experts believe, however, that the potential risk is much less than the benefits for brain development and intellectual and social functions of improved seizure control and reduced dosages of antiepileptic drugs.

The most dangerous potential risk of the ketogenic diet is low blood sugar during the period of starvation. Other potential problems include a deficiency of the B vitamins, vitamin C, and calcium. It is necessary to supplement these nutrients (making sure the supplement does not contain sugar). Now and then, a child may develop a serious decline in the level of protein in the blood (hypoproteinemia) resulting from decreased protein consumption. Other adverse effects that may occasionally occur include abnormal liver function tests and anemia.

Many parents worry about the potential effects of large amounts of dietary fat. We know that high-fat diets in adults can accelerate atherosclerosis, which contributes to heart attacks, stroke, and other disorders of blood vessels. However, there is no evidence that the ketogenic diet accelerates atherosclerosis in children or adolescents. Unfortunately, we cannot be sure that the diet has no long-term effects on the blood vessels. Weight gain is not usually a problem on this diet because caloric intake is carefully supervised.

The ketogenic diet can slightly delay a child's growth, but this is usually made up for when the diet is stopped. Children on this diet also have a small risk of kidney stones, but the risk is minimized by adequate fluid intake. The risk of kidney stones may be increased if the patient is also taking acetazolamide, topiramate, or zonisamide (see Chap. 11).

Other Sources of Information about the Diet

The explosion of interest in the ketogenic diet during the past decade has been accompanied by a greater medical and parental base of shared knowledge (see Appendix 4). Two recent books, *The Epilepsy Diet*

Treatment: An Introduction to the Ketogenic Diet (by John Freeman and others, 2000) and *The Ketogenic Diet: A Complete Guide for the Dieter and Practitioner* (by Lyle McDonald, 1999), remain the best and most comprehensive sources of information on the diet. *The Ketogenic Cookbook* (by Dennis and Cynthia Brake, 1997) is a good source for recipes. The KetoKlub newsletter (e-mail *KetoKlub@aol.com*) is a rich source of parental information, recipes, personal observations, and helpful suggestions. The Internet is also an increasing source of information on the ketogenic diet, but it may be wise to confirm specific recommendations with the doctor or another health care professional before trying them.

VITAMINS, MINERALS, AND OTHER NUTRITIONAL SUPPLEMENTS

Although many books contain lists of vitamins, amino acids, and other nutritional supplements that are said to control seizures, there is little scientific support for such claims. Unconfirmed reports claim that magnesium; calcium; vitamin E; vitamin B_{12}; melatonin; and the amino acids L-taurine, L-tyrosine, or dimethylglycine reduce seizures in some patients. As discussed in Chapter 6, however, no experts in the treatment of epilepsy would recommend the routine use of these substances because there is no scientific evidence that any of them help control seizures. Limited exceptions include magnesium or calcium, which are effective only for patients whose seizures are caused by serious nutritional or metabolic disorders, and vitamin B_6 in cases of the rare deficiency that causes seizures in newborn babies. It is unknown whether any vitamin, mineral, or other nutritional supplement is generally beneficial or detrimental to seizure control, and most so-called authorities who recommend nutritional therapy for epilepsy do not have solid evidence of its effectiveness. Western medicine has not studied the role of nutrition in health as intensively as it deserves, however, and use of a multivitamin or specific vitamin or mineral supplement can have other health benefits.

Alternative Therapies

The gaps in knowledge of doctors who practice Western medicine are matched by the spectrum of alternative health care (also called complementary or integrative health care), which ranges from spiritual to herbal to nutritional to behavioral therapy. People with epilepsy whose seizures are not fully controlled by antiepileptic drugs or who experience troublesome adverse effects may tire of these problems and look for help outside the traditional medical boundaries.

It is fair to criticize Western medicine for studying only those therapies and approaches that it chooses to recognize as being potentially effective. It is also fair to praise it for the care with which it assesses the effectiveness and safety of its treatments. It is difficult for the average person to appreciate the power of bias and placebo effects. Bias refers to the effects of prejudice and expectation. For example, someone who tests a product in which he or she has a financial interest may consciously or unconsciously slant the test to help find a favorable result. A placebo is a substance that has no effect of its own except for that associated with the power of suggestion. For example, when people with chest pain caused by heart problems are given a placebo and told it will make them better, more than a quarter of them report a definite beneficial effect.

When practitioners of any kind prescribe a treatment, they want their therapy to be effective. To find out whether it really is, it should be subjected to a rigorous double-blind controlled study (a study in which neither the doctor nor the patient knows which patients are receiving the "active" drug or other treatment). Mainstream health care professionals have learned over and over that unless the effectiveness and safety of a therapy are demonstrated in controlled studies of this kind, then beware. The best doctor's suspicions, hunches, and experiences over several decades of practice are often dead wrong. So-called alternative therapies are rarely subjected to careful scrutiny (especially a double-blind controlled study), which means we do not know whether most of them are helpful, harmful, or simply ineffective.

HERBAL THERAPIES

Herbal therapies are prepared from the flowers, leaves, stems, bark, or roots of plants. Some of these can be taken directly, but others undergo various forms of processing, such as drying. Herbal therapy is probably the oldest form of medical treatment taken by mouth or applied to the skin. Such substances have been used in all cultural groups throughout recorded history, and some have even been found in prehistoric remains. Many of our modern drugs are derived from plants and were once part of herbal therapy. Textbooks on epilepsy from the 18th and 19th centuries describe many herbal therapies, including mistletoe, foxglove (digitalis), and Cannabis sativa (marijuana), but few were found to be of much help. Unfortunately, none of these therapies has been subjected to proper study; therefore, we remain uncertain as to their benefits or risks.

Herbal preparations are most often recommended for the treatment of epilepsy in Asian and African folk medicine practices. (See Appendix 4 for sources of more information.) The herbal medicines that are alleged, but not proven, to have a beneficial effect on seizures include Ailanthus altissima (Tree of Heaven), Artemisia vulgaris (mugwort), Calotropis procera (calotropis), Cannabis sativa (marijuana), Centella asiatica (hydrocotyle), Convallaria majalis (lily of the valley), Dictamnus albus (burning bush), Paeonia officinalis (peony), Scutellaria lateriflora (scullcap), Senecio vulgaris (groundsel), Taxus baccata (yew), Valeriana officinalis (valerian), and Viscum album (mistletoe). Some of these herbal medicines for epilepsy were used in the Middle Ages or earlier. Most of them are relatively safe in recommended doses. Adverse effects include rash, digestive disturbances, and headache. Overdoses can be dangerous.

RELAXATION THERAPY AND BIOFEEDBACK

Most adults with epilepsy believe that stress can provoke a seizure. Because stress can alter brain chemistry and electrical activity and disrupt normal sleep, it is possible that it can worsen epilepsy in susceptible individuals. It can also cause a person to breathe rapidly (hyperventilate), which makes seizures more likely in some people with epilepsy, especially those with absence seizures.

Relaxation therapy involves a variety of strategies designed to reduce stress and foster relaxation. Breathing maneuvers, hypnosis, and other techniques can be used in relaxation therapy. Biofeedback involves learning to control bodily functions that are usually not under voluntary control. One can learn to control these functions by providing information about them to conscious awareness. For example, the heart rate can be modified by listening to a beep every time one's heart beats and concentrating on lowering or raising the heart rate. Similarly, biofeedback can be used for relaxation by concentrating on lowering the tension in the facial muscles or breathing at a slower rate.

Almost all of us, including people with epilepsy, would benefit from more relaxation and less stress. Relaxation therapy and biofeedback can help to improve seizure control in some people by reducing stress and controlling hyperventilation, but they rarely make someone seizure-free. Unfortunately, because there has been little systematic study of these techniques in people with epilepsy, their role in epilepsy therapy is unclear. In addition to relaxation therapy and biofeedback, tai chi, yoga, and therapeutic massage also are helpful techniques for relieving stress.

ACUPUNCTURE

Acupuncture is used in China and by some practitioners in the West to treat seizures. There is no question that acupuncture can alter brain activity. For instance, many surgical procedures can be performed using acupuncture instead of anesthetic drugs. The ways in which acupuncture works are poorly understood, and its usefulness in the treatment of epilepsy is unconfirmed.

CHIROPRACTIC THERAPY

Some chiropractic teachings suggest that specific nutrients or forms of spinal manipulation can improve seizure control. There is no evidence to support these claims.

Self-Control of Seizures

Many people with epilepsy have warnings of their seizures and have learned techniques to "fight off a seizure." The warnings may take the form of certain symptoms that occur 20 minutes to several days before a seizure. Such symptoms may include irritability, depression, fatigue, "not feeling right," or headache. Patients who have well-defined symptoms of this kind potentially can help prevent a seizure from occurring by getting more sleep or taking additional medication under a doctor's supervision.

Some patients have a simple partial seizure that typically occurs seconds before a complex partial or tonic-clonic seizure. The strategy used to stop seizures from progressing is often hard to describe. It appears to be a very real, but very individual phenomenon. It may involve changing thoughts, repeating a phrase, or attempting to relax. Some patients and doctors have developed specific methods for stopping a seizure. Some patients report that they need to focus on a difficult problem, get up and walk, relax, or keep repeating to themselves "no, no, no." One technique described in the 1800s was used by people who would experience a tingling sensation or jerking movement in an arm or leg. The sensation rose toward the head and would be followed by a tonic-clonic seizure. The seizure could be stopped by vigorously rubbing or scratching the arm or leg or tying a cloth tightly around it. Similarly, some patients with seizures beginning with a smell (olfactory aura) can stop their seizure from progressing by smelling an unrelated strong odor. More examples of self-control of seizures appear in the book *Epilepsy: A New Approach* by Adrienne Richard and Joel Reiter.

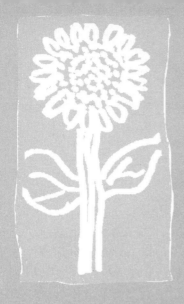

part three

EPILEPSY IN
CHILDREN

Epilepsy in Infancy

A new child is a bundle of anticipation and expectations. Any illness that the child may have, including epilepsy, seems terrible to the parents and family. The stigma that some people still associate with seizures and epilepsy creates unique challenges. Seizures in a newborn usually subside quickly, but may recur as epilepsy in later childhood. The greatest challenge for the parents of a newborn with seizures is fear of the unknown. If the cause of the seizures is understood, the doctor will be better able to make predictions about the baby's development than if the cause is unknown. Even if no cause can be found and all diagnostic tests are normal, however, there is an excellent chance that the baby will develop normally.

Seizures in Newborns

Jane was 2 days old and was on a respirator in the intensive care unit. I was so afraid she wouldn't live, or if she did, that there would be permanent brain damage. Then they told me that she was having seizures and needed to be treated with phenobarbital. It was all very frightening, but Janey is now 2 years old, has been off phenobarbital since the age of 6 months, and has not had any seizures since leaving the hospital at 2 weeks of age.

Seizures in newborns (babies in the first month of life) may appear as fragments of seizures that occur in children and adults. The seizures are fragmentary because the infant's brain is still developing and is unable to make the coordinated responses characteristic of a tonic-clonic seizure. The baby may have jerking or stiffening of a leg or an arm that alternates from side to side, or the whole upper body may suddenly jerk forward, or both legs may jerk up toward the belly with the knees bent. The baby's facial expression, breathing, and heart rate may change. Impairment of responsiveness, which is critical in defining many types of seizures in children and adults, is difficult to assess in newborns. Parents may suspect that responsiveness is impaired when their voices are unable to attract the newborn's attention. Even experts have difficulty recognizing seizures in newborns. Neurologists are often told not to watch their own babies and young children too closely, especially when they sleep, because even they may mistake normal gestures for seizures. Normal babies have many sudden, brief jerks, grimaces, stares, and mouth movements that might suggest epilepsy in an older child or adult. A diagnosis of epilepsy in an infant is more likely if the behavioral changes are not typical of children of the same age (some parents videotape the suspected behavior at home for viewing by the doctor), if repeated episodes are identical in their behavioral features and duration, and if the episodes are not brought on by changes in posture or activity.

The Moro (startle) reflex in babies is a perfectly normal response that can be easily mistaken for a seizure. When a baby is startled—such as by momentary removal of support of its head, a loud noise, or a bright light—its spine will stiffen, its arms and legs will extend outward from the body, and its fingers will fan out. The Moro reflex is present in its full form until age 3 months and in an incomplete form until age 5 months. Jitters are another example of normal behavior in infants that may be confused with seizures. Jitters are shivering movements or tremors; they are not epileptic seizures. They are similar to the shivering that occurs with fever in older children and adults.

Newborns with a rare genetic disorder called benign familial neonatal convulsions begin having frequent brief seizures in the first few days of life. The disorder usually is inherited by an autosomal dominant gene (that is, one parent also had the disorder), but it may also result from a spontaneous mutation in the child's DNA. The seizures usually stop by 6 to 9 months of age.

The electroencephalogram (EEG), which is usually so helpful in defining seizures, is more difficult to interpret in newborns. Although the normal and abnormal patterns of brain electrical activity in newborns are becoming more clearly defined, areas of uncertainty still exist, and only a few neurologists can expertly interpret newborn EEG patterns. To complicate the situation, some seizures seen in newborns are not associated with any specific seizure patterns on the EEG.

Seizures in Infants

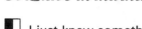 I just knew something was not right. My other children had sudden jerks when they were startled and sometimes when they slept, but Jessie's jerks happened while he was awake just watching a mobile. The pediatrician said not to worry, but when his whole body stiffened, the doctor ordered an EEG, and it showed epilepsy waves.

Seizures in infants (babies age 2 to 12 months) are similar to those that occur in newborns. Because older infants are able to focus their attention briefly, parents and doctors are better able to identify impaired consciousness during seizures. Some seizures can be recognized by episodes of staring from which the infant cannot be distracted. Because all children daydream, however, it may be difficult to distract the healthiest of babies when their minds are focused on an object or a thought, and seizures cannot be diagnosed simply because the child appears to stare. During some staring spells, the infant may make sudden, involuntary movements or jerks or may have a sudden loss of muscle tone and become limp. With other seizures, the baby may make repetitive movements that appear purposeless or semipurposeful. At times, the seizure may be more violent and the baby may fall, or the baby's entire body may stiffen and jerk. Because breathing may be briefly interrupted or irregular, the baby's face may become pale or blue, but the seizure is almost never life threatening.

Nearly all seizures in infants last less than 5 minutes. If seizures last more than 5 minutes or occur in a series, the baby should be taken to an emergency room. If an infant is definitely diagnosed as having epileptic seizures, the doctor should tell the parents when to call the doctor or to take the baby to the doctor's office or a hospital if the seizures worsen.

EEG patterns in infants are more clearly defined than those in newborns. However, the normal range of variability is still quite large; that is, the patterns seen during the waking and sleeping periods can vary considerably between healthy children of the same age. This leads to problems with interpretation. EEG changes are visible during most seizures that occur in infants.

An uncommon disorder called *infantile spasms* (West's syndrome) usually develops during infancy and lasts an average of 5 to 6 months with treatment (see Chap. 4). Many of these children will later have developmental delays and other seizures in childhood. *Febrile seizures* are tonic-clonic seizures that may occur in infants and young children when they have a high fever. They were discussed in detail in Chapter 4.

Diagnosis

Doctors try to identify the cause of seizures in newborns and infants. Commonly recognized causes of epilepsy before the age of 1 year include fever, birth injury and trauma, birth defects resulting from abnormal brain development in the womb, genetic disorders, encephalitis (an infection of the brain), and meningitis (an infection of the membranes covering the brain). Depending on the baby's medical history and examination, the doctor may order a variety of tests or procedures to look for:

- Structural abnormalities in the brain, using an ultrasound, computed tomography (CT) scan, or magnetic resonance imaging (MRI) of the head
- Abnormal electrical activity in the brain, using an EEG
- Metabolic problems, using a variety of blood and urine tests
- Genetic disorders, using chromosomal studies
- Evidence of infection or metabolic disorders, using a lumbar puncture (spinal tap)

The lumbar puncture, which is done to obtain a sample of cerebrospinal fluid, is safe and not very painful. The baby's worst crying usually comes when the doctor cleans the skin with a cool antiseptic solution. An anesthetic cream can be used on the skin for pain relief. General anesthesia is sometimes used.

In many cases no cause of the seizures can be found. Brain injuries causing seizures may be impossible to pinpoint, especially injuries occurring in the womb or those associated with only microscopic damage. For example, seizure disorders in infancy may result from a viral infection in the mother during pregnancy that is undetectable with our current tests (nearly all pregnant women who have mild viral infections have perfectly healthy babies).

Once in a great while, seizures in newborns and infants are caused by a deficiency of vitamin B_6 (pyridoxine). It is important to recognize the deficiency because it is a treatable cause of seizures. The diagnosis can be established by recording the EEG while injecting vitamin B_6. An improvement in the EEG patterns indicates a vitamin B_6 deficiency.

Treatment of Seizures

The treatment of seizures in newborns and infants is determined by the type of seizure and its cause. In some cases, no therapy is needed because the seizure is an isolated event, such as a single seizure associated with a high fever. In other cases, such as low blood sugar levels or a calcium or vitamin B_6 deficiency in a newborn, replacement of a missing nutrient can stop further seizures..

Most of the time, babies who have epilepsy must be treated with antiepileptic drugs. As with any other age group, doctors try to balance the benefits of seizure control against the risks of adverse effects from the drugs. They sometimes prefer to keep the dosage low and let the baby have a brief seizure and several minutes of lethargy once a week, rather than use a high dosage that makes the baby seizure-free but always sedated, listless, and developmentally slow.

This raises an important question if a baby with epilepsy is also developmentally delayed: What is causing the delay? Is it the seizures, the epilepsy waves found on the EEG, the medicines, or the underlying problem? This question is difficult to answer. It can even be impossible to answer for sure because when one factor changes, it can change the others. For example, lowering the dosage and the number of antiepileptic drugs reduces the adverse effects, but may increase the epilepsy waves on the EEG and make the seizures worse. If CT or MRI shows evidence of a brain abnormality, the structural problem is probably a major cause of the developmental delay; however, such babies also may be extra sensitive to the effects of seizures and medications. Despite the difficulties in finding answers, these questions should be addressed. Often there must be a trade-off to get the best results.

Pediatricians and family physicians are often the first to treat babies with seizures, but they usually refer these infants to a pediatric neurologist for consultation or long-term care because epilepsy in the first year of life may be caused by underlying neurologic problems. Especially complex or difficult cases may need further referral to a pediatric epileptologist at a comprehensive epilepsy center.

Epilepsy in Childhood

Children have all types of primary generalized and partial epilepsies. The various types of seizures are described in Chapter 3. Some special types of seizures or epilepsy syndromes usually begin or occur only in childhood. These disorders, discussed in Chapter 4, include febrile seizures, infantile spasms (West's syndrome), Lennox-Gastaut syndrome, absence seizures, juvenile myoclonic epilepsy, benign rolandic epilepsy, and reflex epilepsies.

Causes

Seizures in children have many causes (see Fig. 8). Common causes of childhood seizures or epilepsy include fever, metabolic disorders such as low blood sugar, head injury, infections of the brain and its coverings, lack of oxygen to the brain, hydrocephalus (excess water in the brain cavities), and disorders of brain development. Less common causes of childhood epilepsy include brain tumors or cysts and degenerative disorders (progressive and deteriorating conditions, often associated with loss of brain cells). There is an important difference between something that causes seizures, such as a high fever in a young child, and something that causes epilepsy, such as a severe head injury.

Extensive and careful studies have not found any evidence that immunizations cause epilepsy. However, a seizure may occur within several days of an immunization, especially if it is followed by a fever. In such cases, the child probably had a harmless febrile seizure. When the child receives subsequent immunizations, the parents should ask the doctor about using children's versions of acetaminophen (Tylenol) or ibuprofen (Advil or Motrin) before a fever develops. Children who have a single seizure following an immunization can usually receive further immunizations.

Many childhood seizures are benign; that is, they are self-limited, meaning that they will end without treatment and the child's development and intellect likely will be normal. Other seizures are serious and often are associated with developmental delay or mental retardation and persistent seizures. The outlook for seizures only partially depends on their cause. For example, two children may be infected with the same bacteria and have meningitis (an infection of the membranes covering the brain and spinal cord). One child is left with severe epilepsy, but the other child never has a seizure. How can the different outcomes be explained? The bacterial infection in one child may have been more widespread, involving sensitive areas of the brain. Or the bacteria could have infected a vein in one child and caused a small stroke, which then caused the epilepsy. Or perhaps one child had a genetic (hereditary) tendency to have seizures, and the infection brought this trait to the surface.

All people are capable of having a seizure. It remains uncertain why some children have seizures after incidents such as moderate head trauma while most others do not. *Seizure threshold* refers to the conditions necessary for the production of a seizure. In animals, the seizure threshold can be precisely defined by observing their response to certain chemicals or electrical stimulation. In human beings, the term seizure threshold is used in a more abstract sense. In people who have a tendency to have seizures, the threshold is lower than in people who have a greater resistance, or higher threshold, against seizures. Genetic, hormonal, sleep, and other factors can influence an individual's seizure threshold.

Making the Diagnosis

Epilepsy is the occurrence of two or more seizures that are not provoked by reversible causes, such as very low blood sugar. Epilepsy means that there is a tendency to have recurrent seizures. A detailed and accurate history of a child's seizure-like episodes is the most helpful tool for making the diagnosis of epilepsy (see Chap. 8). The doctor will want to know how the episode began and what happened. He or she will ask some questions:

- Did the spell begin suddenly, shortly after standing, or after an argument?
- Was consciousness lost or impaired?
- Were there jerking movements, automatic chewing or hand movements, eye deviation or blinking, or loss of bladder control?
- Afterward, did the child go to sleep or act confused?
- How long did the episode last? (It is best to time an episode with a watch because 1 minute may seem like 5 minutes to a worried observer.)

If possible, the family should make a video recording of an episode for the doctor to view. All of this information will help the doctor to determine if the episode is a seizure, and if so, what type.

Obtaining an accurate description of symptoms that a child experiences during a seizure is an art. Only the person who feels them can accurately describe them, although in some cases they are easy to identify. For example, the child whose face is suddenly filled with fright and who holds her belly and then begins to stare is most likely experiencing a partial seizure with an emotion of fear and abdominal discomfort. In many children, however, the symptoms cannot be read from behavioral features, and one must rely on the child's description. Many children don't report what they feel because of shyness, embarrassment, inability to put their feelings into words, inability to recognize the relationship of the symptom to a seizure, inability to recall the event, and other less obvious reasons. If simply asked what he or she experiences, a child may just shrug. When given a choice of possible symptoms, however, the child will often say that one or more of them occurred before the seizure. The challenge is separating real from imaginary symptoms. Therefore, all children who are willing or able to talk about their symptoms should first be asked in a nonthreatening way if they feel anything before or during the spell or if they ever have sudden, strange feelings separate from it (which could possibly be a simple partial seizure). If they answer no, inquiries should be made about specific types of symptoms.

Conditions Confused with Childhood Seizures

Not every event that involves jerking, staring, or impairment of consciousness is a seizure. Many kinds of behavior can look like seizures, and certain conditions may be confused with seizures. It may take some time and many tests to sort out which episodes are true seizures.

DAYDREAMING

We all daydream, and children daydream more than adults. Daydreaming in children can be easily confused with absence or complex partial seizures, in which staring is a prominent and common feature. During seizures, lip smacking, eye blinking, or stiffening of muscle groups is common; they are not common during daydreaming. Daydreaming can be stopped by calling the child's name, making a startling noise, tickling the child, or saying something like "Look at the kitty." In The parent also can interrupt daydreaming by turning off the television if the child is watching it rather than listening to the parent. Absence and complex partial seizures seldom can be stopped by such means, although the child may be partially responsive. Absence seizures usually last less than 10 seconds, and complex partial seizures last 30 seconds to 3 minutes. Daydreaming tends to occur when the child is tired, bored, or involved in monotonous activity, such as riding in the backseat of a car; seizures can occur at any time. Another important distinguishing feature is the beginning of the attack. Seizures often begin abruptly. For example, the child may suddenly stop and stare in the middle of a sentence or while playing with a toy. In contrast, daydreaming often represents the continuation of a natural pause in activity. For example, a child may be reading and raise his or her head to reflect on a sentence and then begin to daydream.

"BLUE" BREATH-HOLDING SPELLS

In a classic "blue" breath-holding spell, a young child cries intensely for a long time (usually after some minor upset, such as a bump on the head, being scolded for running into the street, or being told not to play with a toy), holds his or her breath, and then loses consciousness and becomes limp. The child often turns bluish and may sweat profusely. The typical attack lasts 30 to 60 seconds. With more prolonged spells, the entire body may become rigid and jerk, as the lack of oxygen to the brain actually triggers a seizure. Although the seizure looks just like an epileptic seizure, the child does not have epilepsy and is not likely to develop it. The lack of oxygen in breath-holding spells and the occasional seizure that follows do not cause brain injury.

When children cry vigorously, they may exhale and then pause before taking another breath. When the pause is unusually long, it is considered a breath-holding spell. Because of the way they affect the child, breath-holding spells may be confused with atonic, tonic, or tonic-clonic seizures. Distinguishing epileptic seizures from breath-holding spells is based mainly on the typical sequence of a physical or emotional upset, followed by crying and breath-holding, which helps the doctor determine that the spell was an episode of breath-holding, not epilepsy. Breath-holding spells usually begin between 6 and 18 months of age and stop before the child is 6 years old. About 25% of patients who visit the doctor for breath-holding spells have a family history of such episodes.

The outlook for a child with breath-holding spells is excellent, and in most cases no treatment is needed. Parents may try to distract the child during the intense crying to help prevent the breath-holding spell. Parents of children who are prone to prolonged vigorous crying tantrums should try to ignore the behavior (attention and concern seem to reinforce it). In some cases, a psychologist may help in modifying the child's behavior.

PALLID INFANTILE SYNCOPE

Syncope (SIN-ko-pee) means fainting. Pallid infantile syncope may be confused with atonic, tonic, or tonic-clonic seizures. In this nonepileptic disorder, which usually begins between 12 and 18 months of age and ends before age 6, the child suddenly becomes pale (pallid) and then faints. Often family members have had similar spells, sometimes called *pallid breath-holding spells,* in early childhood. In contrast to breath-holding spells, the episodes are not consistently preceded by intense crying. If the spells are prolonged, the entire body may become rigid and jerk as the lack of oxygen to the brain triggers a seizure. These spells may result from sensitivity of the vagus nerve, which controls the heart rate.

The prognosis is excellent. Treatment is rarely needed, although for some patients doctors may prescribe small doses of atropine.

OTHER FORMS OF FAINTING

Fainting is common in children. In many cases, other family members have a history of fainting. Painful situations such as having blood drawn can cause a child to faint. Children also may faint from the depletion of fluids in the body (dehydration) caused by inadequate fluid intake or excessive fluid loss, which may occur with sweating or diarrhea. Excessive sun exposure can also cause fainting. In other cases, heart disorders cause slowing of the heartbeat or a decrease in the force of the heart's contractions, causing the child to faint. Lightheadedness, dizziness, or impaired vision often precede the loss of consciousness, but fainting normally is not followed by confusion or tiredness for more than a minute. Frequent episodes of fainting should be thoroughly investigated by a doctor.

MOVEMENT DISORDERS

Many nonepileptic movement disorders can easily be confused with tonic or motor seizures. Children with these disorders assume abnormal postures (parts of their body are in an unusual position, such as the fingers curled up as if in a cramp or the foot turned inward) or make sudden, unusual movements (such as eye blinking or jerks of a body part). The attacks may begin suddenly, thus mimicking seizures. Most of these movement disorders occur spontaneously, but others are triggered by specific events, such as eating (Sandifer's syndrome).

Tics are involuntary, repetitive, intermittent, brief movements. Although tics are purposeless, they may resemble purposeful movements. The most common tics in children are eye blinks, facial grimaces, shoulder shrugs, and head movements. The most severe form of tics occurs in Tourette's syndrome, which is also associated with vocal tics ranging from grunts and throat-clearing sounds to involuntary cursing and other embarrassing noises. Tics are not seizures.

Sleep jerks (benign nocturnal myoclonus) are brief, involuntary muscular contractions that occur as a person falls asleep. In some cases, they may awaken someone who is drifting off to sleep. Sleep jerks are common in healthy children and adults. These normal movements may be confused with myoclonic seizures.

Taking Medications

Hardly anybody likes taking medications. They are a hassle to remember, and taking them may be embarrassing or may disrupt other, more pleasant activities. When doctors recommend a treatment, they assume that the patient will follow their instructions. Doctors call this "compliance." Noncompliance, or failure to take medications as prescribed, is common for many reasons. Perhaps the most important reason is that the patient and family have not been involved in planning the treatment. They should be told about the possible choices of therapy, their benefits, common minor or troublesome adverse effects, and the rare but serious adverse effects of antiepileptic drugs. Communication is the key to achieving compliance.

Young children often hate taking medications, but can usually be coaxed. It may be necessary to crush the pills and put the powder in the child's favorite foods or give the child a small reward if he or she takes the pills. Even small children can understand the importance of taking their pills. Young children can be told that it will help keep them well. Older children can understand that they are taking their pills so they will not have seizures. Parents may want to use themselves as an example.

They can show their children that they occasionally take an aspirin when they have a headache. They might take a vitamin so the children can copy their behavior. Children love to imitate their parents. *Caution: Keep all medications out of the reach of young children.*

Many children and adolescents feel that they are unable to swallow medication in a tablet or capsule form. Although chewable sprinkle and liquid formulations of most medications are available as a substitute, a child can practice taking tablets or capsules by learning to swallow a whole M&M or Tic-Tac candy with a chewed-up cookie. Alternatively, the pill can be placed on the back of the tongue and taken with water or juice from a glass. Medication can also be mixed with a food or taken just when a mouthful of food has been chewed.

When a child with epilepsy will be away from home, whether visiting the grandparents for the weekend or going to camp for the summer, it is essential to maintain the medication schedule. The child, parent, or both can organize a medication box filled with the necessary number of doses and the times for taking them. Alternatively, a company called Medicine-on-Time (800-722-8824) will bubble-pack individual medication doses and label them by date and time. Whatever procedure is used, it should be one that the child or responsible adult understands and finds easy to use because compliance is vital.

Video Games and Epilepsy

Reports in newspapers and on television have heightened public awareness that playing video games can, in rare cases, trigger seizures, but there is no scientific evidence that video games can cause epilepsy. Playing video games is an extremely common pastime for many children, and they often play them for long periods. Some children who have epilepsy just by coincidence will have seizures while playing video games. How often this happens and to what extent the games trigger the seizures, if at all, is not known.

Stress, fatigue, or hyperventilation may trigger seizures in some children playing video games who have epilepsy. Children who are photosensitive—in whom flashing lights or flickering images can trigger seizures or epilepsy waves on the electroencephalogram (EEG)—may have seizures directly associated with playing video games. Photosensitivity occurs in only about 3% of people with epilepsy, however, so almost all children who have epilepsy should be able to play video games without ill effects. Restricting a child from playing video games simply because he or she has epilepsy is not justified.

Parents who are unsure whether a child who has epilepsy is photosensitive should check with the doctor. Photosensitive children may be able to play some games safely, but may have problems with others. Medication can often prevent seizures caused by photosensitivity.

For parents who are concerned about the possible risk of seizures, it may be helpful to observe the child during the game and watch for brief episodes of blank staring in which the child seems momentarily frozen in place. The parent also should check for rapid blinking or twitching of the mouth or face; jerking movements of other parts of the body; loss of attention; brief inability to talk or respond; or reports from the child that things look, sound, smell, or feel different than usual. Although the presence of one or more of these signs does not necessarily mean that a child has epilepsy or is photosensitive, it is a good idea to tell the doctor.

The following suggestions, adapted from ways of reducing the risk of seizures in photosensitive children while they watch television, may be helpful with regard to video games. Make sure they:

- Play in a well-lighted room to reduce the contrast between the lighted screen and the surrounding area. Reducing the brightness of the screen may also be helpful.
- Keep as far back from the screen as possible.
- Use smaller screens in which it is more difficult to see the horizontal scan lines.
- Avoid playing for long periods.
- Take regular breaks, and look away from the screen every once in a while.
- Cover one eye while playing, alternating between the right eye and the left eye.
- Stop the game if strange or unusual feelings develop.

Consult your doctor if a child has strange or uncomfortable sensations caused by light shimmering on water, sunlight flickering through the trees, flashing strobe lights, or any unusual reaction to sudden or strong light.

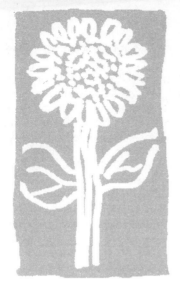

Epilepsy in Adolescence

Adolescence is the passage from childhood to adulthood. It is surrounded by issues of rebellion, independence, heightened self-consciousness, experimentation, dating, driving, and concerns for the future. Communication between adolescents and their parents, who share the highs and lows of this period, is essential to temper the turbulence of adolescence. This is a challenge for both parents and children because adolescence, almost by definition, brings parents and children into conflict. The intense emotions and feelings that come with adolescence are both positive and negative: parents are heroes and villains, best friends and "police officers," and the source of great affection and great frustration. The boundaries of the child's independence, which were tested in early childhood, are tested again in adolescence.

The tidal waves of emotions that consume adolescents also affect those around them. Emotions are infectious. Parents must maintain their perspective and must be sensitive to their child's insecurities, peer pressures, and need for support. Parents must communicate with their children about drugs, smoking, drinking, and sexually transmitted diseases. The key to communication is letting children know that they can feel comfortable talking with their parents. If the parents become too judgmental too quickly, they will harm the trust and openness between them and their children. The balance becomes difficult. Parents need to educate their children and let their feelings be known, but they should try to do it in a positive manner. If adolescents engage in dangerous or irresponsible activities, parents may need to "read them the riot act," but they should try to pause first instead of reacting in the midst of their own emotional storm. Adolescents often know when they have done something wrong, and they are embarrassed and frustrated by their actions.

Adolescence does not need any complicating factors, but epilepsy is just that. In a time of life marked by continuous adjustments to dramatic physical, mental, and social changes, a medical disorder such as epilepsy can upset the tenuous balance. Adolescence is a period of exaggerated concerns over physical and social image. Epilepsy, even if it is well controlled, can torment an adolescent—arousing fears of isolation, ridicule, and humiliation. Restrictions on activities can further accentuate differences from others. For children entering adolescence with good self-esteem and a sense of independence, the impact of epilepsy can be minimal. In adolescents, however, epilepsy can aggravate or create problems of low self-esteem, dependency, or behavioral difficulties. Caring for adolescents with epilepsy requires special patience and understanding.

Children whose intelligence is at least near average and whose epilepsy is well controlled are able to achieve independence during adolescence and adulthood. Children with more severe physical and mental problems confront a different situation as they mature. Parents of adolescents who cannot achieve independence in the community must begin to explore the options for their future living arrangements, employment possibilities, legal and financial security, and social and sexual adjustments.

Puberty

Puberty marks the sexual transition from childhood to adolescence. The sex hormones estrogen and progesterone in girls and testosterone in boys, which were produced in small amounts during childhood, go into a mass-production phase during puberty. These hormones initiate the physical changes associated with puberty, which are a source of anxiety and adjustment. The age at which puberty begins varies considerably from one child to the next, and children who have early or late changes may be concerned (and sometimes teased) about the changes in their bodies compared with those of their schoolmates. Children may be too embarrassed to discuss these concerns with their parents.

The sex hormones affect the body *and* the brain. Sex hormones enter the brain and bind to receptors on nerve cells there, altering the activity of the brain. Changes in brain activity are related to changes in personality and mood. Just as hormones cause some women to experience emotional changes before their menstrual period begins and abuse of steroid hormones related to testosterone causes some athletes to become irritable or aggressive, adolescents also undergo changes in behavior related to hormones. Sometimes these hormonal changes bring out seizures for the first time.

For some children, seizures begin or stop around the time of puberty. This relationship between epilepsy and puberty may be a coincidence, or it may be a result of hormonal changes affecting the brain. Hormones such as estrogen may increase the likelihood of seizures; many women report that seizures most often occur around the time of their menstrual period. There is evidence that seizures occur more frequently during the premenstrual and ovulatory periods in some women.

Other brain changes that may be less directly related to hormones also occur during puberty. Early in adolescence, children gain greater fine motor control and begin to show more mature responses to complex problems. Their ability to think about abstract problems and moral issues is improved. Shortly after puberty, children are much better able to understand the consequences of certain behaviors in a theoretical sense; that is, they can understand the outcome of some behaviors without experiencing the outcome itself. For example, girls can understand that they may become pregnant as a consequence of sexual activity. This ability to consider the consequences of behavior has important implications for health matters such as epilepsy. At this point in their development, children are better able to participate in their own care.

The increased production and release of sex hormones into the bloodstream during puberty is not always a gradual, smooth process. The hormones may be released in large amounts over short periods. The changes in hormone levels can be associated with relatively rapid changes in personality, mood, irritability, and physical features, such as a new crop of pimples. The child is not "bad" or "misbehaving," but simply experiencing natural changes as part of development.

Metabolic changes along with the rapid changes in growth that accompany puberty may be unpredictable and can alter the blood levels of antiepileptic drugs. If seizure control worsens in an adolescent, a decrease in the drug levels should be considered.

Puberty also brings about changes in psychosocial development. The early adolescent is active in three arenas: the peer group (friends and schoolmates), family, and school. The peer group is often the focus of the young adolescent's life. The bonds are usually strongest among members of the same sex, with an emphasis on conformity and joint activities. The child seeks independence from the family. Earlier relationships with parents and sometimes with brothers and sisters are disrupted. As the physical changes of puberty begin, the child often seeks greater privacy, especially with regard to the parent of the opposite sex. The adolescent's testing of parental limits is a conflict between the desire for parental guidance and the desire for autonomy.

School life can also be affected by puberty. Intellectual and behavioral maturation will have an impact on school performance. Adolescents who mature sooner than their peers will usually enjoy higher academic performance, and those with relatively delayed maturation will perform more poorly. Also, adolescents who are very bright may rebel against their parents or react to stressors in their life by getting lower grades at school.

The maturity of children evolves during adolescence, but the changes are often erratic. Behaviors that demonstrate a remarkable degree of maturity may be followed closely by immature actions and reactions. Parents must be available to discuss questions and problems. They must support the child's independence while watching out for his or her safety and well-being. If the child is avoiding some important issues, it is reasonable for the parent to raise them, but if the child is uncomfortable with the discussion, it is best not to push. It is often helpful to enlist the help of an adult outside the immediate family, such as the doctor or someone else who is trusted and liked by the adolescent.

Taking Medications

I know Steve doesn't take his medication regularly. I try to remind him every morning and every night. It's more than forgetting—by not taking his medications, he is saying, "I don't really have epilepsy." I hope he realizes that he won't be able to drive if he still has his occasional complex partial seizures.

The maturity that adolescence brings should make children more aware of the benefits of taking their antiepileptic drugs. For some adolescents, however, rebellion or denial dominates the scene, making them less likely to take their medications as prescribed. When the child reaches early adolescence, it is essential for the parent to repeat the reasons for taking the antiepileptic drugs that were taught during childhood. Adolescents are normally able to understand the consequences of taking or not taking their medications. Education about antiepileptic drugs can come from both the parents and the doctor, but the adolescent should be enlisted as an active partner in his or her treatment. Teenagers with epilepsy should be allowed to take greater responsibility for managing their care. It is often helpful for the adolescent and doctor to be alone for a portion of each visit or even the whole visit. This makes the adolescent feel more in control and more mature and helps to establish trust with the doctor and the parents.

One of the most powerful factors in securing a child's compliance is peer pressure. The adolescent's desire to conform is strong. Seizures can be embarrassing and cause fears of social isolation. Also, uncontrolled seizures can result in restrictions on certain activities, such as driving. Adolescents should know that the longer they are free of seizures by taking medications, the better the chances are that they will be seizure-free without medications.

With older children and adolescents, the easiest and the best assessment of compliance is simply to ask them straight out: "Are you taking your medication?" Measuring the level of antiepileptic drugs in the blood at regular intervals can tell the doctor and the parents if the adolescent is taking the medications as prescribed. It also can reinforce compliance. However, problems with drug absorption or metabolism or a period of rapid growth in height and weight can cause the levels to be low even though the drugs are taken regularly.

Parent-Child Relationships

The nature of the relationships with his or her parents and friends will strongly influence the impact of epilepsy on the adolescent. Parents who have open communication and a strong basis of trust with their child before adolescence will have a much easier time relating to that child during the difficult times of adolescence. For parents who have relationship problems with their child, counseling may be helpful. Parenting is never easy, and parenting of a child with epilepsy during adolescence can be especially difficult. Parents should not hesitate to ask for help. The help can come from a friend, family member, religious leader, social worker, psychologist, or psychiatrist.

Parents must set limits, such as restricting certain activities and setting curfews. Setting limits is difficult for both parents and children. The concern for the child's safety must be balanced against his or her need for independence and peer-group acceptance. All children face some risks. Minimizing the risks does not justify severe restriction of their activities. The parents' goal should be to help their child achieve a mature and independent state. Parents should encourage adolescents to "think things out" and weigh the positive and negative aspects of their decisions. Parents should discuss strategies that can be used to reduce or eliminate negative factors. For example, it may be safe for a child to go on a canoeing and camping trip if certain precautions are taken. Then the child can experience the excitement and adventure of a new activity without the parents and can be included in the peer group. Parents should not see their role simply as protecting their child from danger—the greatest danger may be bringing up a dependent child who has poor self-esteem.

Peer Relationships

The adolescent peer group strongly influences the behavior of its members. In early adolescence, there is a strong need to be part of a group and to conform. Although the bonds at this age appear strong, the relationships are often shallow.

Parents should want their children to be socially active, but the friends they make are often not ideal in the parents' eyes. If friends clearly push a child toward dangerous behaviors, then the parent must intervene. That does not mean forbidding the child from ever socializing with these friends, but it does mean that the child should understand why such behaviors are dangerous and must be avoided. A real problem arises when the child is pressured into participating in repeated undesirable behaviors with friends.

Because acceptance by friends may be especially important for adolescents with epilepsy, parents must be careful in how they react. Often, social isolation is a much more dangerous situation than the rebellious activities of adolescence. However, young people used to rejection can be particularly vulnerable when undesirable groups show a willingness to associate with them. The Epilepsy Foundation (EF) has recently created a TeenChat Internet program that can be accessed through the main EF website (www.epilepsyfoundation.org). The program is open 24 hours a day. The most popular times are between 7 and 10 PM.

Driving

Driving a motor vehicle is one of the greatest acts of independence in our society. There is no other time in life when a certain birthday takes on such meaning as the age at which one can obtain a license to drive. Many people with epilepsy can drive, but there are obvious safety concerns (see Chap. 24).

In most states, a person with epilepsy must submit a letter or form from the doctor about his or her seizure disorder. Many states ask the doctor about compliance with medications. It is often helpful to remind adolescents that a favorable doctor's report depends on their taking the medications as prescribed.

As the age for driving approaches, it is often worthwhile to review the adolescent's medical care. If no seizures have occurred for several years, it may be wise to attempt to lower and eventually stop medications at least 6 months or a year before the driving age is reached. If the adolescent's seizures are poorly controlled, however, approaching the legal age for driving may prompt referral to an epilepsy center for reevaluation and possible changes in the treatment plan.

Adolescents with uncontrolled seizures cannot obtain a driver's license. Alternatives to driving include riding with friends, carpools, or public transportation. Lack of a driver's license should not stand in the way of social activities or holding a job (although it often does).

Dating

Dating does not come naturally to most people. Adolescents are often uncomfortable or uneasy when they start to date, and having epilepsy can complicate an already complicated social situation. Although it is a good idea to discuss epilepsy with a regular boyfriend or girlfriend, it is reasonable to wait until the relationship feels comfortable. The person should not be tested. For example, it is best not to make up "people you know with epilepsy" to see how the other person will react. If the discussion is open and honest, friends will be more willing to ask questions and share their feelings. If the adolescent's seizures are not well controlled, however, it may be a good idea to discuss the epilepsy with the boyfriend or girlfriend sooner rather than later. This situation can be awkward. It is best done in person—not over the telephone. In general, it is wise to wait a bit before talking about epilepsy with new friends. Even if it seems necessary to tell them on the first date, it is best to wait for the right moment.

Every person who has asked someone for a date has known the fear of rejection. It underlies much of the anxiety and discomfort associated with dating. Someone with epilepsy has the added fear that he or she will be rejected because of the epilepsy. This fear is not completely unfounded. Some people who hear the word epilepsy become frightened. They may have little or no knowledge about epilepsy, and fear of the unknown is great. They can be educated by someone who has the disorder. Then, their understanding of epilepsy and feelings about it will reflect the understanding and feelings of the person who lives with it.

Rejection is part of the dating game. No one is spared. People are attracted to others because of physical features and personality. The physical reasons may be more important at first, but the compatibility of personalities and the rapport that develops between people are what keep a couple together. People may be rejected because their nose is too big, their waist is too wide, or countless other physical reasons. People are also rejected because they are insecure, arrogant, obnoxious, lazy, selfish, or have some other personality trait. Most of the time, the reasons for rejection are not clearly defined in the mind of the person who is doing the rejecting. Although epilepsy is one of many possible reasons that someone may reject someone else, often it is not *the* reason. In addition, some people perceive rejection when it is not there; they expect it and therefore imagine it to exist. If the other person is already aware of the disorder before dating begins, the situation is much easier. In this case, there is less to explain and less fear that epilepsy will "turn the other person off."

Sexual Activity

As a couple grows closer in a relationship, there is a natural tendency to want to hold hands, kiss, and have other intimate contact. There are no universal rules about when to kiss or engage in other intimate activities. Religious upbringing; the attitudes of parents, local society, and friends; one's personal beliefs; and feelings about a certain person all influence these decisions. Friends provide the richest source of information about sex and about what other people are "doing." Unfortunately, adolescents, especially boys, often exaggerate their activities. This can lead their friends to have unrealistic expectations. For more information and discussions about dating and sex, it is helpful for the adolescent to talk with a trusted adult, such as a parent, older brother or sister, uncle or aunt, school counselor, or nurse or doctor. If this person is uncomfortable talking about these topics, however, it is best to go to another adult who is more at ease.

There is no reason to fear having a seizure during kissing or other intimate contact any more than at other times. Intimate contact does not protect someone from a seizure, however. Therefore, if a person has uncontrolled seizures, it is possible that one will occur during intimate contact. For this reason, the partner should know about the disorder and what to do if a seizure occurs.

Although most people with epilepsy are able to enjoy sexual feelings and activities, some have less interest than their peers in sexual activity. Libido (interest in sexual activity) may be affected by high dosages of antiepileptic drugs (especially the barbiturates) or the epilepsy itself. In most instances, the person with epilepsy is not aware of a problem. Instead, it may be noticed by a parent or a boyfriend or girlfriend. Because people have a wide range of interest in intimate relationships and sexual activity, the reduced interest may not be a problem. If it does become an issue, it may be helpful to discuss it with a doctor. In some cases, changing medications or reducing the dosage can be helpful.

Use of Alcohol and Illegal Drugs

When adolescents use alcohol or illegal drugs, trouble is not far behind. Their immaturity and willingness to take chances often put adolescents who use alcohol or other drugs in particularly dangerous places, such as behind the wheel of a motor vehicle. Few adolescents understand the potential dangers of illegal drugs. Those who have grown up in homes where alcohol and drugs were never abused may have no idea what intoxication is or what dangers these substances can bring. Those who have grown up in a home where alcohol or other drugs were abused may be more prone toward substance abuse.

The dangers of adolescent substance abuse are clear. Drinking contests continue to kill young people, and alcohol is the leading cause of motor vehicle accidents in the United States. Snorting cocaine and smoking crack can cause strokes, heart attacks, seizures, or death.

The rules concerning alcohol use and epilepsy apply to both adolescents and adults, but greater caution applies to the younger group. Drinking one or two alcoholic beverages causes no meaningful changes in the blood levels of antiepileptic drugs or in seizure control. The problem with one or two drinks for adolescents, whether or not they have epilepsy, is that their understanding of alcohol and their ability to limit its intake is often inadequate. One or two drinks become three or four, intoxication clouds judgment, and serious problems follow. Teenagers often will sleep off a hangover, and those with epilepsy may fail to take their bedtime and morning medications. Therefore, it is a good idea for all adolescents, especially those with epilepsy, to avoid alcohol or use it only under adult supervision, such as having a glass of wine or beer during a family dinner. Adolescents with epilepsy should know that alcohol abuse can worsen seizure control. In addition, the combination of antiepileptic drugs and alcohol can have a strong sedative effect. When excessive amounts of alcohol are consumed, the combination can be dangerous.

Crack and other forms of cocaine can cause seizures in people who have never had one before. Although there are no studies of the effects of crack or cocaine on seizure control, there is an obvious risk that these substances would make the occurrence of seizures more likely. Seizures that occur with cocaine or crack use can be fatal. They are much more dangerous than seizures that occur from other causes or spontaneously. This was clearly demonstrated in 1986 with the case of Len Bias, a basketball star from the University of Maryland who reportedly had seizures and died after using crack. Deadly seizures or heart attacks can occur even after the first-time use of these substances. Crack and cocaine are associated with other serious health problems as well. They should be avoided at all costs.

Seizures can be caused or made worse by the use of uppers (amphetamines), downers (barbiturates or benzodiazepines), heroin, certain pain killers, LSD (acid), PCP (angel dust), or ecstasy. The effects of these drugs on epilepsy are not known with certainty, but they can bring on seizures by causing the user to forget to take antiepileptic medications or to lose sleep. These drugs may also have direct and indirect (withdrawal) effects on the brain. The possession (except if prescribed by a doctor) or selling of all these drugs is illegal, and the severe penalties for even casual association with them, coupled with their numerous health risks, make their use foolish and dangerous.

Thinking about a Career

Most people do not decide on their future career while in high school. Nevertheless, it is often helpful for adolescents with epilepsy to give some thought to the type of career they would like to pursue. Certain classes in high school or college can be aimed toward gaining knowledge and skills related to an area of interest. Guidance counselors and vocational counselors often are available in high school to discuss career plans.

People with well-controlled or infrequent seizures should have few or no limitations on possible careers, but people with uncontrolled seizures may face some career limitations. Adolescents should ask the doctor about their outlook for seizure control. With new medications and advances in epilepsy surgery, it is likely that many people with uncontrolled seizures will become seizure-free in the future.

Adolescents with both epilepsy and developmental disabilities, such as mental retardation, cerebral palsy, or blindness, have never had greater opportunities for employment than they have today (see Chap. 27). Their success in obtaining gratifying employment depends on support from family, school, and medical services. Planning is critical. Adolescents and their families should work with educational, social, and medical resources to develop realistic plans for employment and independence. Vocational planning should focus on the person's ability to learn and master specific technical skills and appropriate social behavior. In many cases, specific training may be less important than self-esteem and personal skills for interacting in a work environment. Realistic but progressive and positive expectations underlie a successful plan.

Part-Time Employment

Part-time work can be rewarding for adolescents who have epilepsy. In addition to the financial rewards, work can provide discipline, skills, education, and a sense of accomplishment and success. A part-time job is often an important step toward independence. It also can be a way of getting some exposure to a career that the young person may be interested in pursuing, and it may even provide an opportunity for future full-time work.

Adolescents can work before or after school or during the summer. When working during the school year, the student must balance the demands of school and job. A job also should not interfere with a healthy personal life. Students who work too many hours often sacrifice sleep while trying to keep up with both schoolwork and a social life. Loss of sleep or the stress of overwork can increase the frequency of seizures, so it is important to limit the number of hours worked at a part-time job.

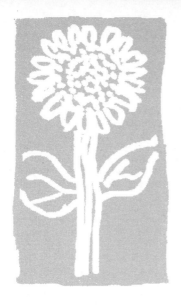

C H A P T E R

17

Outgrowing Epilepsy

Slightly more than half of the children who have epilepsy outgrow it. This simple and positive fact raises important questions: Which children should be treated? How much medication should they receive? How long should the antiepileptic drugs be used? In recent years, doctors have changed their minds about the use of antiepileptic drugs. Several decades ago, the prevailing attitude was that seizures must be stopped at all costs, and once seizures had been stopped, the medications should be continued indefinitely. This outdated approach reflected an overly pessimistic outlook on life with epilepsy. The risks of seizures were overestimated, and the adverse effects of medications were underestimated. Issues such as the quality of life or how patients felt about the frequency and severity of seizures and the adverse effects of therapy were rarely considered, and the natural course of epilepsy in children was poorly understood.

Over the past several decades, there has been a dramatic growth in our knowledge. We are now familiar with the natural history of various seizure types and epileptic syndromes and understand more about the safety of discontinuing antiepileptic drug therapy for specific forms of epilepsy.

215

Stopping Antiepileptic Drugs

Most children who remain seizure-free while taking medications for 1 or 2 years can safely have their medications slowly tapered by their doctors and eventually discontinued. Most of these children will not have another seizure. During the past decade, there has been a trend toward discontinuing medication earlier rather than later because the chances of staying seizure-free after 1 or 2 years of treatment are similar to those after 3 or 4 years. Among children who remain seizure-free while taking antiepileptic drugs for 2 years, approximately 65% will remain seizure-free after the medication is stopped.

The chance that a specific child will remain seizure-free if medications are stopped cannot be predicted with accuracy. Table 7 shows some of the factors that are associated with the risk of having another seizure after medications are stopped in seizure-free children. Favorable signs for remaining seizure-free, based on the study in the table and others, include epilepsy with no identifiable cause for the seizures, normal development and neurologic function, the absence of epilepsy waves on the electroencephalogram (EEG), and seizures that are easily controlled with medication. When all of these conditions are met, the child has an excellent chance of remaining seizure-free after the medications are stopped.

No matter how good the odds, there is a chance that the seizures will recur, and no matter how bad the odds, there is a chance that they will not. Many cases fall between the extremes, making the decision to stop the medications more difficult. As a general rule, it is usually worthwhile

TABLE 7
RISK FACTORS FOR PREDICTING RECURRENT SEIZURE IN CHILDREN

Diagnosis	EEG: No Epileptiform Discharges		EEG: Epileptiform Discharges	
	Neuro Exam Normal (%)	Neuro Exam Abnormal (%)	Neuro Exam Normal (%)	Neuro Exam Abnormal (%)
Tonic-clonic	30	51	47	73
Simple partial	50	75	71	92
Complex partial	58	83	77	96

EEG, Electroencephalogram.
Source: Camfield, PR, et al: Epilepsy after a first unprovoked seizure in childhood. Neurology 35:1657–1660, 1985.

to attempt to discontinue the medication after 2 years. When the child has two or more risk factors for seizure recurrence (first seizure after 12 years of age, neurologic or intellectual disabilities, or complex partial seizures), it may be reasonable to continue the medications until the child has been seizure-free for 4 years before attempting to withdraw them.

Signs indicating less chance of remaining seizure-free without medications are a progressive brain disorder or brain damage such as a birth injury; viral infection of the brain; head injury, developmental delay, mental retardation, or other neurologic abnormalities; the presence of epilepsy waves or moderate to severe slowing on the EEG; and seizures that are not easily controlled with antiepileptic drugs. When all of these factors are present, the chance of seizures recurring after medication is stopped is 50% or more. These are *average* risks, however, which cannot easily be applied to a particular individual. The decision to taper and discontinue medications should be made by the doctor and the parents. The child's opinion is also valuable if he or she is old enough and understands the issue.

Some times are better than others for stopping medication. For example, a girl on a gymnastics team who does difficult routines and dismounts on the uneven parallel bars probably should not begin tapering medications shortly before or during the gymnastic season. Summer camp, when the child will be swimming and boating, presents a similar situation. Also, as discussed in the previous chapter, it is a good idea, if possible, to stop medications at least a year before a teenager is eligible for a driver's license.

When all of these risks are considered, some parents and children may ask, "Why not simply continue to take the drugs? They don't seem to be doing any harm." If there is a moderate to high risk of seizure recurrence, and the medications have few adverse effects, the risks of stopping the drug may outweigh the benefits. However, benefits of stopping the medications make considering their discontinuance worthwhile.

RISKS

> I was frightened when the doctor recommended that we take Katie off the Tegretol. Of course, I wanted her off all medications, but even more, I wanted her seizure-free. We lowered the medication slowly. I slept poorly for months, thinking that any noise in the house was a seizure. She's been off medication for 3 years and has had no seizures.

The most obvious danger of stopping the medications is the chance that seizures will recur. If the medications are stopped abruptly, a recurrent seizure might be more severe or prolonged than the previous seizures. When any drug is withdrawn, the body reacts and undergoes chemical, electrical, and hormonal changes that may cause problems.

Discontinuation of an antiepileptic medication can also cause a withdrawal reaction. The rapid withdrawal of barbiturates (phenobarbital and primidone) and benzodiazepines (clonazepam, clorazepate, diazepam, lorazepam, and clobazam) is associated with the highest risk of a seizure or unpleasant symptoms, such as anxiety, irritability, a racing heart, difficulty sleeping, sweating, abdominal pain, vomiting, and problems with concentration. All withdrawal symptoms are reduced (and in many cases eliminated) when the dosage is lowered very slowly. When antiepileptic medications are properly discontinued, the risk of a withdrawal seizure is very small. Rapid discontinuation of any antiepileptic drug can be dangerous and should only be done under a doctor's supervision. Abrupt withdrawal can cause status epilepticus (see Chap. 6).

When an antiepileptic drug is tapered or withdrawn, seizures may occur simply because the drug was needed to control them. Depending on the type and severity of the seizures, the medications may need to be started again. In some cases, the child may remain seizure-free at a lower dosage than before. Differentiating this type of seizure recurrence from a withdrawal seizure is important because withdrawal seizures can be managed by a temporary increase in the dosage followed by more gradual tapering. Unfortunately, it is usually hard to know whether recurrent seizures result from withdrawal of the drug or the need for medication.

If the medications are stopped, the child, family, and school need to be prepared for the possibility that a seizure could occur. If the child has been seizure-free for 2 years or more, people tend to forget to take precautions. During the tapering and for at least 3 to 6 months after stopping the medications, the child's risk of a seizure is somewhat higher than usual, and simple precautions should be taken. For instance, the child should not swim without close supervision or climb to high places. Table 8 provides some other steps that should be taken to keep the child safe.

Three-quarters of seizure relapses occur within 1 year of stopping the medication. If a seizure recurs after a period of freedom from seizures, it is an emotional setback for both the child and the family. Parents must be prepared for this possibility and discuss it with the child. When people are aware that something is possible, they are much better able to handle it if it happens. Although children often will worry, sometimes in private, about the possibility of having another seizure, their fear diminishes with time.

A rare consequence of discontinuing the medication is the reemergence of difficult-to-control seizures or the development of intolerance to a medication that was previously well tolerated. These situations are very uncommon.

TABLE 8
TIPS ON DISCONTINUING ANTIEPILEPTIC DRUGS

- First-aid management should be reviewed with the child, the parents, and other caregivers.
- The usual medication should be kept on hand in case the child's seizures recur.
- If a seizure occurs, it may be appropriate to give the child a single dose of medication before contacting the doctor.
- If status epilepticus is a concern or access to medical care is a problem, parents should be taught how to administer diazepam rectal suppositories (for all age groups) or lorazepam under the tongue (for an older child or a teenager) when a seizure lasts longer than 5 minutes.
- It is normal for a child who has a recurrent seizure to become depressed, upset, or angry, but if the mood change persists longer than a week, a visit to the doctor is recommended.
- In case of a seizure recurrence, it may be comforting to use an intercom system between the parent's and child's bedrooms or an alerting device, such as the one made by Fisher-Price (costs less than $50), at bedtime or when the child is asleep.

BENEFITS

In the best of all worlds, when the medications are stopped, seizures will not recur and the child will feel better, show improved school performance and behavior, and enjoy the freedom of good health without medication. When a child has been taking a medication for more than 2 years, it can be difficult to estimate the effect that the drug has on the child's behavior. This is particularly true if the dosage was gradually increased over a long period. In many cases, although the medication was thought to have no adverse effect, the child's alertness, ability to concentrate, memory, ability to reason, and behavioral problems such as irritability and hyperactivity improve after the medication is stopped. However, some antiepileptic drugs (such as carbamazepine, lamotrigine, and valproate) can have positive effects on a child's behavior, and occasionally their discontinuation is associated with increased behavioral problems.

In a few people, long exposure to a medication (usually more than 2 to 5 years) can cause problems, such as bone loss. Phenobarbital and phenytoin can cause soft-tissue growths. Phenytoin can also cause nerve injury, excessive hair growth (hirsutism), and damage to the cerebellum of the brain (which affects coordination). Girls who continue taking medication and want to become pregnant later in life will expose their babies to a higher-than-normal risk of birth defects. All of these problems can be avoided by stopping the medications as soon as possible. Because we cannot assess all of the long-term consequences of taking medication, discontinuing the drugs may have other benefits that have not yet been discovered.

Long-Term Treatment

Although most forms of childhood epilepsy are outgrown, some forms are associated with a high risk of recurrent seizures if the medications are stopped. If the EEG shows abundant epilepsy waves or epilepsy waves arising from multiple regions of the brain, the risk of seizures after stopping medications is high. Juvenile myoclonic epilepsy, for example, is associated with a high rate of seizure recurrence after medication is stopped. This epilepsy disorder varies dramatically in its severity, however, and some children have only mild myoclonic jerks a few hours after awakening. For them, stopping the medication may be reasonable. In Lennox-Gastaut syndrome and the progressive myoclonic epilepsies, the seizures are severe and difficult to control. If control is achieved, it is usually wise to continue the medication. For these children, it is more reasonable to try to reduce the dosage of the medication slightly than to discontinue it.

18

Intellectual and Behavioral Development

For parents, watching the growth and development of their child's mind and body is magical. Our society loves to compare things—cars, houses, and, unfortunately, children. Comparing the development of children is unwise because each child's development is a highly individual process. Although certain yardsticks help define a range of developmental milestones in the general population, development is complex. A child must be viewed as an individual, not a statistic or a point on a graph. Delays in one area of development are often accompanied by early advances in other areas. There are no prizes for getting to a certain point first.

Most children with epilepsy do not develop any differently than children without epilepsy. However, children who have frequent or severe seizures that remain uncontrolled, who are being treated with large amounts of antiepileptic drugs, or who have other disorders of brain function may experience some delays in development.

Table 9 summarizes the major milestones associated with large (gross motor) and small (fine motor) movements, personal and social behavior, and language development in babies and young children. It gives a rough estimate of "average" development. It is important to remember that some children attain specific skills somewhat later than indicated and still grow up to be bright and well-coordinated adults.

TABLE 9
MILESTONES IN THE DEVELOPMENT OF INFANTS AND CHILDREN*

Age (Months)	Gross Motor	Fine Motor	Personal–Social	Language
1	Strong suck	—	Smiles responsively	—
3	Rolls over, can pick up head while lying down	Briefly grasps rattle, puts hands together	Smiles spontaneously	Laughs, squeals
6	Sits with support with steady head	Reaches for objects, begins to grasp with one hand (not two)	Feeds self cracker	Turns to voice
9	Sits well, pulls self to sitting position, crawls with arms	Grasps object between thumb and forefinger	Plays pat-a-cake and peek-a-boo	Imitates speech sounds, may say mama or dada
12	Stands alone, walks holding furniture or walls (cruises), may walk without support	Grasps small object (e.g., raisin) between thumb and forefinger	May drink from cup, may play ball, often shy	Says dada or mama (specific person)
15	Walks by self, toddles and falls	Scribbles with crayon, builds tower of two cubes, dumps small items from a bottle	Drinks from cup, indicates wants without crying	Says one to three words other than mama and dada

	Gross Motor	Fine Motor/Adaptive	Personal-Social	Language
18	Walks up or down stairs holding on, throws ball, walks backward	Removes shoes and socks, unzips clothes	Uses spoon well, imitates housework	Combines two words, points to one to three body parts and common objects
24	Walks up steps by self, bends over and picks up objects, runs	Turns knob, kicks ball	Washes hands, puts on some clothing, assists with housework	Uses two- or three-word sentences, points to four or five body parts
30	Jumps with both feet, pedals tricycle, walks on tiptoes	Builds tower of four to eight cubes	Puts on most clothing, uses spoon with little spilling, helps put away toys	Asks questions, knows full name, knows one to six colors
36	Stands on one foot, broad jumps, rides tricycle	Copies "0"	Dresses self except buttons, plays well with others	Recites nursery rhymes, asks "why," uses pronouns correctly
48	Hops on one foot, walks on one foot per step on stairs	Copies "+" and square, picks longer of two lines	Buttons clothing, separates easily from parent, cooperates in play	Tells stories, understands opposites, counts three to four objects

*These milestones are usually reached at the ages shown, but children vary considerably in their development, and some children with average or superior motor and language functions in later childhood may lag in one or more of these early milestones.

If development is significantly delayed, parents should consult a pediatrician or pediatric neurologist about the cause of the delay and what it may mean for the future. In most cases, however, doctors cannot make precise predictions about a child's future development. For children with frequent seizures, who often take high dosages of one or more antiepileptic drugs, it can be difficult to determine whether the slow development is the result of a physical brain abnormality, seizures, or medications. In some children, development slows or stops when seizures become frequent or severe; when the seizures come under better control, their development improves.

Even children with severe cerebral palsy or mental retardation show development. The rate may be slow, and the process may be laborious, but the gains are no less meaningful and exciting. In some cases, the child may lose certain milestones previously achieved. This regression may be brief, lasting weeks or months, or it may persist over years. These losses are sometimes associated with degenerative disorders (progressive and deteriorating conditions, often associated with loss of brain cells), but such a loss does not necessarily mean that the child has one of these disorders.

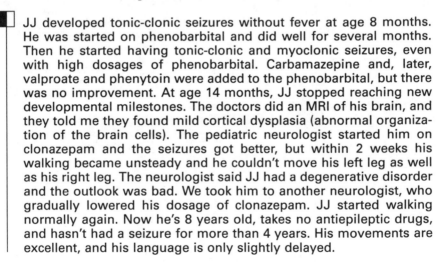

JJ developed tonic-clonic seizures without fever at age 8 months. He was started on phenobarbital and did well for several months. Then he started having tonic-clonic and myoclonic seizures, even with high dosages of phenobarbital. Carbamazepine and, later, valproate and phenytoin were added to the phenobarbital, but there was no improvement. At age 14 months, JJ stopped reaching new developmental milestones. The doctors did an MRI of his brain, and they told me they found mild cortical dysplasia (abnormal organization of the brain cells). The pediatric neurologist started him on clonazepam and the seizures got better, but within 2 weeks his walking became unsteady and he couldn't move his left leg as well as his right leg. The neurologist said JJ had a degenerative disorder and the outlook was bad. We took him to another neurologist, who gradually lowered his dosage of clonazepam. JJ started walking normally again. Now he's 8 years old, takes no antiepileptic drugs, and hasn't had a seizure for more than 4 years. His movements are excellent, and his language is only slightly delayed.

Effects of Seizures and Antiepileptic Drugs on Mental Functions

Single seizures do not permanently impair intellectual or behavioral functions. The long-term effects of numerous or recurrent seizures are still the subject of study and controversy. Most types of seizures do not have permanent effects on mental functions. This is especially true for absence and simple partial seizures. Children who have frequent complex partial seizures may have some memory impairment and behavioral disorders, but it has not been proved that the seizures actually cause the problems. Many of these children have scar tissue in the parts of the brain that are important for memory or emotion, and this scar tissue may be responsible for the cognitive and behavioral difficulties as well as the seizures.

Children who have frequent or prolonged tonic-clonic seizures tend to do less well on tests of intelligence and memory, which suggests that, if frequent or prolonged, this type of seizure may be harmful. In addition, a large number of tonic-clonic seizures (e.g., more than 100 in a lifetime) or episodes of status epilepticus (very prolonged seizures) may be associated with some adverse effects on mental function. However, brain disorders such as cerebral palsy may also be present, and the intellectual problems can be caused by the underlying condition of the brain—not just by the seizures. Children who have frequent atonic, tonic, and tonic-clonic seizures, which make them prone to fall, should wear a protective helmet because head injury (especially repeated episodes) also can impair intellectual function. Separating the contributing effects of underlying brain abnormalities, recurrent seizures, head injury, antiepileptic drugs, and psychosocial factors in intellectual and behavioral disorders is difficult both in clinical studies of patients in general and in individual patients. Any of these factors can be the most important cause of a problem in a specific child, but the role of recurrent complex partial and tonic-clonic seizures has probably been underestimated.

Antiepileptic drugs can also impair intellectual performance and cause behavioral problems. However, among the primary antiepileptic drugs (see Table 3, p. 127), these effects are generally slight, particularly when the drugs are given in the usual dosages. In studies comparing a wide range of cognitive (intellectual) functions of children before and after the discontinuation of antiepileptic drugs, the functions did not improve or only slightly improved after the drugs were stopped. However, the effects of antiepileptic drugs are often dose-related, so children given high dosages are more likely to have significant adverse mental effects. In addition, drugs affect children (and adults) individually. Although group averages may show no statistically significant difference, some individuals may experience real problems, even at low therapeutic blood drug levels.

 The first pediatric neurologist told me that phenobarbital was like water, that we would never know that Brenda was on it. He was wrong. She became cranky, hyperactive, and slept poorly—she was a different child. We were told this would pass, but it only seemed to get worse as time went on. We felt like we had lost our child. If we had to choose between the seizures or the adverse effects, we would take the seizures. We eventually went for a second opinion, and she was changed to Tegretol. She had a rash 2 weeks later. Then she was put on Depakote. She has had no seizures, and we have our daughter back.

The drugs never seemed to bother Allison. She has been on phenobarbital since she was 5 years old. When Tegretol was added to the phenobarbital, she still did well. We eventually got her off the phenobarbital, and now she is just on the Tegretol. She is in the top of her class and on the field hockey team.

Aside from the barbiturates, such as phenobarbital and primidone, and the benzodiazepines, such as clonazepam and clorazepate, there is no convincing evidence that one of the other major antiepileptic drugs is much more likely to cause cognitive or behavioral problems than another drug, although any of the antiepileptic drugs potentially can cause troublesome side effects in one specific child. The barbiturates and benzodiazepines are most likely to cause intellectual and behavioral problems. The behavioral problems most often include hyperactivity, irritability, decreased attention span, memory impairment, sleep alterations, aggressiveness, and mood changes (including depression). Children and adolescents who have a close family member with major depression may be at special risk for becoming depressed when treated with a barbiturate. Nevertheless, barbiturates and benzodiazepines are useful in treating seizures, and many children do well while taking them. The antiepileptic drug topiramate has been found to cause impaired word retrieval, slowing of mental processes, and depression in some patients, but it's not certain whether the rate of these problems is higher with topiramate than with other antiepileptic drugs.

As the dosage and blood levels of antiepileptic drugs increase, the adverse effects also increase. Excessive drowsiness and need for sleep, slowed thinking and movement, decreased initiative and motivation, memory lapses, and other cognitive problems become more pronounced with higher blood levels.

Combinations of antiepileptic drugs are also more likely to cause cognitive problems and other adverse effects. As discussed in Chapter 10, when high doses or combinations of antiepileptic drugs are used, there must be a careful balance between the beneficial effects and the adverse effects of the therapy. The goal of treatment is freedom from seizures without adverse effects. If this goal cannot be attained, the adverse effects of the seizures must be weighed against the adverse effects of the drugs. For example, the doctor probably would not choose to increase the dosage to the point of sedation or emotional and intellectual dulling just to reduce complex partial seizures from three a month to one a month. After all, a complex partial seizure may be disruptive only 1 to 3 minutes during the seizure and perhaps 20 minutes afterwards, but the adverse effects would be present, in varying degrees, throughout every day of the child's life.

Difficult decisions about the use of antiepileptic drugs come when the adverse effects are subtle and intermittent. A description of the child's behavior, based on the parent's observations and supplemented by reports from teachers and others who are familiar with the child, is invaluable to the doctor. It is extremely important to record the adverse effects and relate their occurrence to the time medications are taken. Both adverse effects and seizures often can be reduced by changing the medication schedule. For example, the medication can be given after meals to reduce adverse effects caused by rapid absorption of the drug. In other cases, more frequent but smaller doses can help to maintain steadier blood levels of the drug, thereby reducing adverse effects and improving seizure control. When adverse effects are bothersome in the daytime, or seizures are most likely to occur during sleep or shortly after awakening, the bedtime or after-dinner dose can be increased and the daytime doses can be decreased. Midday doses of medication during the school day may be able to be avoided if the child feels embarrassed by going to the nurse for medication.

When a child has taken antiepileptic drugs for years, it may be difficult to detect the adverse effects of the medication. It is often impossible to untangle the effects of the normal turmoil of youth, an underlying neurologic disorder, the recurrent seizures, and the medications. Also, if the child has been taking medications from an early age, it is impossible to know exactly what his or her behavior would be like without them, and asking the child how a drug makes him or her feel won't be helpful if the child can't remember what it was like to be free of medications. In some cases, it is only after the medications are discontinued or changed that a difference can be recognized, making everyone realize how the medications were affecting the child.

Some children with epilepsy have associated neurologic disorders. Although these disorders affect intellect and behavior, it is common to blame the antiepileptic drugs or seizures for the problems. In fact, these children may be more susceptible to the adverse effects of both seizures and antiepileptic drugs.

Building Self-Esteem in Children with Epilepsy

It seems strange that it took a social worker at the epilepsy center to make me realize what I had been doing. By doing everything for Tricia, I was making her more dependent on me—making her bed, helping her dress, clearing her dishes, always staying within a few feet in case she were to have a seizure, and everything else I was doing because I'm her mother and I love her. I never thought she could put her own sneakers on until she did it at the hospital. It is hard to let go, but it is exciting to see what Tricia can do.

Of all the things that parents can give children, the opportunity to develop self-esteem and self-confidence is among the most important. For children to develop, learn, and interact at school—and to grow successfully toward independence and adulthood—they must have a strong and positive sense of self. Building self-esteem requires a parent to be patient, use educational discipline, provide opportunities for children to do things independently, and praise them for their initiatives and progress.

The parents of a child with epilepsy must first maintain their own self-esteem (see Chap. 20). Having a child with an illness, especially one that has been associated with negative attitudes, punctures the balloon of perfection that parents like to imagine for their children. Before they can help their child to build his or her own self-esteem, the parents should reflect on their own feelings about the child's disorder. Even very young children can sense and understand their parents' feelings.

Parents must emphasize the positive and minimize the negative aspects. They should focus on the things that the child can do and build on those achievements. Negative messages can limit self-esteem and motivation. Parents should try hard not to show their frustration at what the child cannot do or compare their child negatively with brothers or sisters, relatives, or other children. Talking about "the problem" in front of the child is not a good idea. This is not to say that parents should not discuss the epilepsy in a supportive fashion, but they should not focus on the child as a problem. Discussing financial problems and the burden of the medical care in front of the child should be avoided. The child's condition should not be used as an excuse for avoiding family activities. It is not a good practice to say, for example, "We'd love to come over for the party, but Judy's seizures have really been a problem lately, and I think we should stay home." Brothers and sisters should not be made the child's caretakers because this may limit their independence and activities and breed resentment. The child's condition must not be used as an excuse for limiting his or her participation in activities, such as school clubs or scouts because this will send the message to the child that the parents do not have confidence in him or her.

No parent is perfect. All parents get frustrated and say things and show emotions they later wish that they had not. Children are resilient. It is important for parents to recognize ways in which they can be more positive and encouraging to their child who has epilepsy. Parenting of children with special needs is an exceptional challenge, and resources are available for parents who need support (see Appendixes 4 and 5).

ENCOURAGING PERSONAL RESPONSIBILITY

Children can understand epilepsy. That includes children with epilepsy and children without it. Children should be told about the condition in words they can understand. They should know why taking medication on time is important, why tests are done, and why certain activities may have to be restricted. Children usually understand more than adults give them credit for. The Epilepsy Foundation (EF) has pamphlets for children that explain the condition in simple terms.

If possible, a child with epilepsy should know the name of their medication, the color of the pill, the dosage, and the schedule for taking it. Certainly an attentive parent can do everything needed to manage the condition and make the child a passive participant in his or her care, but this should be resisted. The earlier trust and knowledge are given to the child, the sooner the disorder will cease to be a disability.

AVOIDING OVERPROTECTIVENESS

There is a fine line between healthy caution and overprotection. Parents have a strong and natural tendency to direct their children's behavior. They want them to do the things they think are right and not to do the things they deem wrong or dangerous. For children with epilepsy and other related disorders, this tendency may become exaggerated, and parents may drift into being overprotective. They are often unaware of their directive behavior, or they fiercely defend it. Doing everything for children and restricting their exposure to the usual challenges of childhood takes away independence, slows their social growth, and lowers their self-esteem. They see their peers maturing while they remain children.

Overprotectiveness can take many forms. In the extreme form, children may never be told they have epilepsy; they are given medications by their parents, who refuse to tell them why they are taking them. They may try to figure out what the problem is by going to the library and reading about medical disorders. There are still some children and even young adults who are largely confined to their houses because of the parents' fear that they could be injured if they go out. Fortunately, mild overprotectiveness is much more common. In this case, children are encouraged to do things and to take responsibility, but their parents are still too fearful of dangers and show their love by doing and restricting too much. Sometimes, less is better.

The excessively dependent child is in danger of becoming overly attached to the person who cares for him or her most of the time. Prolonged dependence and over-attachment foster separation anxiety. This can make it difficult for the child to adjust later to play groups and school settings. In addition, it may leave the child vulnerable if the caretaker and child become separated. A clinging, overprotective parent does not produce a happy, secure child. Instead the child is anxious, dependent, and frightened of the rest of the world.

Children usually survive their parents. Most children will become independent long before their parents are gone. However, some children with severe epilepsy and associated neurologic disorders remain dependent and will require some degree of supportive care throughout their lives. Because the parents of these children will not be around forever, they must plan for the child eventually to live in some type of supportive environment, such as a residential home or "independent living center." Such planning should begin early so that the young person gets into the system while the parents are able to oversee the conditions and make sure the living arrangement meets their son's or daughter's medical and social needs. Parents who have cared for a severely affected child may feel reluctant to let go in this way, but when they do, they assure a smooth transition for the young adult. Regardless of the severity of the epilepsy or associated neurologic and physical disorders, young people should be encouraged toward independence and self-care.

ENCOURAGING SOCIAL CONTACTS

One of the most important parts of childhood is learning to relate, play, disagree, share, make friendships, and grow together—in other words, to socialize. Perhaps the greatest cost of overprotection and isolation is limited social contacts. No matter how loving and giving parents are, they can never replace the joys and lessons that children bring to each other. Although children can inflict upon each other the cruelest insults and most painful taunts and teasing, the parents must move beyond the fears of possible problems. Children, even those with epilepsy, need other children.

Parents should encourage their child's participation in activities with other children. These activities can range from play groups and play dates, where parents and children get together, to "mommy and me" classes for 18- to 36-month-olds; preschool programs; nursery and kindergarten classes; school classes; extracurricular activities, such as sports, dancing, singing, or crafts; and, for older children, independently playing with other children after school and on weekends. Parents should emphasize the principle of inclusion, not exclusion. Epilepsy is not a reason for excluding a child from the social world of children. Although the parents may believe some activities are unsafe, it is often worthwhile to speak with the doctor and the child about such activities. In some cases, special precautions, including supervision by parents, can be taken to make these activities safer.

Children with epilepsy may benefit from meeting, talking, and playing with other children who have epilepsy. Local EF affiliates frequently offer camps, buddy systems, and other programs that provide ways for children with similar conditions to get together. For a child to learn that he or she is not alone can be enormously comforting; there is something special about a comrade. The chance to see someone else who has a similar problem can change a child's entire outlook on the disorder. If an area has no groups for children with epilepsy, a motivated parent is the perfect person to get one going. Parents can work with the pediatrician, neurologist, and local EF office to help establish a group for children with epilepsy or even a simple buddy system of two kids getting together regularly.

If a child wishes to join a group for children with epilepsy, the parents should inquire about the range of neurologic and other handicaps among children in the group. Many groups have a mix of children—some who have had only one or two seizures and have normal physical and neurologic development and others who have severe cerebral palsy with multiple physical challenges and mental handicap. In such cases, the child should be told that the group includes other children with more serious problems and should be reassured that these difficulties will not happen to him or her.

USING EDUCATIONAL DISCIPLINE

Susie has always been impossible. She does what she wants, when she wants. Nothing worked—taking away her favorite toys or foods, sending her up to her room, or raising my voice. We wanted to give up. Then a friend with a child who has cerebral palsy and hyperactivity told me what she thought we were doing wrong. We were inconsistent, often giving in to her tantrums. We reacted to Susie with frustration, never really understanding her needs. It took a lot of hard work. Before Susie could change, we had to change. Now Susie's favorite book is *Clifford's Manners* (see Appendix 5).

Some parents of children with epilepsy overindulge them and ignore bad behaviors as a way of "making up" for the epilepsy or because they fear that sterner punishment will cause more seizures. Although seizures can occasionally be brought on by emotional stress, there is no evidence that they are caused by *educational discipline*. Educational discipline means explaining why the child's behavior was wrong and withholding something the child desires or using the technique of "time out," in which reinforcement is withheld. For example, the child must go to the corner of the room and stand quietly for a minute or so because of bad behavior. There is ample evidence that an undisciplined child can face serious problems in learning to socialize in a healthy fashion with other children, to behave and learn at school, and to grow up to be an independent and well-functioning adult. If a child has epilepsy, the problems will be compounded by allowing the child to have and do whatever he or she wants.

Caring for children causes some frustration. Even the best-natured child gets ornery, cranky, mischievous, jealous, angry, or even aggressive. Children reflect the emotions and behaviors of those around them. When a child requires discipline, it is often best to pause before reacting. Most children respond well to a quiet and calm explanation of why their behavior was wrong or why they cannot have what they want. However, any child can challenge even superhuman patience at times.

For children with epilepsy, who have to deal with more problems than average, educational discipline is critical. Because of their seizures, medications, and, in some cases, their associated neurologic disorders, these children are more likely to have certain behavioral problems. The unwanted behavior can be prevented or controlled by taking the time to explain things—not by spankings or other types of corporal punishment. If behavioral problems develop after a new medication is started or after the dosage is increased, the doctor should be told because the medication may be causing or aggravating the problems. Even "harmless" drugs, such as gabapentin (Neurontin), can cause dramatic adverse behavioral effects.

Managing Behavioral Problems

Although someone has both a problem, such as irritability, and a disorder, such as epilepsy, it does not prove that the disorder causes the problem. Nevertheless, behavioral problems are more common among children with epilepsy. As mentioned earlier, determining the cause of behavioral or intellectual disorders in children with epilepsy can be difficult. Parents may think their child is misbehaving when, in fact, the problems are caused by absence seizures, partial seizures, or other disorders (such as tics). It is natural for parents to assume that a child who "doesn't listen," for example, is misbehaving. When the behavior is accounted for by a diagnosis of epilepsy, parents may feel guilty for scolding the innocent child. This guilt is natural, but it is neither justified nor productive. Children with epilepsy have seizure-related problems— that is, disturbances occurring before, during, and after their seizures. Additionally, in some cases, they have other behavioral disorders that may or may not be related to the epilepsy.

SEIZURE-RELATED PROBLEMS

Although behavioral disorders preceding seizures by hours to days have been described by doctors for more than a century, there is still a scarcity of information about these problems. Many family members and older children with epilepsy describe changes in personality, mood, and other symptoms, such as a headache, that reliably precede a seizure by hours or days; these are called *premonitory symptoms.*

Behavioral problems are most often seen shortly after seizures, but they can also occur during seizures. During complex partial and absence seizures, children are inattentive and cannot understand or remember what is happening in the world around them. Some parents and teachers may feel that the child is not paying attention, is purposely ignoring what they say, or has a learning disability. During complex partial seizures, some children act in a strange way (automatisms). For example, the child may laugh or cry for no apparent reason, scream, shout, kick, spit, run, make rocking movements, or partially undress. Such actions are easily confused with a behavioral disorder.

Simple partial seizures can cause a variety of symptoms that are upsetting for adults and bewildering or frightening for children. The symptoms include experiencing bodily sensations and discomforts; feeling powerful emotions, such as fear, anxiety, depression, or embarrassment for no apparent reason; feeling as if the mind and body are separating; having strange thoughts suddenly racing through the mind; seeing objects and people get larger or smaller or appear distorted; seeing things that are not there (visual hallucinations); smelling things that are not there (olfactory hallucinations); and hearing things that are not there (auditory hallucinations). Many children have great difficulty describing these symptoms to their parents or the doctor. In many cases, they are only discovered when someone specifically asks about them. Even then, it may be hard to determine whether some children are simply saying "yes" to the questions or whether their answers relate to what they have actually experienced.

As occur in most children with complex partial and tonic-clonic seizures, temporary behavioral changes observed after seizures include confusion and tiredness. Also, verbal or physical aggressiveness or running away may occur if the child is confronted or restrained after the seizure. These difficulties can often be avoided by speaking in a soft and comforting manner and not restraining the child. The confusion that follows certain seizures may be mild but can cause difficulties with memory, understanding language (including parental instructions), and ability to do schoolwork. If a seizure goes unnoticed, the parents may think that the child has misbehaved when he or she fails to do as the parent has asked.

Children with epilepsy are like all other children. When kids with epilepsy misbehave usually it is simply because they are kids. Often they do not do what their parents ask them to do, or they do the exact opposite. Parents should not blame every little thing on seizures and epilepsy.

OTHER BEHAVIORAL PROBLEMS

The period between seizures is the time when children with epilepsy live most of their lives. Behavioral problems that may occur in this period often have a serious affect on them. In many cases, the epilepsy itself is probably unrelated to the problem behavior. The types of problems include learning disorders, difficulty with concentration (attention deficit), hyperactivity, and language and cognitive impairments, as well as anxiety, irritability, aggressive verbal or physical behavior, depression, mood swings, poor social skills, lack of motivation and energy, and inability to plan and organize behavior.

Learning Disorders

In children with learning disorders, there is a discrepancy between intellectual level and academic achievement; that is, intelligence outpaces achievement. A major cause of learning disorders is a neurologic disorder. Children with epilepsy, by definition, have a neurologic disorder and thus have an increased risk of a learning disorder. However, although the rate of learning disorders is higher among children with epilepsy than among the general population, most children with epilepsy do not have learning disorders.

To learn is to absorb, remember, and apply information. It requires a complicated series of brain processes. The absorption process requires paying attention and perceiving (seeing and hearing the material). The memory process requires actively comparing the newly acquired information with previously learned information and recalling it when necessary. These are but a few of the many complex steps in the process of learning.

The learning process can be disrupted in many different ways. The most extensively studied learning disorder is *dyslexia*, a developmental reading disorder. The cause of dyslexia is not understood, but it may result from some microscopic abnormality in the structure and functions of the left temporal and parietal lobes—brain areas that are critical for reading and language comprehension. Seizures can arise from these areas.

Many things can impair reading. Children who are unable to focus their attention for more than a few seconds can have reading problems. Poor vision that is not corrected can impair reading. Reading will also be impaired if there is a problem with sending visual information from the eye to the brain, with the areas of the brain that process visual information, or with the language areas of the brain. Reading also can be disrupted by abnormalities on the right side of the brain that allow someone to see only the right half of the page or the right half of individual words.

Reading is only one of many specific functions that can be impaired in people who have learning problems. Some people have problems with arithmetic, spoken information (because of impaired hearing or processing of sound by the brain), visual information other than reading, relating visual information to movement components (visuomotor disorders), or relating objects in space (disorders of visuospatial analysis). Other children have difficulty understanding social rules and emotionally relating to peers or adults.

A child who is suspected of having a learning disability should be evaluated by specialists, such as school psychologists, neuropsychologists, or child study teams. Such services can be requested through the child's school (see Chap. 21). The evaluation can often identify the cause of a learning disorder. Testing should not be limited to measuring the intelligence quotient (IQ test), an achievement test, and measures of emotional function. A common scenario is that a child is found to have a normal IQ, substandard achievement, and some emotional difficulties. With a diagnosis of "behavioral disorder," the child is placed in a classroom for "children with behavioral disorders." To avoid misdiagnosis, neuropsychological testing must include assessment of language, memory, attention, and other cognitive functions not adequately assessed with an IQ test.

Seizures can affect academic performance and learning. Brief staring spells, whether they are absence seizures or complex partial seizures, can lead to missed information. When the seizures are frequent, the child can miss large amounts of information; the child is essentially "tuned out" and does not hear or absorb what is being taught. In the case of complex partial seizures, memory is often affected for minutes or longer after the seizure has ended. In the case of tonic-clonic seizures, memory can be affected for hours after the seizure has ended. Epilepsy, especially when it is severe or associated with other medical and neurologic disorders, may require medical treatment or hospitalization that causes the child to miss school, which can affect learning. In some children, antiepileptic drugs can contribute to learning problems. In other cases, the ability to learn can be impaired temporarily by frequent small epilepsy waves on the EEG that do not cause obvious symptoms, by frequent minor seizures, or by occasional tonic-clonic seizures.

Attention Deficit Disorder

A little more than a century ago, the American psychologist William James wrote the following description of attention: "Everyone knows what attention is. It is the taking possession by the mind, in clear and vivid form, of one out of what seem several possible objects or trains of thought." Attention is the cornerstone on which intellectual functions rest. If we do not pay attention, we cannot efficiently understand, learn, or remember. We are all confronted by a swarm of sensations, feelings, and thoughts at any one moment. Only a small fraction of these reach our conscious awareness. Attention is the filtering process that allows us to focus on the important things. Without the complex attentional systems of our brains, our minds would be overwhelmed by the bombardment of images and sensations coming at us from the inside (our mind and body) and outside (our environment). We take for granted the amount of filtering out of unimportant information that our brains do every moment we are awake. The filtering system develops in children just as the systems that control fine movements and the ability to learn abstract mathematical relationships develop. A 3-year-old simply cannot sit quietly for 3 hours and read; his or her attentional system is too immature to filter out distractions such as the sound of the television or the sight of a friend.

A common problem in schoolchildren is attention deficit disorder (ADD). It is characterized by the inability to maintain attention, poor concentration, distractibility, and impulsivity. These problems clearly exceed the normal behavior for the child's age and interfere with learning. Teachers and parents usually notice them. ADD usually begins before the age of 5 years and is thought to be more common in boys. Girls have similar rates of ADD but often their behavior is not disruptive so their disorder goes unrecognized.

Hyperactivity (discussed later) and ADD often coexist in the same child. The two disorders are separate, however, and one may occur without the other. ADD refers to cognitive behavior; hyperactivity refers to motor behavior. Children with epilepsy may have higher incidences of both ADD and hyperactivity. In some children with epilepsy and ADD, the attentional (and hyperactivity) problem is related to the underlying neurologic problem that also causes epilepsy.

The cause of ADD is unknown. Genetic factors appear to contribute. Parents of some children report that consumption of sugar "sets them off" and "winds them up," reducing their attention span. Medical studies, however, have generally not found dietary restrictions to be effective, other than the possibility that eliminating foods with colorings and additives may improve 5% to 10% of cases. ADD may be a disorder of brain maturity or a chemical imbalance. Most children adapt to their

ADD, although many continue to have attentional problems in adolescence and adulthood.

Medications can cause or intensify attentional problems. Any drug that makes a person tired has the potential to impair attention. Among the medications used to treat epilepsy, phenobarbital and primidone are the most likely to impair attention and cause hyperactivity; the benzodiazepines (i.e., diazepam and clonazepam) can also have the same effect. If attentional problems develop or worsen after a drug is started or the dosage is increased, the doctor should be informed. In some children, the problem may lessen within weeks or a few months, but for others the dosage may need to be reduced or the medication changed.

When ADD causes learning or social problems, treatment with drugs may be helpful. The drugs used to treat ADD are classified as stimulants because in adults they increase alertness and decrease the need for sleep. In children with ADD, however, the stimulants act in an opposite manner, leading to a more relaxed and focused state of mind. The drugs most commonly used are methylphenidate (Ritalin and Concerta) and amphetamines (Adderall and Dexedrine). They can be used safely in children for prolonged periods, but a doctor must carefully supervise their use. Short-term use of these drugs may cause decreased appetite and weight loss, stomach discomfort, difficulty sleeping, depression, and irritability. As the child grows older, gradual reduction of the ADD medications should be considered because the disorder may be outgrown. Also, there is a growing problem of abuse of stimulants by adolescents, who crush the pills into a powder and snort it. When consumed in this form, these drugs are dangerous to the heart and brain.

The drugs used to treat ADD and hyperactivity can be used safely in nearly all children with epilepsy. Sleep deprivation from any cause, including stimulants, can potentially increase seizure frequency or severity, however. Methylphenidate can occasionally worsen seizures, especially if the child's seizures are not fully controlled by antiepileptic drugs. More studies are needed regarding the safety of stimulants in children and adolescents with epilepsy, but when therapy is clearly indicated, most children with epilepsy and ADD can experience improved attention with no worsening of seizure control.

Impulsiveness is another problem that can affect a child's social relations and academic achievements. Impulsiveness is characterized by a tendency to act automatically in response to surrounding situations, without considering the results of the actions. The ability to reflect on one's actions and consider both short-term and long-term effects is only fully achieved in adulthood. Even then, we all regret certain things that we say and do on the "spur of the moment." Some children are much more impulsive in their words and deeds than others of their age.

Stimulants and clonidine (Catapress) are used to treat impulsivity. Clonidine can cause sedation, but it does not worsen seizure control.

Hyperactivity

Children by nature are very active—much more so than adults. A 4-year-old child, for example, is always moving and doing things. His or her arms and legs never seem to hold the same position for more than a few seconds.

In some children (usually boys), excessive movement—or hyperactivity—causes problems. The increased activity may take the form of excessive fidgeting, an inability to stay seated for more than a minute, or running around endlessly. Hyperactivity prevents the child from staying in one place for long. It is disruptive in both the classroom and at home and is exhausting for teachers and parents.

As with ADD, immaturity of the brain may contribute to the cause of hyperactivity. In general, young children are more active than older children and adults. Therefore, hyperactivity may reflect relative immaturity of the brain. As the brain matures, the hyperactivity lessens.

Hyperactivity is slightly more common among children with epilepsy. It is also more common among children with tic disorders and mental handicap. The drugs that can improve ADD, which have already been discussed, have the same desirable effects on hyperactivity.

Severe Language, Cognitive, and Behavioral Impairments

Some children with epilepsy have severe language and cognitive impairments. Social and behavioral problems may further impair their intellectual development because socializing is the primary process by which children obtain language skills. Similarly, language impairment can severely hinder social play. Most children react positively to a voice or smile, but to many children with severe developmental disabilities (such as autism or "pervasive developmental delay," which affects motor, language, and nonverbal behaviors), these sounds and gestures can be threatening and confusing. Their reactions to stimuli are inappropriate, unpredictable, and sometimes destructive.

The parents' reaction to this situation is sympathy and pity, leading them to make their child's world as pleasant and comfortable as possible. This attempt to foster trust and comfort may be successful, but often it is not. Some children may only communicate *on their own terms*. Fortunately, behavior management techniques are available to change the child's avoidance patterns and create new patterns of interaction, which can provide the child with a base of trust in our complicated world (see

Appendix 5). For example, the child is presented with a simple social choice: either control his or her behavior or the adult will control it. Through time and effort, the child chooses self-control. Initially, a simple social world must be created. As the child's behavior improves, the social world is steadily and slowly made more complex.

In this behavioral management technique (which is one of many possible approaches), the first step in controlling the child's behavior is the establishment of routines. The initial routine must be simple and demands must be minimal, but the adult must insist that the child comply with them. This means that the child must limit behavior that interferes with desired activities or attentiveness. For example, the child must lift up or put down his or her arms on command when getting dressed and undressed, sit in a chair without doing things to excite himself or herself (such as waving a hand back and forth in front of the light), or pick up objects on request.

These routines are then modified, and the child is required to adapt to the variation. To maintain and increase the child's sense of stability, everything that is taught must be preserved even as new tasks are being added. The child must feel the comfort of practicing well-established skills while new demands are being introduced. These techniques are often difficult and time-consuming. Yet, if they are consistently incorporated into the child's daily routine, key behavior patterns will be established that may allow the development of cognitive and language skills.

Severe behavioral problems are difficult to remedy. Multiple interventions are often needed, which can address the child's actions and help the parents recognize and react to inappropriate behavior. Help may be needed from social workers, mental health therapists, psychologists, pediatricians, and psychiatrists. Often the behavioral problems pose long-term issues that can be improved, but not fully controlled.

Telling Children and Others about Epilepsy

Epilepsy was once shrouded in secrecy. The word, like "cancer" or "leprosy," evoked fear and isolation. Those days are gone for the most part. The more the word "epilepsy" is used, the more children and adults can learn to understand the condition. The more openness surrounds it, the more the secrecy and fear about epilepsy will disappear.

Telling Children

Children should be told about epilepsy. I recently met a woman who was never told about her disorder, which began when she was 6 years old. She finally went to a library at age 20 to research her symptoms and recognized that she had been treated for epilepsy, but was never told about it. She was furious at her parents and doctors.

It is always a balancing act when deciding how much to tell children about their epilepsy. The child must not be overwhelmed with words and ideas that are either incomprehensible or frightening, but "protecting" the child by withholding the truth can be the worst choice of all. There is no script detailing what to say to children at different ages. Parents should be guided by common sense. In general, children under 3 years of age do not need to be told anything. After age 3, children can usually understand if epilepsy is explained in simple language without the use of medical words. Parents need to keep it simple and be positive about the condition.

The book entitled *Lee, the Rabbit with Epilepsy* is about a rabbit that has a seizure (see Appendix 4). This brightly illustrated book for young children describes how the rabbit visits the doctor, takes medication, and most importantly, continues to enjoy life. This book and other materials designed for children are available through the Epilepsy Foundation (EF). Parents can show these materials to their children or study the materials themselves and use them as a model.

Telling Others Who Need to Know

Anyone who is teaching, caring for, or closely associated with a child with epilepsy should know about the child's disorder. If someone responsible for a child's health or safety doesn't know that the child has epilepsy, the door is opened for potential problems.

In some cultures, parents may be especially reluctant to discuss their child's epilepsy. These are often the same cultures in which there are strong concerns about epilepsy and marriage. For example, some members of the Asian and Orthodox Jewish communities have strong reservations about disclosing the presence of epilepsy in a family member. This attitude is mostly based on realistic concerns regarding the stigma and discrimination still associated with epilepsy in some groups, embarrassment for the family and the family name, and future concerns about the child's ability to find a spouse. However, a child's health should take precedence over other concerns. For this reason—and to help break down the cultural walls of the stigma—all people caring for a child with epilepsy should be informed about the disorder.

RELATIVES

Relatives can be the most supportive and helpful people in the world; they also can be the most difficult. As a general rule, relatives should be told about a child's epilepsy. Who and how much to tell should depend on whether the relatives are likely to be alone with the child and how they may react to the news. Practically speaking, however, if one relative has been told, they have all been told.

A potential problem with relatives is that they love to give advice. Advice is often helpful, but the primary caregivers (usually the parents) must do what they feel is best for the child. Just as it is important that one doctor manage a child's care, it is important that parents assume primary responsibility for their child's disorder. As the child gets older, he or she should begin to assume some of this responsibility.

SCHOOL NURSES, TEACHERS, AND CLASSMATES

School is a major part of the child's day. If the child has daytime seizures, school nurses and teachers should be told about the child's epilepsy. The school nurse is an important part of the child's health care team and serves as the advocate for the child in the school and a resource for teachers who need information about epilepsy. The school nurse is most likely to be called on if the child has a seizure or experiences adverse effects from medication. The nurse should be informed about the nature of the child's seizures and the medications being used. He or she should be kept up-to-date on any changes. The nurse should also have the parent's and doctor's telephone numbers. In some cases, the school nurse may confer with the gym teacher or sports coach to discuss possible precautions during some activities.

The teacher should always know the type of seizures the child has and what they look like. Teachers who are not familiar with epilepsy or with the child's seizure type can be given a pamphlet from the EF or chapters from a book such as this one that explain how to recognize seizures, first aid for seizures, and adverse effects of medications. The teacher should be asked to observe the child carefully for possible seizures or adverse effects of medication. If the teacher notices any unusual behavior, such as staring, lip smacking, repetitive hand movements, or involuntary movements, the parents and the doctor should be told. These behaviors may represent seizures. Also, certain problems—such as tremor, lethargy, nausea, or double vision —may occur only when the medication levels reach a peak during school hours. In this case, the teacher's observations will be critical in adjusting the dosage to relieve these symptoms. Thus, the teacher is an extension of the parents' and doctor's eyes and ears.

The teacher must balance the careful observation of the child with the need to treat him or her just the same as the other children. The teacher is a powerful role model for children's attitudes toward epilepsy. How the teacher responds to the occurrence of a seizure in the classroom can have a strong influence on how it is perceived by the other children. A calm and matter-of-fact manner and openness to questions can do much to lessen classmates' fears and encourage acceptance.

If daytime seizures are frequent, it is important to discuss the disorder with the rest of the children in the class. A time can be set aside to discuss epilepsy and the child's seizures. (See Chap. 32 for resources for in-class education on epilepsy.) By discussing it openly, all of the children can be educated and a sense of community can be fostered. A staff member from the local affiliate of the EF or an epilepsy center may be asked to conduct an educational program for the child's classmates or the whole school. These open forums can be helpful in shifting the other children's perspective from fear and teasing to respect and friendship.

THE CHILD'S FRIENDS AND THEIR PARENTS

More than anything else, Pete just wants to be one of the kids. He has overcome a learning disability and is now in mainstream classes and doing well. He has a few good friends and loves intramural basketball. Although his seizures are now well controlled, he doesn't want anyone at school to know about his epilepsy. We have tried to convince him to tell his close friends, but he refuses.

Children with epilepsy should be encouraged to pursue friendships and social activities. Healthy socialization with other children is essential for self-esteem and future success. The decision to tell a child's friends about epilepsy is often difficult. Children are immature and can be insensitive. In addition, if the friends' parents are uninformed about epilepsy, they may unnecessarily fear for their children's safety or be afraid that they will suffer "psychological trauma" if they witness a seizure.

The child's friends and their parents should be carefully told about the child's epilepsy; it should not just be casually mentioned. It may be a good idea for the young person to discuss the epilepsy with his or her close friends and for the parent to discuss the disorder one-on-one with the friends' parents. The discussion should explain the type of seizures, their frequency, how the seizures affect the child, and what to do in case a seizure occurs. Most important, they need to know that epilepsy is just another episodic medical problem, like asthma, which affects otherwise healthy, active children, and it is not something that a person can "catch." The other children and their parents also should be given a chance to ask questions.

The need to conform and belong to a group makes many adolescents (starting at around age 12) want to hide their epilepsy. Therefore, whether to tell their friends about epilepsy can be a difficult decision. *The adolescent must always be involved in the decision to reveal his or her disorder—whom to tell, how to tell, and how much to tell.* Older children, perhaps as young as 8 or 9, should also be involved in decisions about who is told and what is said. Because the maturity of teens and preteens varies, some friends may be frightened by the disorder; others may react with teasing and try to isolate the young person with epilepsy. For adolescents whose seizures are not fully controlled, it is especially important that their friends know about the epilepsy and what to do in case a seizure occurs, but the decision to confide still should be the adolescent's, not the parents' decision. For adolescents with well-controlled seizures who have few or no adverse effects from medications, it is less important to tell other people about epilepsy.

Although such negative reactions are becoming less frequent, ridicule remains a part of life for many children with epilepsy, especially in the lower grades. When a child makes fun of another child with epilepsy, the most effective strategy is to pay little heed. It may be worthwhile to respond calmly that epilepsy is a medical disorder or ask if they would make fun of their own mother or grandfather who had a heart condition or an athlete who broke a bone. Most children are understanding and supportive.

BABYSITTERS

Babysitters allow parents to have some independence from their children. Babysitters who are educated about the disorder can care for children with epilepsy. Although parents are correct in thinking that no one will watch and care for their children the way they do, mature and responsible babysitters can do a very good job. It is also important for children's maturation for them to learn that their parents cannot be there every minute. This will pave the way toward successful separation from the parents when it comes time to go to school or camp.

Babysitters should be told that a child has epilepsy before they agree to watch the child. Because babysitters are left alone with the child, they should be knowledgeable about the epilepsy and basic first-aid measures. They should be reassured that dangerous situations and emergencies are extremely uncommon, but they must be prepared. They should know the type and frequency of seizures, medication dosage, where the medication is stored, and the telephone numbers of those to call in an emergency (including the doctor's number). For children with seizures associated with incontinence, keeping a change of clothing on hand for the child (and the babysitter) can be helpful.

The EF has an educational pamphlet for babysitters. It gives basic information about children with epilepsy and describes first aid.

THE DENTIST AND ORTHODONTIST

Although children with epilepsy rarely require special attention during dental procedures, dentists should be made aware of the child's seizure disorder. The dentist may want to speak briefly with the child's doctor about the condition. For children who have frequent tonic-clonic, myoclonic, or atonic seizures, it may be helpful to take a low dose of a benzodiazepine, such as lorazepam before dental procedures. Children with epilepsy who are taking medications that affect gum growth should receive regular dental care and should be taught to brush with care and, when old enough, to use dental floss.

Children with severe epilepsy, cerebral palsy, or associated neurologic disorders may require general anesthesia for major dental work. Before such procedures, it may be helpful for the dentist and doctor to discuss the medications and precautions. Finally, the orthodontist using braces or other equipment should know that the child has epilepsy because special precautions or procedures may be needed when braces are fitted.

20

Living an Active Life

The effects of epilepsy on children's behavioral, intellectual, and social development are extremely variable. Most children with epilepsy lead normal lives and have few or no restrictions on social or physical activities. Even if the seizures are well controlled, however, the diagnosis of epilepsy and the medical visits can be frightening to them. For some children, seizures and the effects of the antiepileptic drugs cause many difficulties. Other children have additional medical and neurologic problems that affect their lives. Regardless of the severity of the condition, children with epilepsy need special attention to ensure that their outlook and self-esteem are positive.

Children with epilepsy see the disorder through the window of their parents' eyes. How the epilepsy affects the child often depends on how the epilepsy affects the parents. On hearing the diagnosis of epilepsy, parents are likely to go through a series of responses: shock, bewilderment, disappointment, hopelessness, guilt, anger, and grief (not necessarily in that order). The adjustment period is followed by the realization that life goes on—the child and family can enjoy life and flourish. If the parents take a positive outlook, the child will, too.

Family and Social Life

A child's illness complicates the challenges of family life. The epilepsy of a child with minor seizures that are fully controlled should not unduly affect the family. But when a child's seizures are more disabling, or when the child also has other physical or neurologic disorders, family life is affected. All relationships in the family are changed—the relationship of the parents with each other, the parents' relationship with the children, and the relationship of brothers and sisters to the child with epilepsy.

The changes that epilepsy in a child bring to a family deserve careful attention. The child with epilepsy has special needs, but so do the other children in the family. As their age and maturity permit, siblings should be educated about epilepsy. They should not be neglected. They should be given honest information that they can understand, and they should be encouraged to ask questions and express their fears and feelings. Because the child with epilepsy will draw time and attention like a magnet, parents must make special time for their other children. This action may help prevent later resentment directed at both the parents and the child with epilepsy.

Just as it may be helpful for the child with epilepsy to join a group of children or have a buddy with epilepsy to share experiences with, it may be helpful for the parents to join a parents' group or to have other parents to talk with and share experiences with occasionally. The parental "grapevine" for children with medical disorders is one of our most powerful communication networks. Parents share problems, frustrations, coping strategies, achievements, and joys, as well as information about doctors, hospitals, medications, and educational and recreational programs. In the process, parents also build strong bonds. The local Epilepsy Foundation (EF) affiliate may have parent groups. A pediatrician, neurologist, or comprehensive epilepsy center may be able to put parents in touch with other parents of children with epilepsy. If there is not a local group, a motivated parent can easily be the force to create one.

It is important to be aware that information gathered from conversations with other parents in person or on the Internet is often based on the experience of a single child, the results of a single drug trial, or "gut reactions." These perspectives may be accurate in a specific instance, but are often the exceptions or are incorrectly interpreted. Parents should be skeptical of "interesting" results that have not been subjected to rigorous scientific testing.

GETTING ON WITH LIFE

Initially, Jim and I were so consumed by Anthony's epilepsy that nothing else seemed to matter. Between the seizures, medications, doctor visits, tests, meetings with teachers, and our jobs, there was no time for anything else. It took us 6 months or so, but we have finally realized that life goes on for Anthony, for his older brother Paul, and for us. We do special things with Paul to let him know how much we love him. We also have our parents come every few months to spend the weekend with the kids so that we can just get away. Now we can give Anthony the attention he needs without resentment or guilt.

Once the child's epilepsy has been diagnosed, treatment has begun, and some time has passed for understanding and accepting the disorder, it is time for the parents to get on with their lives. In the mildest cases, this is easy. In the cases of moderate severity, with intermittent seizures and some adverse medication effects, resuming normal life is a challenge. In the most serious cases, especially those with other neurologic disorders, assuming a normal life may seem impossible, but it is not. For families with children who have frequent and intense seizures and associated developmental problems, life can never be exactly the way it would have been if the child did not have these problems. The situation does not mean that the parents can never spend time alone together or enjoy their life. They can. They will just have to work harder to get the time.

There are two steps toward resuming the life the parents want. The first step is all about attitude. Parents must accept the condition and the associated disorders for what they are. They should understand the needs of the child with epilepsy and their other children as well as their own needs and those of their partner. It means that parents must search for the best care for their child, decide how they want to live their lives, and most important, decide that they can do it. Some parents feel as if they are swept up in a current, and the current is pulling them. That is true for everyone at the beginning. It is important that parents not passively ride the current, however, or they will find themselves in a place they do not want to be. Instead, they must determine the direction.

The second step is acting on the commitment to a satisfying life. Parents must work toward a balance between their needs, the needs of their child with epilepsy, and the needs of other family members. Their happiness and the soundness of the other relationships in the family will positively affect the child with epilepsy. Unfortunately, divorce is much more common among parents who have children with developmental disabilities than among couples in general. Early recognition of the additional stress and open communication about feelings and responsibilities can be invaluable. For some parents, it is a good idea to investigate family support, getting help around the house, community programs, respite programs, and the local EF affiliate.

COUNSELING

I thought that Jake told us everything. We were positive and supportive about the epilepsy, and it seemed like he was doing great. We never suspected that things were bothering him—the epilepsy, feeling pressure to get good grades, and other kids in his school. It was building up inside for a while. When the school called to ask how he was doing, we realized that he had been missing classes for a while, telling the teachers he had seizures. It was all too much for him. The counselor has been a godsend. Jake needs us, but he also needs someone else.

Parents, brothers and sisters, grandparents, and teachers provide children with role models, advice, guidance, and support. They offer a nurturing environment and a positive outlook, but usually none of them has epilepsy. Despite their best intentions and loving support, they often do not ask important questions: "How do you feel about having epilepsy?" "How do you think other kids react to you because you have epilepsy?" "Do you understand what the doctor said?" "What are your greatest fears?" If the diagnosis and treatment of epilepsy are confusing for the parents, they will certainly be bewildering to the child. In addition, the social impact of epilepsy is often psychologically painful for the child (as mentioned in Chap. 19).

Most children with epilepsy do not need formal counseling, but all of them require education about the disorder and help in learning to adjust to it. Counseling can be important support for children with epilepsy. The counselor provides the outside perspective that is often lacking. Parents are well-meaning, but their concern can be misdirected into telling the child how to feel and how to act. Although all parents feel that they know what is best for their children, it can be difficult to determine what is truly best. A dialogue is often much more helpful than a suggestion or an order. The successful counselor can help "open" the part of the child that epilepsy can hide. The essence of counseling is to provide understanding and help the person cope with the medical and social impact of the disorder. Counseling can be beneficial for the entire family or the child alone.

Referral

The recommendation for counseling can come from a doctor, social worker, teacher, or school guidance counselor. Counseling is of no benefit unless the child or family wants it.

Finding the right counselor is usually not difficult. The doctor, school guidance counselor or psychologist, social worker, and local EF affiliate are potential sources of information and referral. The counselor must have some knowledge of epilepsy. In addition, there must be a good relationship and trust between the counselor and the child. If the "chemistry" between them is not good, it is not wise to pursue the relationship too long. It is better to find another counselor.

Benefits

Counseling is helpful if there is a need for the child or family to gain a greater understanding of the disorder, accept the diagnosis and treatment, regain a sense of control over one's own life, or talk to someone about concerns. Counselors can help in a variety of ways. For some children and adolescents, understanding their epilepsy may be most important. They often have fears and misunderstandings that go unaddressed. Fear of dying or serious injury during a seizure is a fairly common hidden concern, but children often will not bring the subject up to parents or doctors because they are too frightened, shy, or protective of their parents or do not know how to ask the question.

The relationship of stress to seizures is poorly understood, but seizures often are more common during or shortly after stressful times (see Chap. 6). The counselor can help identify sources of stress, such as family or school problems. The counselor also can offer simple techniques of stress management, which can be helpful even for a child.

Poor self-esteem may be an obvious concern or an undiscovered problem. The parents and teachers of children with epilepsy may see them as "doing remarkably well," but deep inside, the children may remain insecure and have low self-esteem. To protect their parents and their own image, they may hide their feelings or overcompensate. Although this may be the exception rather than the rule, parents and others must look beyond what they want to see. Counselors can identify home and school situations and issues that have an impact on the emotional well-being of children with epilepsy.

FRIENDSHIPS

Like other children, children with epilepsy should be encouraged to pursue friendships and social activities. Perhaps the most negative effect of epilepsy on children is the isolation and rejection that may accompany the disorder. Vigorous pursuit of regular social activities is the best protection against negative social effects and is important for normal intellectual and behavioral development (see Chap. 18 and Chap. 19).

A child must be given independence to pursue healthy friendships. Parents may face conflicting desires: they want the child to play with other children, and they also want to protect the child from danger. Such conflicts are inherent in parenthood, but they are exaggerated for parents of children with epilepsy. Physical injury can be caused by seizures, and parents are often the best at recognizing a seizure and protecting their child. However, the emotional trauma of isolation is probably more painful and more long-lasting than a seizure-related physical injury.

Many parents would like their child to be more active in friendships and social activities, but find that the child is fearful of rejection or that the opportunities are limited. The social activities of some children are limited by other neurologic and emotional disorders. For these children, community programs and networking between parents can be helpful. It also can be beneficial for children to meet other children with epilepsy through camping or similar programs available through the local EF affiliate.

GOING TO CAMP

All children with epilepsy can enjoy camp. Those with well-controlled or occasional seizures should be able to attend a regular camp. The range of activities and precautions must be individually specified, but these children can usually enjoy a very full and active camp experience.

Children with frequent seizures, or children who have never met another child with epilepsy, may benefit from going to a camp with other children who have epilepsy. The EF provides information about these camps, some of which include educational sessions on epilepsy for the children.

Some camps specialize in programs for children with severe epilepsy, cerebral palsy, or emotional disorders. They provide a wonderful social opportunity for the children and an important respite for parents.

Physical Activities and Sports

The balance between a child's safety and the ability to enjoy a full range of activities is tested when it comes to recommendations regarding sports and other physical activities. Because epilepsy affects each person differently, the approach must be individualized. The seizure type and frequency of the seizures, the type of medication and its adverse effects, the child's ability to follow instructions and act responsibly, and the nature and supervision of the activity must all be considered.

Common sense should be the guiding force in making these decisions. The goals should be safety and a lifestyle that is as normal as possible. No activity is completely safe. Making safety the exclusive concern will unnecessarily limit the child's activities. Restriction and isolation foster low self-esteem and emphasize the disability. Nevertheless, certain activities and sports can be dangerous for some children with epilepsy, and safety concerns require that these activities be forbidden or carefully supervised. In the past, doctors and parents tended to strictly limit physical activities. Today, children with epilepsy are allowed to be children and to pursue as full a range of activity as reasonable.

The type of seizures and their frequency are critical in determining which activities are safe. Children whose motor control or consciousness is impaired during seizures are at higher risk for injuries. Children who have uncontrolled, frequent seizures should know that certain activities are restricted. For example, they should not swim alone (in fact, *no* child should swim alone) or play on high bars or climb ropes without a proper mat and supervision. Climbing a rope higher than 5 feet is also dangerous if seizures are not well controlled. Other activities, such as riding a bicycle in traffic, should be forbidden. However, bicycling may be permitted in safer settings, as discussed later in this chapter. If a child's seizures are more common at certain times (e.g., within 2 hours of awakening), activities can be scheduled for the times when seizures are less likely to occur.

Seizures are only rarely provoked by exercise, but when this pattern is identified, physical exertion should be limited. However, it may be possible to devise a satisfactory program of exercise in which the level of exertion is gradually increased. Prolonged physical activity in a hot environment may provoke seizures in some children. In such cases, plenty of cool drinks and frequent rest periods can help reduce the risk of seizures.

Children with epilepsy should be encouraged to participate in group and competitive sports, such as Little League baseball, community sports, and varsity sports at school. These activities are usually well supervised and require appropriate safety gear. Most children with epilepsy can safely participate without special accommodations. Most important, group activities are part of childhood and foster a sense of "belonging," high self-esteem, and independence. These benefits are extremely valuable, and the risks of participation must be serious to warrant prohibiting a child from joining group activities. Most potential hazards can be overcome. In fact, players with epilepsy can be found in major league baseball, ice hockey, and other professional sports.

Serious injuries in children with epilepsy are uncommon and rarely occur during participation in sports. Believe it or not, bathrooms are much more dangerous to children than playing soccer or ice skating.

STAIR CLIMBING

Our world is filled with stairs. For most children with epilepsy, stairs should not be barriers to getting around. However, seizures that impair motor control or consciousness can cause serious injuries if they occur while the child is on a staircase. If a child has an aura (warning) before a seizure, he or she may be able to sit down until the seizure is over. If the child has frequent seizures that cause falling, it is not unreasonable to have him or her use elevators instead of stairs. In school, however, this restriction can cause the child to be late for classes or to stand out from schoolmates. In these unusual cases, a buddy who is aware of the epilepsy may be able to accompany the child from one class to the next.

BATHING

Children with epilepsy should not bathe in a bathtub unsupervised. Children should take tub baths only when they can be supervised moment to moment. Any child can drown in a bathtub with only 2 inches of water. As children get older, however, they need privacy, and this means that they must take showers. Bathroom doors should never be locked.

SWIMMING AND WATER SPORTS

Swimming is a pleasure children should be encouraged to enjoy. Although water poses special dangers for children with epilepsy, the condition is not an insurmountable barrier to swimming. The issue of epilepsy and water safety is really a question of how much supervision is necessary. No matter how severe or frequent the epilepsy, a child can enjoy the water. A parent can hold a child in a shallow pool with little risk, for instance. If the child's seizures are well controlled, swimming should be encouraged, although it is necessary to make sure that at least one person who knows the child has epilepsy and who knows basic lifesaving is nearby. (This person can be a teenager.)

The most difficult decisions about swimming arise when children have occasional seizures that impair motor control or consciousness. These children should be allowed to swim, but they must be closely supervised. There should be a lifeguard on duty who is responsible and aware of the child's disorder. There also should be another child in the pool who is the buddy. Unfortunately, lifeguards are often adolescents who may be easily distracted. The lifeguards should know that they *must* keep their eyes on the pool while the child is swimming. The buddy system, used by many camps for young children who swim (and by adult scuba divers), is another precaution to ensure a child's safety. The buddy should be responsible and understand the need for keeping an eye on the child. He or she should never go far away in the pool.

Swimming in a lake, bay, or ocean is much more dangerous than swimming in a pool. A person swimming in open waters can disappear in seconds and may be impossible to locate quickly. Therefore, extreme caution must be exercised when a child with epilepsy, especially one with poorly controlled seizures, swims in open waters. The wearing of a lifejacket is recommended in this setting.

The child with epilepsy who wants to swim competitively should be encouraged. Competitive swimming practices and matches are usually well supervised. The coach should be aware that the child has epilepsy, however, and everyone involved, including the child, should recognize that there is some additional risk to this activity and make an informed decision about whether it is worth it.

Older children with well-controlled seizures can snorkel and scuba dive. Children with uncontrolled seizures that impair consciousness or motor control should not scuba dive and should only snorkel in relatively calm water, very close to someone who has lifesaving skills.

Jumping from the high dive poses clear dangers for children with epilepsy. Only children with well-controlled seizures should consider high diving.

BICYCLING

Bicycles are a part of childhood. Yet a bicycle, if ridden on or near the street, presents a serious potential danger for a child with epilepsy. Even if a parent rides just behind the child on the sidewalk, during a complex partial seizure the child may suddenly veer off into the street, out of the parent's reach and protection.

Despite the dangers, children with epilepsy can learn to ride and enjoy bicycles. Because most serious bicycle injuries involve the head, everyone who rides a bicycle should wear a helmet. If seizures are under control or do not impair motor control or consciousness, bicycle riding should be unrestricted. When the seizures pose a danger, bicycles can be ridden in a park or other place where there are no motor vehicles.

Stationary bicycles for exercise pose no serious danger for children with epilepsy. Ideally, the floor should be carpeted or padded. Low-seated bicycles are the safest.

HORSEBACK RIDING

Horseback riding can be safe and fun for children whose seizures are well controlled or always preceded by an adequate warning. Those who have seizures that could cause them to fall off the horse can ride, but they must be closely supervised. Someone may need to walk alongside the horse. The risks and benefits of horseback riding must be carefully weighed for these children. Competitive horseback riding often involves galloping and jumping and should only be considered for children with mild or well-controlled epilepsy.

CONTACT SPORTS

Contact sports—such as football, basketball, soccer, rugby, and ice hockey—are generally safe for children with epilepsy. The principal concern with contact sports is the chance of head or bodily injury, but children with epilepsy are not necessarily more likely to be hurt than other children. If an absence or complex partial seizure were to occur during a game, there is a small chance of injury if someone were to tackle the child, for instance, during the spell. Tackle football, rugby, and ice hockey have a higher incidence of injuries than most other sports, and participation in them should probably be limited to children with well-controlled seizures. There is nothing wrong, however, with a child who has occasional or even frequent seizures playing touch football in the back yard. The risks must be weighed against the benefits of the sport. The chances of serious injury are small compared with the positive effects of team participation.

It would be hard to recommend boxing for any child, and even less for a child with epilepsy. The goal of boxing is to inflict an injury, especially to the head. Because participation can mean taking a hard hit directly to the head, children with absence seizures or complex partial seizures are at particular risk of injury from boxing. Head injuries also can aggravate a seizure disorder. Children with epilepsy should avoid boxing, as well as fights with other children.

Wrestling may be safe for children with well-controlled seizures or seizures that do not impair consciousness or motor control. It can be dangerous for other children with epilepsy.

GYMNASTICS

Some forms of gymnastics are dangerous for children with epilepsy. Only children with well-controlled seizures should consider performing on the high bar, uneven parallel bars, vaults, or rings. Other gymnastic events, such as floor routines and the pommel horse, pose little risk. The parallel bars are of intermediate risk; the risk reflects the specific exercises being done. Climbing a rope higher than 5 feet is also dangerous if seizures are not well controlled.

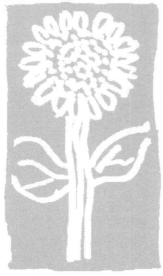

CHAPTER

21

Education of Children with Epilepsy

Children with epilepsy usually are of normal intelligence, but some do not do well academically. When this happens, it is important to find out why. Neurologic impairment, frequent seizures, or adverse effects of antiepileptic drugs can affect school performance. If a child is doing well in school, there is no reason to worry about the effects of epilepsy on learning. If the teacher reports problems or if parents become aware that their child's performance is slipping, it may be worthwhile to consider interventions. First, the problem must be identified. The child may have an attention deficit with frequent distractibility, may be excessively tired from medications or poor sleep, or may have a specific learning disability that may or may not be related to the epilepsy (see Chap. 18). After talking with the child's teachers, obtaining an educational assessment is the next step. Parents have the right to request an assessment of their child's problems and needs.

The Individuals with Disabilities Education Act (IDEA), discussed later, provides legal guarantees for educating children with handicaps. The law states that the child has the right to be taught in a regular (mainstream) classroom environment as much as possible. The child has the right to be included in social activities and other activities provided by the school. Parents have the right to be directly involved in the process of planning the child's education.

In urban and suburban areas, parent advocacy groups are often active, and school systems recognize the special needs of children with handicaps. In these settings, parents may need to be assertive—a behavior that is not foreign to the urban environment. In contrast, in small rural communities, where there is often only one school system and one education "czar," children with handicaps and their parents face greater challenges. Parents are often extremely reluctant to question the school personnel and system. Suggestions from parents about their child's special needs or their desire to have their child attend regular classes can be met with indignation and ridicule. Knowing the child's rights under the law and being cautiously assertive can go a long way toward ensuring that the child receives the best possible education.

Attending Regular Classes

Most children with epilepsy attend regular classes, although in some cases they need special aides to work with them. Regular classes offer the opportunity for children with epilepsy and other disorders to enjoy their education and to be in the social environment of other children, most of whom do not have disabilities. By attending mainstream classes, a child with epilepsy will be exposed to a wider array of educational opportunities, will have the chance to develop lasting social relationships with other children with and without disabilities, and will be more likely to feel like a regular child instead of a child with a disability. That is not to deny the existence of the epilepsy, but it emphasizes that most children with epilepsy have the potential to learn and accomplish the things that other children can.

Regular classes do present potential problems for a child with epilepsy. Children can be cruel. They may tease the child. Other parents may forbid their children to play with a child who has epilepsy. If teasing or cruelty becomes a problem, it may be worth asking the school to conduct an educational program so that the children can better understand epilepsy. The "Kids on the Block" puppet show, sponsored by the Epilepsy Foundation (EF) affiliates and other groups, is an entertaining and effective means of educating children about epilepsy. These and other programs help other children understand the human and medical sides of a health problem, and through that process, teach them to be more accepting of the child with epilepsy.

Special Education

Special education programs are designed to meet the special needs of children with disabilities by supplementing or adapting the regular curriculum. Instruction may take place in regular classrooms or in separate facilities for all or part of the day. Students may also be assigned to special programs in physical education, occupational and physical rehabilitation, music education programs, home instruction, or instruction in hospitals and other institutions.

These classes and programs recognize that some students can be educated, but have mental or physical impairments that make it essential to tailor their education to their special needs. The variety of special education programs offered by each school system reflects the types and severity of the children's disabilities, the educational emphasis, the student-to-teacher ratio, the funding for quality teachers and equipment, and other factors.

Most children with epilepsy are best served by mainstream classes. Many receive special education services partly or entirely in the regular classroom. Children with frequent and severe seizures who also have orthopedic and emotional problems, however, obviously need a specialized program. Many children fall between these two extremes. If a child is not doing well in mainstream classes, it is often helpful for parents to meet with the teachers to learn if the cause of the problems can be identified, through special testing if necessary. In addition, consultation with the child's doctor may provide insights. For example, attention deficit disorder may be causing the problems in school.

Just because special education is recommended does not mean that it is necessary. In most cases, the recommendation is valid and should be followed, but if parents disagree with the school's placement, they can appeal or seek an outside assessment by a psychologist or neuropsychologist. It may also be helpful for parents to observe the child in mainstream or special education classes to better judge the proper balance.

As discussed further in the next section, schools are required to deliver services in the "least restrictive environment." This means that a child has the right to be educated in the classroom with children who do not have disabilities, to the maximum extent that such placement meets the child's educational needs. Some children do require many special classes or a special school, and emotional issues often arise when children are assigned to special education programs that remove them from the mainstream. Sometimes the children are placed with other children who have severe emotional or behavioral problems and thus provide poor behavioral models. For some parents, the recommendation that their child attend special classes signals that the epilepsy or associated problems are severe and that their child is "not normal."

Children who attend special education programs are aware that they are not in the mainstream, particularly if they were formerly enrolled in regular classes. The word "special" is key. Parents and teachers should emphasize that the child is special—not handicapped, disabled, or less bright. They should not deny or avoid discussing the epilepsy or other disabilities; they should emphasize the positive. Parents may wish to discuss with the child why he or she goes to a certain school while brothers and sisters or other children on the block attend another school. The parents can highlight some of the advantages of the special school, such as more teachers, more enjoyable activities, and more children who are like him or her.

Individuals with Disabilities Education Act

The Individuals with Disabilities Education Act (IDEA), formerly known as the Education of All Handicapped Children Act (Public Law 94-142), was passed by the U.S. Congress to ensure that all handicapped children receive appropriate education at no cost and in the "least restrictive environment." All states that receive federal funds under this Act must follow the rules for identifying, evaluating, and providing services to eligible children between 3 and 21 years of age. Federal funds are also provided to the states to develop early intervention services for infants and toddlers who have physical or mental conditions that are likely to cause developmental delay.

This Act recognizes the special needs of children with disabilities. This group includes children with epilepsy, mental retardation, hearing and visual impairments (including, but not limited to, deafness and blindness), serious emotional disorders, orthopedic impairments such as scoliosis or immobile joints, autism, traumatic brain injury, learning disabilities, and other impairments that require special education and related services. Children may qualify who have only epilepsy or epilepsy and another disabling condition, such as mental handicap. However, to qualify for service, the presence of a potentially disabling condition is not sufficient. The impairment must adversely affect the child's educational capacity to the degree that special education or related services are required.

In some children, although their epilepsy is not disabling and their intelligence is normal, other problems may require special attention. These include impairments of attention, reading, arithmetic learning, motor skills, memory, and behavior. They are often identified at a young age, which permits early intervention and treatment.

Most children with epilepsy and other disabilities can be educated in the regular classroom with the use of supplemental aides and services. For example, a child with a disability may attend homeroom and four regular classes, but also attend a special tutorial for a reading disorder and physical therapy instead of gym. In this case, the child enjoys the benefits of the mainstream environment and the benefits of special education.

IDEA requires that schools provide all the additional services needed to help children with disabilities benefit from special education. These related services include transportation, audiology and speech therapy, psychological evaluation and treatment, physical and occupational therapy, recreation, therapeutic recreation, social-work services, counseling, early identification and assessment of disabling conditions, and medical evaluations.

For children with epilepsy, related services include education for teachers and school nurses about epilepsy, how to administer medications, and first aid for seizures. Ideally, this education will be extended to include classmates because social acceptance may be one of the greatest challenges for children with epilepsy.

IDEA states that a child with disabilities must have a written individualized educational plan (IEP) constructed jointly by the parents and school personnel. The IEP is a written report describing the child's present level of development, the short-term and annual goals of the special education program, the specific educational services the child will receive, the date services will start and their expected duration, standards for determining whether the goals of the educational program are being met, and the extent to which the child will be able to participate in regular educational programs.

The IEP is usually developed during a series of meetings involving the parents, teachers, and representatives of the school district. Because a child with epilepsy has special needs, it is essential that the IEP be written with care to meet those needs. Unless the parents request specific services such as physical therapy, speech therapy, or a barrier-free school, such needs may be overlooked.

Before or during the IEP process, parents should explore available educational programs, including public, private, federal, state, county, and municipal programs. They should observe classes and see for themselves which program is best suited for their child. Parents may bring a spouse, doctor, teacher, advocate, and others for support if they do not wish to attend the IEP meeting alone. They should be aware of the actions of everyone involved in their child's case. They must be assertive and persuasive advocates for their child during the IEP process. This does not mean that all school officials are adversaries, but it does mean that parents are a child's most important advocates; they know their child best.

Parents are entitled to a copy of the IEP, and they should request it if it is not offered. Parents also have channels for filing an appeal if they do not agree with their child's plan.

The Rehabilitation Act of 1973, Section 504

Section 504 of The Rehabilitation Act of 1973 provides education rights for children and adults with disabilities. Although provisions of Section 504 and IDEA overlap somewhat, Section 504 is primarily an anti-discrimination law, which says that it is illegal for any program or activity receiving federal funding to exclude or discriminate against qualified people with handicaps. It also requires that reasonable accommodations be made by educational institutions.

Note that Section 504 covers "qualified" people with handicaps—not only children of school age, but also other people if they are at an age during which state law requires that such services be provided to people with handicaps. In many cases, this includes elementary and secondary education and adult educational services. It also may include college, graduate school, and technical schools. Section 504 prohibits schools of higher education from inquiring before admission whether an applicant has a disability. However, if academic or other accommodations are necessary, the student must request and justify them. Examples of such accommodations include adjustments in the class schedule to allow for rest and recuperation after medical treatment, modified test arrangements such as oral tests for those with certain learning disabilities, and transportation services for people with impaired mobility.

Mental Handicap and Cerebral Palsy

Children with epilepsy who also have mental handicap (a term preferred over the older term "mental retardation") or cerebral palsy experience a wider range of problems than do children who have uncomplicated epilepsy. Children with mental handicaps have below-average intellectual ability and are often impaired in their ability to understand, communicate, solve problems, and function in social settings. Children with cerebral palsy have muscle spasms, difficulty standing or walking, or postural problems. Their intelligence may range from average to below average. Mental handicap and cerebral palsy can also be associated with vision, hearing, and speech problems and possibly some physical deformity or emotional disturbance. Management of children with epilepsy and mental handicap or cerebral palsy requires the combined effort of doctors, therapists, and parents.

Acceptance and Adjustment

When a handicapped child is born, the parents' distress may be severe. The feelings of guilt, shame, despair, and self-pity may be overwhelming, and the agony of longing for a way out may be excruciating. Torturing questions may flood the parents' minds: What did I do wrong? Why did this happen to our family? The turmoil may give way to sadness; a feeling of desolation and isolation; and a longing for the lost, healthy baby.

The way in which the parents adjust to the situation is crucial for the future welfare of the child who is handicapped and the whole family. A handicapped child needs to be loved and accepted as any other child would be. When mutually enjoyable relationships develop between the child and the family, the child's personality is allowed to develop in the most favorable environment. Whether a child is healthy or handicapped at birth, he or she will most easily achieve happiness and a satisfying adult social role if brought up in a loving, contented, and united family.

Adjusting to the shock of the child's handicap is difficult, but families can receive assistance, support, and education from United Cerebral Palsy (www.ucpa.org) or The Arc of the United States (www.thearc.org), a national organization for people with mental handicap and related developmental disabilities and their families. As the distress lessens, the family must prepare for the task of doing its best for the handicapped child. The child with mental handicap or cerebral palsy and epilepsy has the same emotional needs as other children. He or she needs love but not smothering, care but not overindulgence, and above all, opportunities for achievement, self-control, and social growth toward an independent place in adult society.

The parents of a handicapped child are faced with the question of what to tell relatives, friends, and neighbors. As discussed in Chapter 19, the best answer is the truth. Friends and neighbors are going to visit when the baby comes home from the hospital, and failure to tell them at once of the child's disability will only make it more difficult later. As naturally as they can, parents should tell all who ask, including their other children, that the doctors think the baby has weak arms and legs, or is severely mentally and physically handicapped, or has seizures, and treatment has begun. Few people will fail to be helpful and sympathetic. If the child's disorder only becomes apparent and clearly diagnosed months or even years after birth, it is still wise to tell the truth.

Mental Handicap

Mental handicap is a term loaded with fear for parents. In the past, "mental retardation" usually implied mental incompetence, and the child was often placed in an institution. Mental handicap means slowed or delayed mental development. Children with mental handicap are not incapable of learning; they just do not learn as rapidly as other children.

Until recently, about two-thirds of children with cerebral palsy were thought to have mental handicap. Epilepsy was also frequently associated with mental handicap. Now, thanks to early medical intervention and advanced technology, the incidence of mental handicap among children has fallen markedly. Approximately 2% of children in the general population are affected by mental handicap; up to 25% of children with cerebral palsy are affected. Among children with epilepsy, mental handicap occurs in 9%. For those children who have epilepsy, mental handicap is more common when the following factors are present: early age when seizures begin (especially before age 2 years), prolonged duration of epilepsy, multiple seizure types, and use of several antiepileptic drugs in high dosages.

Parents need to keep in mind that the usual intelligence quotient (IQ) test is based on an established method of measuring a broad range of cognitive functions such as math, reasoning and logic, and spatial skills, as well as the fund of knowledge. Many children with cerebral palsy are penalized on IQ tests because their movement impairments can interfere with test-taking performance. Children with epilepsy may be slowed by medication or by seizures that are not obvious to others. Therefore, intelligence testing may not accurately indicate a child's true potential.

Mental handicap is classified as mild (IQ of 69 to 55), moderate (IQ of 54 to 40), severe (IQ of 39 to 25), and profound (IQ of less than 25). If a child with epilepsy scores in the mentally handicapped range, his or her development will probably be slower than that of other children of the same age. However, as with children without physical or mental handicaps, children with mental handicap have a wide range of abilities.

The IQ score is only one measure of intelligence. Psychologists can also measure a child's adaptive level (ability to manage common daily activities, such as feeding, dressing, toileting, and social interaction). Children with movement problems may be delayed in these areas. The accuracy of these tests depends on the expertise and experience of the test administrators. Obtaining an accurate picture of a child's potential requires an assessment by professionals from different fields. By integrating the different observations and test results, these professionals can reach a depth of understanding that could not be provided by one person. What mental handicap means for a child depends on the nature and severity of the problem.

Although a child's IQ may place some restrictions on what he or she learns and the rate at which he or she learns it, early intervention and special education programs can reduce the impact of mental handicap. Programs can tailor the curriculum so that children can learn at a rate that gives them confidence in their emerging new abilities. Therefore, parents must recognize their child's developmental strengths and weaknesses so they can help plan an educational program that will help achieve their child's potential. When the curriculum is appropriate, a child is less likely to experience stress and more apt to appreciate his or her own achievements (see Chap. 21). Skill development—not high scores on intelligence tests—should always be the goal. Although a handicapped child's pace of learning may be somewhat slower than other children's, the achievements are just as meaningful.

Parents of children with epilepsy who also have mental handicap must remember that they learn new skills more slowly than other children and find it harder to master advanced skills such as reading, math, and complex problem solving. They also may not be as motivated as other children to learn new skills, but it does not mean that they cannot learn. Given a good educational program and support from family and friends, almost all children can make important, steady progress in intellectual abilities.

Cerebral Palsy

About 25% to 35% of all children with cerebral palsy have epilepsy. A much smaller proportion of those with epilepsy have cerebral palsy. Epilepsy and cerebral palsy are separate disorders, but both can result from the same abnormality of the brain. Epilepsy does not cause cerebral palsy. Cerebral palsy does not cause epilepsy. The two conditions simply coexist.

Cerebral palsy is not a specific medical diagnosis; instead, it is a descriptive name given to a group of disorders that affect control of movement and result from an abnormality of the central nervous system (the brain and spinal cord). The disorder is referred to as "stable" or "static" because the condition does not worsen over time. The abnormality may occur while the fetus is in the womb, during or shortly after birth, or during the first year of life. Even when an injury occurs in the womb or at birth, not all children born with cerebral palsy show any clear signs of the disorder immediately after birth, and the symptoms vary in severity depending on the type and degree of abnormality involved.

Usually, the child's intellectual functioning is not diminished by the disorder. However, mental handicap occurs in approximately one third of children with cerebral palsy, and some children with cerebral palsy and epilepsy are also mentally handicapped. The major problems for children with cerebral palsy are poor muscle control (e.g., difficulty sucking or holding up the head), delay in rolling over, delay in walking or inability to walk, incoordination, muscle tightness, and muscle spasms.

Cerebral palsy is classified according to six principal abnormal movements, all of which are not under a person's voluntary control; that is, they are involuntary movements. Many children with cerebral palsy have a combination of the movements, and their symptoms may vary from time to time. The abnormal movements are the following:

- *Spasticity:* Tense, stiff, contracted muscles.
- *Ataxia:* Poor sense of balance and impaired coordination. For example, when walking, the child may sway or lose balance; when reaching for an object, the child's hand may stop before reaching it and then move past it before finally arriving in the desired place.
- *Rigidity:* Tense, stiff, contracted muscles that resist movement. Both spasticity and rigidity are forms of excessive muscle tightness. The difference is based mainly on other abnormalities: athetosis and dystonia (see the following) with the rigid form, and weakness and increased reflexes with the spastic form.
- *Athetosis:* Uncoordinated, writhing, or wormlike movements of the head, limbs, and eyes that occur without deliberate effort.
- *Dystonia:* Unnatural, sustained postures of a body part such as the hand, leg, or neck.
- *Tremor:* Trembling or shaking.

There are two main types of cerebral palsy: *pyramidal* and *extrapyramidal.* The pyramidal and extrapyramidal systems are the two principal systems of the brain and spinal cord that control movement. The pyramidal system is primarily concerned with strength and control of fine movements of the arms and legs, especially the hands and feet. The extrapyramidal system is primarily concerned with more basic aspects of movement and exerts greater control over muscles of the body, shoulders, and hips, although it also controls muscles in the arms and legs. Many children with cerebral palsy and epilepsy have overlapping features of these two types. Children with either type of cerebral palsy may have ataxia, tremor, or other impairments such as mental handicap.

PYRAMIDAL CEREBRAL PALSY

More than 80% of children with cerebral palsy have the spastic form, a pyramidal type of cerebral palsy that occurs either alone or in combination with the extrapyramidal type. These children usually have weakness, increased muscle tone (spasticity), and increased reflexes (e.g., when the doctor taps the knee and the leg jumps forward). The injury in this disorder is either to the brain cells in the frontal lobe area that control voluntary movement or to the nerve fibers that pass from this area into the spinal cord. Different patterns of damage give rise to different types of impairment: spastic hemiparesis, diplegia, and spastic quadriparesis.

Spastic Hemiparesis

Hemiparesis refers to weakness on one side of the body (hemi = half; paresis = slight or incomplete paralysis). This is the most common form of spastic cerebral palsy, and it most often results from an injury to the opposite side of the brain. The damage may affect the motor area of the brain, the nerve fibers, or both. Stroke from blockage of a blood vessel or bleeding in the brain is the most common cause of hemiparesis. Other causes include traumatic injury or an abnormality in brain development. In most children with spastic hemiparesis, the arm is weaker than the leg, and the hand often is severely impaired. (As shown in Fig. 4, the hand and fingers have a large representation in the motor area of the brain.) Depending on how severely the leg is affected, children with spastic hemiparesis can usually walk, but with a limp. Braces for the ankle or an operation to release tight tendons can improve the child's ability to walk. Because the injury is relatively restricted to one area of the brain, most children with spastic hemiparesis are not mentally handicapped.

Because the cerebral cortex of the brain is often damaged in children with spastic hemiparesis, they usually have epilepsy. The seizures are partial seizures and are treated with medications for partial epilepsy. The seizures usually can be controlled with antiepileptic drugs, but if not, surgery can be considered.

Diplegia

In children with diplegia, both legs are weak and stiff (di = two; plegia = paralysis). The arms usually function well and may be entirely normal. Diplegia most often occurs in children who are born prematurely. It usually results from injury to the nerve fibers in the deep parts of the brain. Because the cerebral cortex is usually not affected, neither seizures nor mental handicap are common.

Walking is the main problem for children with diplegia. Physical therapy, leg braces, orthopedic surgery, or the use of a wheelchair can improve function and the quality of life.

Spastic Quadriparesis

Quadriparesis refers to weakness of all four limbs (quadri = four). In this severe form of cerebral palsy, the injury often affects multiple and widely distributed areas of the brain. The weakness is often severe and affects not only the limbs, but also the muscles of the trunk, neck, mouth, and face. In addition to a severe movement disorder, the children have epilepsy and mental handicap, which often are also severe.

The seizures in children with the spastic quadriparetic form of cerebral palsy usually begin early (during the newborn period or in the first year of life) and are difficult to control with drugs. The first seizures are often infantile spasms, followed later by Lennox-Gastaut syndrome, with various types of seizures that are only partially controlled with high dosages of medications.

EXTRAPYRAMIDAL CEREBRAL PALSY

The extrapyramidal type of cerebral palsy is characterized by involuntary abnormal movements, which include dystonia (sustained postures, such as the fingers curled up), athetosis (wormlike, writhing movements), chorea (irregular, minor jerks or dancelike movements), and tremor. The extrapyramidal motor system is deep within the brain. Because it is so far removed from the cerebral cortex, mental handicap and seizures are uncommon in children with this type of cerebral palsy. They do often have impaired balance and coordination, however.

In the past, this type of cerebral palsy often occurred when babies born with blood types different from their mothers' (Rh incompatibility) had severe metabolic changes that injured the extrapyramidal parts of the brain. Better care of this problem has now made extrapyramidal cerebral palsy less common. Extrapyramidal types now account for about 20% of children with cerebral palsy. About half of these have only extrapyramidal problems; the other half also have the pyramidal type. Those who have both types are said to have mixed cerebral palsy.

TREATMENT

Treatment of children with cerebral palsy and epilepsy varies according to their age, the severity of their symptoms, and the type of cerebral palsy. Common steps include corrective lenses, braces, and corrective surgery for affected limbs; injections of tiny doses of botulin toxin to relieve spasticity and treat movement disorders; drug therapy to reduce spastic tension in muscles; speech and physical therapy; psychological counseling to assist with adjustment issues; and referrals to appropriate resources. Comprehensive child development clinics (centers for neuromuscular and developmental disorders) can help with many parts of this treatment. They can identify, assess, and diagnose children's general health conditions; identify emotional and learning problems; refer children with particular problems to specialists; provide instruction and counseling for parents; serve as a source of referrals to other programs; and provide physical, occupational, and speech therapy.

Exercise is an essential part of the therapy for children with cerebral palsy. Babies who are developing normally are seldom still; their arms and legs are in almost continuous motion. As they roll, crawl, get into and out of sitting positions, and reach for objects and manipulate them, they are exercising without making a conscious effort. For babies with cerebral palsy, this kind of healthy, spontaneous exercise is more challenging. Some may be capable of only a few movements, so these babies are often relatively inactive. Children with cerebral palsy must have exercise, however. Movement through all ranges of motion can prevent contractures or joint limitations and help the child's body maintain its potential. Weight-bearing exercises can prevent bone loss. Also, the input from exercise is an important building block for the future development of motor and cognitive skills.

The parents of a child with epilepsy and cerebral palsy must make sure the child gets enough exercise. If the child is passive and content to lie back and watch the world go by, the parents need to encourage activity. For young children with cerebral palsy, one of the best ways to do this is through the roughhouse play that other children instinctively make a part of their regular exercise. The touch and movement that are so much a part of this type of play are essential to the development of touch, balance, and the sense of head and body position. A child can enjoy roughhousing if the parents keep in mind the principles of good handling and pay attention to the child's body. For example, if rapid movements such as playfully lifting and lowering make the child stiff, it is better to try a slower activity involving some trunk rotation and leg separation, which should decrease the child's muscle tone (the firmness and consistency of muscles at rest and with movement) and reduce the child's stiffness. A good alternative might be the "merry-go-round," in which the parent holds the child face-to-face with the child's legs straddling the parent's waist and twirls around. In general, children with increased muscle tone (stiff or rigid muscles) respond better to a slow pace, and those with low muscle tone, who are floppy or hypotonic, generally respond well to fast movements.

Ideally, the child should get much of his or her exercise from the daily routine of diapering, dressing, and feeding. Two general guidelines in accomplishing this goal are to place objects far enough away that the child needs to reach for them or crawl to them and to encourage the child to do all the physical activities he or she is capable of, even if it sometimes seems easier for someone else to do them. The child's occupational and physical therapists can provide additional tips on increasing the exercise the child gets in the daily routine.

In addition, some parents of children with epilepsy and cerebral palsy enroll the child in formal physical fitness programs. Gym classes, movement experiences, and other programs for young children are blossoming, and many are quite receptive to children with special needs. It is not absolutely essential to find a program with a staff trained in dealing with these children, although the instructor should be helpful and cooperative. Generally, it will be up to the parent to apply the correct principles to reduce or increase muscle tone and encourage normal movement. The physical or occupational therapist can tell parents whether the child might benefit from any program they are considering.

As the child grows older, it becomes increasingly important for the exercise routine to include outdoor activities. Walks with the child in a stroller or in a carrier on the parent's back provide fresh air and opportunities for learning about the world outside the house. For some children, just lying or sitting on the grass while parents do yard work can be a special event. Outdoor smells, sights, and sounds all stimulate the child's developing sensory system. With proper precautions, the child may also enjoy riding on the back of the parent's bicycle. Parents may have to be creative in thinking of outdoor play activities that are within the child's abilities, but because playing outdoors is the most enjoyable form of exercise for many children, the more activities parents can come up with, the better. For example, horseback riding can provide both good physical therapy and fun for children with cerebral palsy. As with many other aspects of raising a child with cerebral palsy, much trial and error is involved in finding enjoyable exercises that are right for the child.

Independence

Some children with epilepsy and cerebral palsy have average or close-to-average intelligence and mild to moderate physical problems. These children usually achieve independence during later adolescence and adulthood, but others are not so fortunate. Children who are also mentally handicapped and whose physical problems limit their mobility or prevent the mastery of self-help skills will continue to depend on others to some extent for the rest of their lives. The parents of these children should try to help them become as independent as possible.

The need for special education or other services depends on how the disorders affect the person with epilepsy and cerebral palsy. These services can be provided through the school system, employment programs, and residential or community-based programs. In addition, programs such as the Special Olympics (www.specialolympics.org) can allow children with epilepsy and cerebral palsy to participate in athletics, excel at their own level, and enjoy the excitement and self-esteem of accomplishment.

EDUCATION AND TRAINING

The education of children with cerebral palsy and epilepsy may begin shortly after birth. Many children begin receiving services through infant stimulation programs soon after the diagnosis is made. The best infant stimulation programs almost always involve the parents as teachers of their own children. These programs stress stimulation of the child's visual, auditory, olfactory, and tactile senses and include activities that promote language, cognitive, social, and self-help development. Some programs include specialists such as physical or speech therapists in addition to specially trained teachers. Most parents are very receptive to infant stimulation programs because their involvement fulfills their need to "do something" to help their children.

Children with cerebral palsy and epilepsy are often educated in regular classes, but they are eligible for special education programs, if they need them, under the Individuals with Disabilities Education Act (IDEA) (see Chap. 21).

Vocational Training Programs

In the past, people with epilepsy whose cerebral palsy was severely disabling were excluded from receiving vocational training services because they were unlikely to achieve the goal of competitive full-time or part-time employment. Those who had only epilepsy were often excluded for the same reason. IDEA has made services and training available to people with severe disabilities. They are eligible even if the most they will achieve is "supported employment," which means employment in a setting with a job coach, special training, or other services that allow an individual to perform work.

The department of vocational rehabilitation in each state, sometimes called "DVR," "OVR," or "Voc Rehab," is charged with carrying out the law (see Chap. 27). Under these programs, adults with epilepsy and cerebral palsy can continue to receive vocational education after they reach age 21. The state vocational rehabilitation department, United Cerebral Palsy (UCP), or a local UCP affiliate can be contacted for specific information on available services.

The Workforce Investment Act of 1998 established "one-stop shopping" resource centers for employment services, educational services, training and placement, and vocational rehabilitation. These may also be useful resources for people with cerebral palsy and epilepsy who are seeking employment.

LIVING AND WORKING IN THE COMMUNITY

New trends are emerging to help enable people with epilepsy and other disabilities to live independently and productively. The focus of these efforts is to help people with disabling conditions to overcome the physical limitations that in the past too often meant lives spent in institutions.

Personal assistance services are available for those who need help with daily care and mobility. In some programs, a personal assistant can help with cooking meals, cleaning house, and grooming so that a person with cerebral palsy can live independently. The extent to which Medicaid will help fund these programs varies from state to state.

Another trend is the movement away from caring for people with severe cerebral palsy and epilepsy in large public or private facilities, called intermediate care facilities. Instead, funding and services are provided for independent living within the community. State-run programs for adults with epilepsy and cerebral palsy should provide a variety of community living and working arrangements.

Protecting the rights of people with epilepsy and cerebral palsy to employment and equal opportunity in the community is of utmost importance. In 1990, the Americans with Disabilities Act was passed to protect people with disabilities from discrimination in employment, public accommodations, transportation, telecommunications, and other areas (see Chap. 27). The Epilepsy Foundation may be helpful in providing additional information.

DRIVING

Persons with cerebral palsy and epilepsy have the same right as everyone else to obtain a driver's license if their seizures are completely controlled by medication for a specific period (usually 3 to 12 months). If they can pass the written test (given verbally if the person is unable to write) and the driving test, persons with these disorders can obtain a license to drive (see Chap. 24).

INCOME MAINTENANCE AND MEDICAL ASSISTANCE

Two federally funded income maintenance programs can provide additional income to persons with cerebral palsy, mental handicap, or both: Supplemental Security Income (SSI), a public assistance program, and Social Security Disability Insurance (SSDI), a disability insurance program (see Chap. 31). Both provide a monthly income to qualified persons with disabilities. The regulations of the Social Security Administration (www.ssa.gov) prescribe a set of tests for making the determination of disability. The test of severity is somewhat different for children and adults. A child with epilepsy and cerebral palsy meets the test of severity if he or she has severe motor impairment (dysfunction) *or* less severe motor impairment with cognitive impairment (IQ of 69 or less) *and* a seizure disorder (major motor seizures with disabling episodes, major motor seizures with a significant communication deficit or a significant emotional disorder, or minor motor seizures with loss of consciousness).

Under current rules, an adult with epilepsy may qualify as having a disability if the Social Security Administration determines that he or she has more than one major motor seizure (loss of consciousness and convulsions) per month or one minor motor seizure (alteration of awareness or consciousness) per week. In either situation, the seizures must persist for at least 3 months after treatment begins and must be documented by a health care professional. Some persons with both epilepsy and cerebral palsy can qualify without meeting these frequency requirements. In any case, there are income restrictions on who can receive payments. An adult must earn less than the current level of an official statistic called the substantial gainful activity level. Because regulations may change, it is always wise to check with the Social Security Administration on the rules presently in effect.

The Medicare and Medicaid programs (see Chap. 31) are important to people with epilepsy and cerebral palsy. Each program has its own eligibility requirements and rules for recipients. Both of these programs may be available to children with disabilities who are under 18 years of age. Medicaid provides medical assistance to people who are eligible for SSI and to other people with incomes that are insufficient to pay for medical care. Because eligibility is based on financial need, placing assets in the name of a child with epilepsy and cerebral palsy or providing the children with income through a trust may mean disqualification. However, trust funds designed to supplement benefits may not be disqualifying if they are properly drawn up (see Chap. 23). Medicare is not based on financial need. Anyone entitled to receive Social Security benefits is also entitled to Medicare coverage after a 2-year waiting period.

OUTLOOK FOR SUCCESS IN LIFE

The outlook for children with epilepsy and cerebral palsy has never been brighter. Advanced therapeutic and surgical techniques are helping to minimize the effects of cerebral palsy and its complications, and new medications and treatment methods are helping to control seizures. In addition, special equipment is helping children with these disorders to unlock their potential as never before. For example, computers are giving voices to children who might not otherwise be able to speak, and devices made from lightweight plastics and metals are granting new freedom of movement to children with limited motor skills.

Increased opportunities in education are helping these children make giant steps toward conquering the effects of their disabilities. Another bright spot is that their parents are taking increasingly larger roles in helping the children reach their potential. For example, therapists now routinely train parents to reinforce their child's movement and speech skills at home. Teachers usually confer with parents when deciding how and what these children should learn in school. Most professionals recognize that parents are the experts on their child's special needs and are often able to help the child receive the most appropriate services. These parent-professional partnerships naturally foster greater progress.

Some children with epilepsy and cerebral palsy graduate from regular academic high school programs and go to college. Others succeed in completing vocational high school programs. Still others spend their school years in programs designed to help them become as self-sufficient as possible. Likewise, some children with epilepsy and cerebral palsy grow up to hold jobs that enable them to support themselves. Others need varying amounts of financial help throughout their adult lives.

Today, all children with epilepsy and cerebral palsy have the potential to live rich, fulfilling lives and to enjoy good health, good friends, and good feelings about themselves and their accomplishments. The right therapeutic and educational programs will start these children on the road to a rewarding future; motivation and support will keep them on track.

After the Parents Are Gone

No one wants to think about the reality of growing old or dying. For parents of children with uncontrolled seizures and serious physical and neurologic disabilities, planning for the future is critical. The more the child depends on the parent, the more necessary planning becomes.

All adults should have a will. A will is especially necessary for parents of young children and adolescents with epilepsy and for parents whose older children are unable to fully care for themselves. A will allows parents to designate someone to take care of their children, manage the money they leave behind for the children, and supervise the proper distribution of their estate. A will can be drawn up inexpensively. It is the only way that parents can guarantee that their children will be cared for in the way the parents desire and that their assets will be distributed in accordance with their wishes.

If there is no will, the state's rules for the situation—called intestacy rules—will apply. The intestacy rules, rather than the individual's desires, will govern the distribution of assets and the ultimate guardianship of any children who are minors.

Choosing a Guardian

Guardians have the legal responsibility for a child (or a legally incompetent person) if the child's natural parents die or are unable to care for the child. Whether a guardian is required depends on the child's age and ability to manage his or her own affairs.

Choosing a guardian is one of the most difficult decisions any parent has to make. A guardian has awesome responsibilities. Parents should consider their own values and how they would want their child to be brought up. The guardian should share the parents' values and principles about raising a child or overseeing the well-being of an adult with severe seizures and related disabilities. Parents should discuss their concerns and wishes with the potential guardians. Even after talking things over, it is a good idea for the parents to put their thoughts in writing.

Family members and close friends are usually considered possible guardians. The guardians should be responsible and mature, but they should also love, or at least have the capacity to love, the child. The guardians should have a stable family structure. If the guardians have children, parents should make sure that their child will not be an added burden and a source of resentment.

A grown sister or brother may be the best person to look after an older child or mentally handicapped adult with epilepsy after the parents are gone. As participants in family life throughout the years, they should be taught that, like their parents, they have responsibilities for their disabled sibling. These responsibilities may continue throughout their lifetimes, and one of the other children in the family may expect to eventually assume the role of parent for the dependent person. That is an enormous commitment, but most sisters and brothers lovingly and willingly accept it.

Trusts and Estate Planning

After deciding on the guardian, parents must next decide on the trustees and executors of their wills. The executor oversees the administration of the estate and the distribution of the assets. The trustees are responsible for administering trust funds for the child. Attorneys who specialize in estate planning can help create trusts with terms that parents find in their child's best interest.

The terms of a trust vary depending on the amount of assets, the immediate and long-term needs of the child, the maturity and age of the child, and other factors. A trust instrument can be very flexible. It can provide that the trustee have the discretion to distribute money as required for the health, welfare, and maintenance of the child. In some cases, the child can be given the interest earned in addition to these discretionary distributions. In other cases, the child can receive the interest until a certain age and then, if the trustee feels the child can manage the money, the entire assets or a fraction of the assets can be given to the child.

When parents write their wills, it is often a good time to consider estate planning. No one wants to pay more taxes than legally necessary. As much as $675,000 can be passed from parents to children without incurring federal estate tax. (This will increase to $1 million over the next several years.)

When there is a child with special needs, assets assume even greater importance. Parents can do several things to protect the amount of money their child receives from their estate. First, every year, each child can receive a gift of up to $10,000 from each parent. This money, and the interest that it generates over time, can go into a carefully drawn trust fund designed to supplement the child's other benefits. This money will not be subject to estate taxes when the parent dies. The gift to the child's trust can be in the form of cash, investments, or insurance policies. For example, a parent can purchase a whole-life insurance policy that is owned by the child's trust. The cost of the premiums can be paid as part of the child's yearly gift. If structured correctly, the death benefit goes to the child when the parent dies without being subject to estate taxes.

Similarly, whole-life policies can be obtained that are payable to the trust only when both parents have passed away. These policies are often much less expensive than policies on a single parent, and the benefits from these policies can be used to pay estate taxes, leaving the assets to the children.

A variety of other strategies may be worth considering. The laws regarding estate taxes and exemptions are complex; parents should consult an attorney who is knowledgeable about estate taxes.

When an adult child needs assisted living arrangements and cannot be self-supporting, he or she will qualify for a range of services through state and federal agencies. Such funding can often provide resources for long-term placement in a residential facility. However, eligibility for these programs can be lost if there is a transfer of funds when the parents pass away. Trusts must be set up to *supplement* the benefits, not to replace them. It is important that the proper legal steps are taken and that the family knows that bequests to the affected family member must go to the trust, not directly to the person.

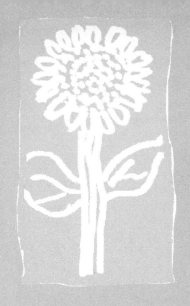

part four

EPILEPSY
IN ADULTS

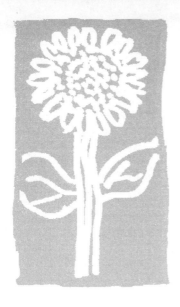

Living with Epilepsy

One of the biggest concerns for adults with epilepsy is whether and how much to restrict their activities of daily living. There must be a balance between safety and the need to pursue employment, fulfill household responsibilities, and enjoy leisure activities. That balance can best be achieved by using common sense. For people with rare or fully controlled seizures, most activities can be safely pursued. For those who have frequent seizures with impairment of consciousness and a period of confusion afterward, certain activities must be restricted. The restrictions may be able to be lifted if seizure control improves.

Risk-Benefit Decisions

Life is never free of risks for anyone. Making decisions about the risks and benefits associated with different activities is not unique to people with epilepsy. High-risk activities like skydiving, scuba diving, motorcycle riding, or firefighting can potentially cause injury or death, yet millions of people participate in them every year. Those who do so feel that the benefits—enjoyment, economical transportation, or employment— outweigh the risks. Many more of us engage in lower-risk activities, such as driving a car or snorkeling.

Our decisions ultimately reflect our personal philosophy of life and how we define the benefits and risks. The risk-benefit decisions of people with epilepsy should be influenced by their seizure control. For people whose seizures are well controlled, the situation is essentially no different from that of someone without epilepsy. For people with frequent, uncontrolled seizures, some activities, such as swimming and bike riding, can be carried out with precautions, but other activities, such as driving a car or flying a plane, are simply unsafe. The most difficult decisions involve people who have occasional seizures.

It is important that people with epilepsy consider how having a seizure during a specific activity affects themselves as well as others. For example, cigarette smoking by people with epilepsy can present dangers other than the well-known ones that affect all smokers. If someone is smoking and has a seizure, the fallen cigarette can start a fire.

Prevention of Seizure-Related Injuries

Most seizures do not cause physical injury. However, serious injuries can occur during tonic-clonic and tonic or atonic seizures. During these attacks, people usually fall and may bruise or cut themselves, fracture their bones, chip their teeth, dislocate their shoulders, or sprain their joints. Because of the dangers, people with frequent, uncontrolled seizures that cause them to lose control of their muscles or become unaware of their surroundings should take special precautions, especially in the kitchen. They should not work in places where they could be injured by heat, electricity, or dangerous equipment (such as an electric saw), unless special safety features are in place or unless they *always* have a warning (aura) of an approaching seizure.

SPECIAL PRECAUTIONS

Prevention is the best strategy for avoiding seizure-related injuries. When cooking, for example, people with frequent seizures may be safer using a microwave oven or putting guards around an open flame. Whenever possible, they should bring individual dishes to the source of hot food rather than carrying kettles or saucepans across the kitchen. Other safeguards in the home include carpeting the bathroom, putting a temperature monitor on showerheads, lowering the temperature of the water heater, putting guards around radiators, taking clothes that have to be ironed to the cleaners, and avoiding electric carving knives and slicing machines. It may even be a good idea to live in a single-story house or a first-floor or elevator-served apartment to avoid falls on stairs.

SEIZURE-ALERT DOGS

Some people with epilepsy have reported that their dogs are able to "sense" when a seizure is coming. The dog may then respond in a variety of ways, such as whining, pawing, or remaining close to the owner. This distinctive behavior can warn the person or their family that a seizure may soon occur. This behavior has been reported in a number of different breeds. It is possible that dogs can detect some change (e.g., an odor or tone of voice) that warns them of an approaching seizure, similar to the way that certain symptoms warn some patients.

No scientific studies of seizure-alert dogs have been completed so it remains uncertain whether dogs can reliably "sense" an impending seizure. It is also unclear how often they are correct when they indicate that a seizure is coming and how often they fail to indicate an approaching seizure. It is likely that the accuracy of the dog's predictive skills will vary considerably for different patients and different dogs.

Public and press interest in seizure-alert dogs has led several commercial groups to begin training and selling dogs for this purpose. In many cases, the cost exceeds $2000. There is little information on the quality of the different services and the ability of different breeds. Some services are training dogs to protect their owners in the case of a seizure. This could be dangerous if the dog prevents emergency medical services or other assistance from treating an individual during a seizure that is prolonged or associated with injury.

Quality of Life

A 40-year-old married man with two children was referred to an epileptologist after he asked his neurologist to recommend a doctor who could give a second opinion on his care. He had juvenile myoclonic epilepsy, had had seizures for more than 15 years, and was being treated with high doses of two antiepileptic drugs (which caused him to sleep 12 hours a night, yet feel constantly tired). He complained that he was "always a bit foggy, a little down and depressed. It's not me, I know it's the medications." Despite the therapy, he continued to have two or three tonic-clonic seizures a year. The epileptologist took the old drugs away and prescribed another antiepileptic drug. The man has been seizure-free for more than a year and has almost no adverse reactions to the new drug. He says, "I feel as if I have been reborn. I am another person. Everyone at work and at home can see the difference. I am awake. My spirits are great. I can think. I am so happy."

The concept of "quality of life" is relatively new in medicine. Quality of life is difficult to measure. Simply stated, it reflects the patient's, not the doctor's, perspectives on an illness and its effects on life. Although it would seem that the patient's and doctor's views on the quality of life would be similar, they can be quite different. In various fields of medicine, quality-of-life studies have provided new insights into the effect of disorders and treatments on patients and have offered ways of improving their lives.

There has been increasing recognition that the quality of life is often impaired in people with epilepsy, but doctors still may not be aware of it. Many doctors who care for people with epilepsy consider occasional seizures "acceptable" and minor adverse effects of medications "tolerable." Of course, in some cases, the seizures cannot be entirely controlled, and adverse effects invariably occur despite the doctor's best attempts to adjust the medications. Too often, however, the doctor does not aggressively try to control the seizures further or to reduce the adverse effects of the medication. The problem is often one of perception: the doctor does not see a problem worthy of attention, but the patient does.

A person who has occasional seizures may have restrictions on driving; difficulties with getting a job or advancing in their career; and problems with finances, social and family life, and self-esteem. Fear of another seizure may be the person's greatest disability. The stigma of epilepsy, which unfortunately is still too often encountered, may have altered the person's view of society and affected his or her possibilities of employment. In some cases, however, the person's perception of the stigma may be greater than any actual discrimination. Others may find that tolerating an occasional seizure offers a better quality of life than the adverse effects that accompany more aggressive treatment.

Achieving the best possible quality of life for people with epilepsy is a challenge. On the one hand, doctors must pay greater attention to patients' expectations and their actual experiences of living with epilepsy. On the other hand, patients must help doctors understand how epilepsy and its treatment affect their lives.

Driving

A driver's license is a passport to adulthood in the United States. In both rural and suburban areas, access to a motor vehicle is often essential for independence and employment. Even in many urban areas, driving is required for employment or to reach certain locations for work or pleasure.

Driving is a privilege, and applicants must meet the criteria set forth by their state to qualify for a driver's license. Applicants in all states must be older than a minimum age (usually 16 or 17 years); must not have a medical disorder that would make driving dangerous; and must pass a written test, a vision test, and a driving test.

LICENSURE OF PEOPLE WITH EPILEPSY

The laws determining which medical conditions disqualify someone from obtaining a driver's license vary from state to state. In many states, the laws have become more liberal in recent years, resulting in fewer restrictions for people with epilepsy. The laws are written to protect public safety and to grant the privilege of driving to people who are the least likely to have an accident. Compared with those of most European nations, American driving restrictions are quite liberal. In some European countries, for example, a single tonic-clonic seizure in adulthood prohibits holding a license for the rest of the person's life.

Many people do not recognize that absence or complex partial seizures while driving can be just as deadly as tonic-clonic seizures. Furthermore, the risk of injury or death is not restricted to the driver and passengers; it also applies to pedestrians and people in other vehicles. Studies have shown that the rate of motor-vehicle accidents for people with epilepsy is higher than the average rate, but nowhere near the rate for those who drink and drive. Accidents involving epilepsy usually are caused by people (especially men) who are driving without a license or who fail to report their epilepsy when applying for a license.

To obtain a driver's license in most states, a person with epilepsy must be free of seizures that affect consciousness for a certain period and must submit a doctor's statement of opinion that the person can drive safely. The seizure-free period varies from state to state. The recent trend is away from requiring an "absolute period" of being seizure-free toward a shorter interval of freedom from seizures. Although some states still require a period of at least 1 year during which the person with epilepsy is seizure-free, most consider exceptions that would permit someone to drive after a shorter seizure-free interval. A recent conference of professional and lay epilepsy organizations recommended a seizure-free period of 3 months for driving privileges. In most states, the doctor who cares for the person with epilepsy must fill out a form stating that it is safe for the person to drive and recommending licensure. This recommendation is used as one of several factors in making a decision. In states that do not require a specific seizure-free period, the doctor's recommendation often carries considerable weight.

REVIEW AND DECISION PROCESS

In most states, the medical information submitted by the applicant and the doctor is reviewed by personnel in the state's Department of Motor Vehicles (DMV) or equivalent department. In complex cases, or in those in which the decision is uncertain, the information is usually forwarded to a consulting doctor or the state's medical advisory board. Most states have such a board, which may also hear appeals concerning decisions to deny or revoke drivers' licenses.

Decisions made by the DMV can be appealed by requesting an administrative hearing before the medical advisory board or another designated body. If the administrative decision is not favorable, the applicant can request a review by a judge. Such requests must be made within a specified period.

In some states, someone with persistent seizures may be allowed to drive if the seizures do not impair consciousness or control of movement, occur only during sleep, are consistently preceded by an aura, are restricted to a certain time of the day (e.g., within an hour after awakening), or occur only when the antiepileptic medications are reduced or stopped on the advice of a doctor. A letter from the doctor confirming the presence and consistency of these features is often required by the state DMV. If a driver's license is revoked because of a breakthrough seizure surrounded by extenuating circumstances (e.g., reduction of medication on a doctor's advice or unusual stress, such as the death of a loved one) the driver may appeal the decision. Evidence that the person takes the prescribed medications is often required, and the level of the antiepileptic drug in the blood is usually provided as confirmation of compliance.

In many states, people who do not meet the requirements for a regular driver's license may be granted a restricted license. This license may allow a person with epilepsy or other disabilities to drive under certain conditions (e.g., during daytime only, to and from work within a certain distance from the home, or only during an emergency).

COMMERCIAL DRIVER'S LICENSES

The U.S. Department of Transportation (DOT) prohibits anyone with a history of epilepsy from having a commercial driver's license. They are not allowed to drive a truck between states. These regulations are currently under review, however. For advice about the current rules, a person with epilepsy should contact the DOT.

The blanket denial of a commercial driver's license to any person with a history of epilepsy is unfair for several reasons. Some childhood epilepsies, such as benign rolandic epilepsy, are associated with a high remission rate; the seizures in some people may have been fully controlled for years; and some types of seizures are not dangerous if they occur while driving.

Regulations for driving a truck or bus within one state vary from state to state. Some states have restrictive policies that prohibit any person with a history of epilepsy from driving a commercial vehicle. Others take a more reasonable approach and review each case individually.

MAINTAINING A DRIVER'S LICENSE

Most states that grant driver's licenses to people with epilepsy require periodic medical reports. These reports document that seizure control has not deteriorated and that the person is taking or does not need to take medications. If the seizures have stopped or have been controlled for more than 3 to 5 years, most states will no longer require periodic medical reports.

Regardless of the reporting requirements, if seizures recur and impair consciousness or control of movement, it is imperative to stop driving and consult the doctor, who may be able to suggest changes in lifestyle (such as more sleep) or adjustments in medications that may restore seizure control.

POTENTIAL LIABILITY AND PHYSICIAN REPORTING

A person with epilepsy may be civilly or criminally liable for a motor-vehicle accident caused by having a seizure while driving. Liability may occur when a person drives against medical advice, without a valid license, without notifying the state DMV of the medical condition, or with the knowledge that he or she is prohibited from driving.

In 2001, six states (California, Delaware, Nevada, New Jersey, Oregon, and Pennsylvania) had "mandatory reporting laws" requiring that doctors report people with epilepsy and other disorders that may make driving hazardous. These laws generally order the doctor to notify the DMV of the person's name, age, and address. In these states, doctors may be liable for negligence if they fail to report a person with epilepsy who is later involved in a motor-vehicle accident. In states without such laws, however, the question of whether a doctor should report a patient who may be driving unsafely presents a difficult conflict between public safety and the doctor's need to respect the privacy of the relationship with the patient. In theory, a physician who reports a patient's condition could be sued for disclosing confidential information. As discussed later, the state of Connecticut has attempted to establish a middle ground in this conflict.

In states that do have mandatory reporting laws, the specifics of when a doctor must report someone can be vague. In New Jersey, for example, the law states that the doctor must report any person 16 years of age or older for recurrent convulsive seizures *or* for recurrent periods of unconsciousness *or* for impairment or loss of motor coordination due to conditions such as, but not limited to, epilepsy in any of its forms when such conditions persist or recur despite medical treatments. This law is open to some interpretation. For example, it remains unclear what constitutes "medical treatments." The plural usage indicates that more than one treatment has failed to control the seizures, but does not specify how many dosage adjustments or medications must have been tried.

Mandatory reporting laws should be repealed, as was done by Connecticut in 1990. However, the current law states that if a physician in Connecticut cares for a person whose seizures are so poorly controlled that driving would present a serious risk to public safety and there is evidence that the person continues to drive, the doctor can report the person with immunity from lawsuit by the patient. Such cases are rare. Connecticut's approach to mandatory reporting is a reasonable middle ground because it strikes a balance between the rights of the individual and the public's safety.

The chief problem with mandatory reporting is that it can destroy the doctor-patient relationship. In many cases, those who believe that they "must" drive will lie to the doctor about their condition to avoid mandatory reporting and potential loss of their driver's license. This is the worst of both worlds: the person is not receiving the best medical care and is driving. If the doctor and patient can work together, the seizures are likely to be better controlled and the person can drive more safely.

The most common penalty for a physician's failure to report a patient under mandatory reporting laws is a fine, usually ranging from $5 to $50. However, an accident can lead to a lawsuit charging wrongful death or injury, with a large judgment against the doctor. In states that require mandatory reporting, compliance varies widely among doctors.

Doctors who state that it is safe for a person with epilepsy to drive and recommend licensure could also face some liability in case of an accident, although it appears to be minimal. Very few cases have been brought against a doctor by a third party who was injured in a motor-vehicle accident allegedly caused by a person with epilepsy. Doctors should not be liable for recommendations made to the DMV if their opinions are reasonable and consistent with good medical care. Some states grant immunity from liability to doctors who make recommendations about driving privileges.

Sports and Other Physical Activities

Common sense must prevail in making decisions about sports and other potentially dangerous physical activities. The discussion in Chapter 20 about sports and other activities for children and adolescents also is relevant to adults. There must be a balance between an active, full life and safety. The balance is easily achieved because most sports can be safely pursued by adults with epilepsy. People with well-controlled seizures, seizures occurring only during sleep, or seizures that are always preceded by a warning should have few or no restrictions on physical activities. For people who have complex partial or tonic-clonic seizures, even if they are preceded by warnings, some restrictions should apply. In skydiving, for example, even if the person is able to pull the ripcord, a seizure may prevent control of the descent, increasing the risk of landing in trees or power lines or hitting the ground at high speed. Restrictions also apply to scuba diving, unless the dive depth is less than 15 feet and, as with any scuba dive, the person is accompanied by a buddy.

Most sporting activities can be pursued by people whose seizures are not fully controlled. These activities include water skiing, sailing, wind-surfing, snorkeling, bicycling, gymnastics, soccer, football, baseball, handball, squash, tennis, basketball, volleyball, archery, skiing, sledding, hiking, and many others. None of these activities should be pursued by a person with epilepsy unless someone is nearby who is familiar with the condition and has basic lifesaving skills. When a person is engaged in any of these activities, precautions can be taken to minimize the risk of injury. For example, when participating in water sports, wearing a life vest reduces the risk of drowning if the person ends up in the water; its use is required of all water skiers in many states. Snorkeling can also be enjoyed by people with seizures, but they must use caution about where they snorkel. In some areas, the rocks, coral, and sea urchin spines form a maze close to the water's surface. If the water stirs, even an experienced snorkeler can get cut or injured. Such areas should be avoided by people whose seizures are not fully controlled because their ability to navigate through the sharp objects in the maze could be impaired. Although diving from the edge of a pool, dock, or low diving board is generally safe, diving off a high diving board is dangerous for people with epilepsy. For all of these activities, people with epilepsy must weigh the benefits and risks.

Although hiking can be safely pursued by people with recurrent seizures, mountain climbing can be dangerous for them. Using ropes or climbing along difficult paths can be dangerous even for the most alert and agile climber. A brief lapse of concentration or a small problem with control of movement could be deadly. Nature is not forgiving. Climbers should carefully consider the specific trail or mountain before starting and remember that there is no glory in proceeding if they reach an unexpected and dangerous obstacle.

Hunting can be safely pursued by people with epilepsy. When hunting, someone else should stay close by a person whose seizures are not fully controlled. If the person has a warning of a seizure, he or she should lay the gun down immediately. If a warning does not always occur, it may be best only to load the rifle shortly before shooting and then unload it if no shot is taken.

People with frequent, uncontrolled seizures can also vigorously pursue sporting activities, although the safety issues assume even greater importance. They must use greater precautions and more carefully consider the risks.

Smoking

Smoking contributes to the death of approximately 500,000 people each year from heart disease, stroke, and cancer. Smoking tobacco is not known to have any definite effects on seizure control. However, people with epilepsy not only are susceptible to all the usual effects of smoking, but also are at increased risk of injury or death from fire.

Consider what happened to one of my patients and her daughter. The patient, a 35-year-old woman with absence and tonic-clonic seizures, shared an apartment with her lively 5-year-old daughter. One evening, the woman had a tonic-clonic seizure while she was smoking. When she awoke in the hospital, she had first-degree burns on a large part of her arms and body. Her daughter suffered severe smoke inhalation and brain damage. The girl, now 18 years old, is severely mentally handicapped, uses a wheelchair, and is in an institution. The woman stopped smoking and has gone through a long emotional process of dealing with what happened.

Unlike many other activities, smoking presents risks for the person with epilepsy as well as for others, who can be severely injured or killed. Therefore, any person with epilepsy who has episodes of impaired consciousness should stop smoking. There are a variety of programs and methods (e.g., acupuncture) that can help a smoker stop smoking. The use of nicotine patches to help break the smoking habit is safe for people with epilepsy. The use of buproprion (Zyban) tablets as an aid to stop smoking can increase the seizure frequency or intensity, but at the usual dosage of 300 mg/day, the risk of worsening the seizures is small. If the seizures are well controlled and the blood levels of antiepileptic drugs are adequate, the benefits of Zyban are likely to outweigh the risks. For those who find it impossible or unacceptable to stop smoking, the risk of a dangerous fire can be substantially reduced by smoking only when another adult is nearby. All places where people smoke should be equipped with working smoke detectors.

Romantic Relationships and Marriage

People with well-controlled or infrequent seizures should have no serious problems dating or developing and maintaining a stable, intimate relationship. For people with uncontrolled seizures, dating and romantic relationships can be more difficult. Nevertheless, some people with frequent seizures have adjusted well to their condition and are successful in pursuing an active romantic life.

People with epilepsy in a relationship sooner or later face some important questions: Do I tell this person that I have epilepsy? When should I tell him or her? How much should I tell? There is no reason to rush the disclosure of epilepsy. Unless the seizures are so frequent that one might occur on the first date, it is best to wait until the ice is broken and trust and openness have developed in the relationship. These developments may happen on the first or the tenth date, or they may never happen. If the two people are obviously incompatible, there is no reason to discuss the disorder. If the relationship is developing slowly but is promising, it is reasonable to discuss the epilepsy earlier rather than later. It is best to tell the other person face to face, not over the telephone or by letter.

The way in which the disorder is presented is often how the other person will see it. The person with epilepsy should tell the truth about the disorder and how he or she has been affected by it. The other person should be allowed to react to what he or she has heard. The person with epilepsy has had time to adjust to the disorder, but the friend needs time to ask questions and to think about it.

Epilepsy need not be made the focus of all conversation. The two people should be able to discuss it and then move on to other subjects. Like everyone else, a person with epilepsy is defined by many traits and attributes; epilepsy need not be the defining feature.

Anyone who dates and gets involved in romantic relationships is likely to experience rejection at some time or another. Some prospective partners may refuse the first date or the second date, and others may break up the relationship after an extended period of dating. Rejection is part of dating and relationships for everyone; it is not unique to people with epilepsy. People are rejected for a variety reasons, including physical characteristics, personality traits, and social beliefs. Numerous observations and feelings about other people merge in the subconscious parts of our minds, and we are attracted to some people and not to others. Epilepsy may contribute to the reasons for rejection by some people, but it may be "attractive" to others who have a need to nurture or care for someone. However, a healthy and long-term relationship is more likely to develop when the other person is attracted to the individual's unique qualities and is able to put epilepsy in its rightful place—as a medical condition.

SEX LIFE

People with epilepsy can enjoy all the sexual feelings and pleasures others enjoy. Epilepsy is not generally associated with restrictions on sexual activities. Most people with epilepsy have normal sex lives. There is no convincing evidence that seizures are more likely to occur during sexual activities. Rarely, seizures may be more likely to occur during or shortly after physical exertion and intense emotional experiences. In this case, some modifications may be needed for the enjoyment of an active sex life.

Sexual dysfunction, a common problem in the general population, refers to an inability to experience sexual feelings and arousal or to perform sexual activities. For example, the failure of a man to achieve an erection (impotence) or the inability of a man or woman to achieve an orgasm (anorgasmia) are forms of sexual dysfunction. In the general population of people without epilepsy, many women do not routinely achieve orgasm and intermittent impotence is a problem for young men and even more of a problem for older men. Impotence is more common among men with epilepsy than for men in the general population. Antiepileptic drugs, mainly the barbiturates (phenobarbital and primidone), can cause or aggravate the impotence. The epilepsy itself, and not antiepileptic drugs, *may* contribute to sexual dysfunction, especially if the seizures are poorly controlled. If depression is present, its treatment may lead to resumption of normal sexual functioning. Sildenafil (Viagra) appears to be safe for epilepsy patients and does not interact with antiepileptic drugs.

Studies suggest that some people with epilepsy have a reduced libido (a lower level of interest in sexual activity) compared with people in the general population. Only a few people with epilepsy have such a problem, and they are not usually concerned about it. More often, one partner feels that the other partner's interest in sex is less than expected. Women with epilepsy are more likely than other women to experience painful intercourse and sexual dissatisfaction. If sexual dysfunction is a problem, a person should not hesitate to discuss it with the doctor; visiting a gynecologist, urologist, or other specialist may be helpful.

FAMILY PLANNING

Adolescent girls and women with epilepsy should be aware that antiepileptic drugs can cause birth defects (see Chap. 25). They also need to be educated about the different types of birth control and the effects of antiepileptic drugs on birth control pills (see Chap. 10). Adolescent girls with epilepsy have a higher frequency of unplanned pregnancy than females their age in the general population. The reasons for the increased rate of pregnancy in these women is uncertain. In one study, approximately 30% of females with epilepsy who were age 24 years or younger experienced unplanned pregnancy.

Men with epilepsy who are potential fathers also need to know about family planning, but they should be reassured that in general they are just about as likely as other men to father healthy babies. The rate of epilepsy among children whose fathers have epilepsy but whose mothers do not is only slightly higher than the rate in the general population. Some studies show a slight increase in birth defects among babies whose fathers took antiepileptic drugs, but others show no increase at all.

FERTILITY

Most men and women with epilepsy have normal sex lives, are fertile, and are able to have perfectly healthy children. Nevertheless, epilepsy, its treatment, and associated disorders may affect fertility and reproduction. Men with epilepsy may have slightly reduced fertility. Hormonal changes associated with the seizures may contribute to the problem. In addition, sperm production may be reduced in men who take antiepileptic drugs. Women with epilepsy also have somewhat higher rates of infertility than women in the general population. Antiepileptic drugs and irregular menstrual cycles probably contribute to this infertility.

The polycystic ovary syndrome in women is characterized by high levels of testosterone in the blood, increased hair growth on the body (hirsutism), multiple ovarian cysts, irregular menstruation, and lack of ovulation. Many of the affected women are obese. This syndrome is more common among women with epilepsy. Some evidence suggests that it occurs more often in women who take valproic acid.

Infertile couples in which one member, or both, have epilepsy should consult with an infertility specialist. Common causes of infertility, such as endometriosis (abnormal location of the lining of the womb) in women or a varicocele (abnormal collection of veins in the scrotal sac) in men, should be investigated and treated. Infertility should never be dismissed as simply a problem resulting from epilepsy or the antiepileptic drugs used to treat it.

Pregnancy and Menopause

The Childbearing Years

Planning a family and expecting a child should be joyous activities, but some fear also may be associated with these events. The fears that accompany pregnancy and parenthood are compounded for people with epilepsy, especially for women with epilepsy. Although taking certain medications during pregnancy is unsafe, most women with epilepsy are unable to safely stop their antiepileptic drugs during pregnancy. The risk of stopping medications may outweigh the risks of taking them.

PLANNING BEFORE PREGNANCY

In recent years, much attention has been focused on epilepsy in women of childbearing age. It has been realized that planning for pregnancy is essential—but which people with epilepsy should plan for pregnancy? Most people answer this question incorrectly, saying that women with epilepsy who want a family should make plans. The correct answer is that *all* women of childbearing age who have epilepsy should learn about pregnancy. Many babies are born each year to women with epilepsy who were not planning on becoming pregnant. As noted in Chapter 24, some studies have found higher rates of unplanned pregnancies among young women with epilepsy, and some antiepileptic drugs may reduce the effectiveness of birth control pills. (See Chapter 10 for details.)

Defining the potential dangers and ways of reducing risks is a starting point for family planning. The risks associated with pregnancy for women with epilepsy are fairly well defined. Many of the steps to reduce the problems for the mother and the child must be taken before the pregnancy begins. There should be good communication among the couple, the neurologist, and the obstetrician to ensure that the need for seizure control and the desire for a healthy baby are met to the highest degree possible and are well balanced. Potential parents should know that more than 90% of women with epilepsy have healthy babies.

Risk of Epilepsy in the Baby

Children whose parents have epilepsy have a slightly higher risk of developing epilepsy. The lifetime risk of developing epilepsy in the general population is approximately 3%. If the father has epilepsy and the mother does not, the risk to the children is only slightly higher than 3%. If the mother has epilepsy and the father does not, the risk is somewhat higher, but still less than 5%. The highest risk in this group is in women with primary generalized epilepsy. If both parents have epilepsy, the risk is a bit higher than if only one parent has the condition.

A couple in which one or even both partners have epilepsy should not decide against having children because of fear that the children will have epilepsy. The risk of epilepsy is low, many children outgrow epilepsy, and in most people with epilepsy, the seizures are well controlled by a single drug.

Birth Defects and Antiepileptic Drugs

The healthiest women have a 2.5% chance of having a baby with a major birth defect. The chance increases to approximately 6% in women with epilepsy. The reasons for this increase are not fully understood. We know that the risk is heightened by the use of anticpileptic drugs before or during pregnancy. Genetic factors definitely contribute to an increased risk of birth defects in the general population. It remains uncertain, however, whether genetic factors increase the risk that women or men with epilepsy will have children with birth defects. A few studies suggest that certain birth defects are slightly more common among children of parents who have epilepsy, even if the parents did not take antiepileptic drugs. If there is a family history of birth defects, then the parents should seek genetic counseling.

Antiepileptic drugs taken by the mother shortly before conception and during the first 3 months of pregnancy clearly present the greatest danger to the developing baby. The danger of antiepileptic drugs taken by the father is less clear. Some studies show a slight increase in birth defects among babies whose fathers took antiepileptic drugs, but others show no increase.

Women with epilepsy are faced with a difficult decision. The use of antiepileptic drugs during pregnancy has risks for the baby, but most women need to continue taking them. It is an understandable but misguided and dangerous practice to reduce or stop taking the medication without a doctor's recommendation. Seizures can be dangerous to both the woman and the baby (and perhaps to others if the woman continues to drive).

The first trimester (first 3 months) of pregnancy, especially days 21 to 56, is the critical period for development of the baby's major organ systems. The second and third trimesters (the last 6 months) are critical for the baby's growth and maturation. In a relatively small number of cases, exposure to antiepileptic drugs during the first trimester may cause major birth defects, such as cleft lip and cleft palate (a gap in the middle of the lip or palate) or structural defects of the heart. Other major malformations affect the central nervous system, the gastrointestinal system, the reproductive system, the urinary system, and the skeletal system. These defects are serious, but often the child can live normally after surgical correction or other forms of treatment. Minor malformations may result from exposure to antiepileptic drugs during the last 6 months of pregnancy. These include widely spaced eyes, a small and upturned nose, and short fingers and toes. Minor defects are common in the general population and may disappear after the first year of life.

The new antiepileptic drugs (felbamate, gabapentin, lamotrigine, levetiracetam, oxcarbazepine, tiagabine, topiramate, and zonisamide) have not been adequately studied in pregnant women, and their safety remains uncertain. Information about their safety will eventually come from a North American registry for women taking antiepileptic drugs during pregnancy. Pregnant women who are taking antiepileptic drugs are strongly urged to contact the registry (888-233-2334 or www.aedpregnancyregistry.org) and provide information that may help define the safety of their future pregnancies and the pregnancies of other women. Communication with the registry is confidential.

Treatment with one antiepileptic drug in the lowest dosage that will control the seizures presents the least risk for the baby's development. Any woman of childbearing age who is taking two or more antiepileptic drugs and who would consider having a baby if she became pregnant should ask her doctor if she could be treated with one medication. More than one drug may be necessary for some women because of the difficult nature of their seizure disorder, but many can be safely treated with one drug, and some can remain seizure-free with lower dosages than usually taken. Women who are thinking of discontinuing their antiepileptic drugs may find no better time to try it, under a doctor's supervision, than before pregnancy.

Knowing the approximate risks is not always reassuring. Some couples are relieved to learn that the risk of major birth defects is only slightly greater than if the woman did not have epilepsy. Others focus on the relative percentages, noting that the risk of birth defects is approximately double that of the general population, although the percentages are still small. It is important for couples to discuss pregnancy ahead of time and to feel comfortable with family-planning decisions. Most experts recommend that women and men with epilepsy should feel free to have babies.

Taking Vitamins

Taking vitamins before and during pregnancy can help reduce the risks of birth defects in the baby. Folate (folic acid) appears to be the most important vitamin, but the best dose remains unknown. The recommended daily minimum in the general adult population is 0.4 mg—the amount of folate found in most high-potency vitamins. For women taking antiepileptic drugs, a supplemental dose of 0.4 to 2 mg per day is reasonable. A dose of 2 to 4 mg per day is reasonable for women with a history of birth defects in their family or in a previous pregnancy.

In addition to folate, women with epilepsy who may become pregnant should take a high-potency multivitamin pill. During pregnancy, women with epilepsy may have an additional need for vitamins, which can be discussed with the obstetrician. Some evidence links very high doses of vitamin A or D with birth defects, but the doses in a standard high-potency multivitamin should be safe. Also, for women taking antiepileptic drugs that increase vitamin D metabolism, supplementation with low to moderate doses (up to 800 IU/day) is safe.

CARE DURING PREGNANCY

Regular medical care is essential for all pregnant women. With regular visits, the doctor may be able to identify common problems of pregnancy before they become serious. Because of the increased risk of problems during pregnancy and the potential for problems with seizure control, regular visits to both the obstetrician and the neurologist are crucial for women with epilepsy.

Vaginal bleeding is the most common obstetric problem in women with epilepsy. Other problems that are more common among women with epilepsy include abnormalities of the placenta (the organ that nourishes the baby) and complications around the time of birth, such as high blood pressure (pre-eclampsia) and premature delivery. Some (but not all) studies have found that the infants of women with epilepsy have had more problems after birth (including a higher rate of death), but with modern care for pregnant women with epilepsy adverse outcomes of this kind are becoming less likely.

Effects of Pregnancy on Seizure Control

Pregnancy brings about dramatic changes in the body. It affects metabolism, fluid balance, hormone levels, and other physical functions. It also has a psychological and emotional impact. The net result of all of these changes makes seizure control unpredictable. Of women with epilepsy who become pregnant, one-quarter have an increase in seizure frequency, one-fifth have a reduction, and more than half have no change. Good seizure control during one pregnancy does not necessarily predict that seizures will not increase during subsequent pregnancies. Women can help keep their seizures well controlled during pregnancy by taking their medications as prescribed. If nausea and vomiting become a problem, the doctor should be informed immediately because the absorption of antiepileptic drugs can be seriously affected.

Doctors and pregnant women face difficult decisions about adjusting drug dosages during pregnancy. Monitoring blood levels of the drugs may be helpful, but the patient's condition should be the principal guide for maintaining or changing therapy. If the seizures have been well controlled before pregnancy, most doctors do not increase the dosage of antiepileptic drugs during the first 3 months, even if the blood levels of the drugs decline. If the frequency of the seizures increases, however, a higher dosage may be needed.

The blood levels of antiepileptic drugs usually decline during pregnancy, even if the drugs are taken as prescribed. Causes for declining blood levels include decreased protein binding (see the following), increased metabolism, and increased blood volume and weight gain. Because the pregnant woman has more blood, the concentration produced by a certain dose of a drug will be less, just as a teaspoon of sugar will be sweet in a small cup of tea but hardly noticeable in a large pitcher.

The decline in blood levels of antiepileptic drugs during pregnancy is associated with the amount of "total" and "free" drug in the bloodstream. As discussed in Chapter 10, the total amount of drug consists of two parts: drug that is bound, or attached, to proteins in the blood and drug that is unbound, or floating freely, in the blood. Only the unbound, or free, drug crosses from the blood to the brain and helps to control seizures. When a blood drug level is monitored, the results are usually reported as the total drug level rather than the free level. Although the total blood levels of all antiepileptic drugs are moderately reduced during pregnancy, the free levels of most drugs (phenobarbital is the major exception) are usually reduced by a smaller percentage. A doctor who considered only the total drug level in the blood might predict that seizure control would worsen, but if he or she considered the more meaningful free level, the prediction for a change in seizure control would be more realistic.

Women who are taking enzyme-inducing antiepileptic drugs (e.g., carbamazepine, phenobarbital, phenytoin, primidone, topiramate) should take 10 to 20 mg per day of vitamin K by mouth during the last 4 weeks of pregnancy. This is taken to prevent the possibility of internal bleeding in the newborn. Although intramuscular vitamin K is given to most babies at delivery, use of oral vitamin K by the mother is still recommended.

Effects of a Woman's Seizures on the Baby

Absence seizures, simple partial seizures, or complex partial seizures during pregnancy pose no danger to the baby unless the woman injures herself during the seizure (which is rare). Convulsive (tonic-clonic) seizures in the woman, however, can be dangerous for the developing baby. Most women who have one or two tonic-clonic seizures during pregnancy have healthy babies, but during a convulsion, there is a risk of trauma to the abdomen, which could injure the baby. Also, the temporary interruption of breathing that accompanies tonic-clonic seizures, which is rarely of any significance for the woman, can lead to oxygen deprivation in the baby. The baby's heart rate slows for as much as 30 minutes after a tonic-clonic seizure. The greatest dangers are prolonged or repetitive tonic-clonic seizures, which can seriously impair the supply of oxygen to the baby's brain and other organs. Tonic-clonic seizures are probably most dangerous to the fetus during the last trimester, when the brain is larger and needs more oxygen. Women who are pregnant should avoid the stressors that are known to provoke seizures (see Chap. 6) as well as drinking alcohol, taking illegal drugs, having caffeine, and smoking.

Labor and Delivery

Women with epilepsy have cesarean deliveries ("C sections") much more often than women without epilepsy. The reasons for this difference are poorly understood. Women with epilepsy who are taking high dosages of antiepileptic drugs may have slightly weaker contractions of the womb (uterus) during delivery. Or perhaps the high rate of cesarean deliveries in women with epilepsy may have more to do with the perceived risks of complications in a vaginal delivery than with the actual risks.

The use of drugs to induce labor is approximately three times more common among women with epilepsy than among women in the general population. The reasons for this are not fully defined. Very few women with epilepsy need drugs to induce labor. Epilepsy itself is not a reason to induce labor because most women with epilepsy are able to have normal, spontaneous labor and deliveries. In selected situations, however, it may be prudent to induce labor in women with epilepsy. The potential benefits of an induced labor must be weighed against the risks, which include prolonged labor and uterine and physical exhaustion, which can lead to the need for a cesarean section.

For women who have only simple or complex partial seizures, myoclonic seizures, or absence seizures, there should be no problems with a vaginal delivery. Similarly, well-controlled or infrequent tonic-clonic seizures present no reason not to try a vaginal delivery. However, for women who have uncontrolled tonic-clonic seizures during pregnancy or those with tonic-clonic seizures during labor and delivery (approximately 1–2% of women with epilepsy), a cesarean delivery may be indicated.

The frequency of seizures increases slightly during labor and delivery and the first 2 days after delivery. An additional 1% to 2% of women may have tonic-clonic seizures during this period. This increase may result from the failure or inability of the women to take antiepileptic medication, sleep deprivation, hyperventilation, stress, physical pain, and other medications such as meperidine (Demerol). Women should prepare for labor with a reminder to take medications as scheduled, and they should tell the doctor if they are unable to take them because of nausea or pain. Fortunately, despite many of these problems, most women do not have tonic-clonic seizures around the time of delivery.

Spinal anesthesia is safe for women with epilepsy. If general anesthesia is required, it also can be given safely. The anesthesiologist should be informed about the woman's history of epilepsy and the antiepileptic drugs she is taking (as well as about other medical disorders and medications).

COGNITIVE DEVELOPMENT IN CHILDREN OF MOTHERS WITH EPILEPSY

Do children of women with epilepsy have higher rates of cognitive problems? If they do, are the problems associated with genetic or nutritional factors, specific drugs, certain seizure types, or other factors? Current knowledge does not provide clear answers. Although more than 10 studies have been completed, none of them provides definite answers and the findings vary considerably from study to study. Some studies did not find higher rates of cognitive disorders in children of women with epilepsy. Among the studies that did find an increased frequency of cognitive impairments, some found that such problems were associated with partial or generalized seizures or antiepileptic drug use during pregnancy. It does appear that children born to mothers with epilepsy may have slightly higher rates of mental handicap and learning disorders than do the children of mothers without epilepsy. For now, the principles of using the lowest effective dose of a single drug and controlling seizures during pregnancy may help minimize any potential risks.

Menopause

Menopause, which occurs in women usually between ages 44 and 56 years, is marked by a set of changes in body function. The most dramatic change is a decline in the production of hormones by the ovaries, which causes menstrual cycles to cease. Changes in brain activity regulating the endocrine system likely contribute to the transition into menopause. The time around menopause is called perimenopause. The most common symptoms during the transition into menopause include hot flashes and mood changes.

In menopause, the body reduces its production of the hormones estrogen, progesterone, and androgen (such as testosterone). The effects of menopause on the frequency and intensity of seizures in women have not been extensively studied, but we know that hormones can influence seizure activity. In experiments with animals, for example, giving estrogen has increased seizure activity and giving progesterone has decreased it. For most women, seizure activity does not significantly change, although it can worsen or improve. As in other stages of life, care around the time of menopause for women with epilepsy should be individualized.

The benefits and risks of hormone replacement therapy for women after menopause are uncertain. Estrogen replacement can help reduce hot flashes and prevent cardiovascular disease and osteoporosis. However, some (but not all) studies suggest that estrogen replacement can increase the risk of breast and uterine cancer. The effects of hormone replacement therapy on seizure activity in women with epilepsy have not been well studied. In theory, use of a combined estrogen and progesterone therapy rather than estrogen alone could minimize the risk of increasing seizure activity (and certain other adverse effects). Some authorities recommend the use of natural progesterones, rather than synthetic ones, for women with epilepsy.

Some antiepileptic drugs (e.g., carbamazepine, phenobarbital, phenytoin, and topiramate) increase the liver's metabolism of steroid hormones. Thus, they can decrease the effectiveness of hormone replacement therapy, similar to their effect on contraceptives, making higher doses of estrogen or progesterone replacement therapy necessary.

Androgens, such as testosterone, are occasionally used to improve libido (sexual desire), emotional well-being, and bone density in women during and after menopause. However, androgen supplementation after menopause may have adverse effects and is not recommended routinely. Long-term follow-up studies are limited.

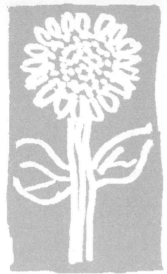

Parenting by People with Epilepsy

Few other joys equal those of parenthood. Epilepsy should not be viewed as a restriction on becoming a parent. Early in the 20th century, many states had laws against marriage and parenthood for people with epilepsy, but all these prohibitions have been repealed. There are no legal barriers between epilepsy and parenthood, except for those associated with custody suits. Chapter 30 addresses legal rights related to adoption by people with epilepsy.

Parenthood is not for every person or couple, however. Becoming a parent is a major commitment of time and resources. The responsibility of caring for a child is difficult to understand before the child is born. A baby is completely dependent on parents or caregivers for food, clothing, diaper changing, and protection. Caring for a child can be as frustrating as it is joyful.

Caring for Infants and Children

Caring for a baby or child means loss of freedom and personal time and a new sense of responsibility. Maternal and paternal instincts are strong. After having made it through the potential hazards of a pregnancy with epilepsy, the parents may sigh with relief, feeling that the dangers of epilepsy have passed. People with well-controlled epilepsy have no restrictions on child care, but those with episodes of impaired consciousness or control of movement must take special precautions when caring for a baby or a young child. The precautions will depend on the child's age and nature and other circumstances.

If at all possible, a parent with uncontrolled seizures should not bathe the baby alone. The baby should be placed in a safely designed baby bath and transferred to and from the bath as close to the floor as possible. If the baby bath is placed inside a larger tub, the drain should be open. The room where the bath is given should be carpeted if possible. The parent should always heed an aura, or warning, of a seizure while bathing the baby.

A parent with uncontrolled seizures should be extremely careful when carrying the baby. That is not to say that persons with epilepsy should not carry a baby, but care must be exercised. Some get enough warning of a seizure that they have time to place the baby in a safe place. Others have no warning, and must be especially careful when caring for a baby. Breast-feeding and diaper changing by women who are at risk of having a seizure are best done on the floor or on a low, soft surface where the baby would be safe from falling.

The baby or young child of a parent who has epilepsy is better off sleeping in his or her own crib or bed. There is a chance the child could be injured if the parent had a seizure, especially a tonic-clonic seizure, while sleeping.

As the baby becomes a toddler, other potential dangers confront a parent whose seizures are not fully controlled. For example, walking or playing near a busy street with an impulsive, active 2-year-old could be potentially dangerous if the parent had a complex partial seizure. During the minute or two of the parent's impaired consciousness, the child's ball could bounce into the street and the child might run after it. Although events such as this are rare, it is worthwhile to consider ways of reducing the risk. In this case, the child might be given another toy that is less likely to bounce into the street, or the child's hand and the parent's hand might be linked by a colorful plastic coil that will keep them close together.

If a parent's seizures are not fully controlled, the disorder should be discussed with older children. Children understand more than adults give them credit for, and they may be aware of the seizures and frightened by them. Explaining to the children what a seizure is, why the parent takes medication, and why the children should not worry is comforting to them. As the children get older, they should be told more about epilepsy and what to do if first aid is needed.

Missed medications, sleep deprivation, and stress can aggravate seizures. For new parents, some sleep deprivation and stress are unavoidable, and dramatic changes in the daily schedule can easily lead to missed medications. It is important to recognize these potential problems and plan to reduce their impact. A mother with epilepsy who chooses to breastfeed, for example, might want to use a formula supplement or pump breast milk so that she can sleep while her husband or another person feeds the baby during the night. Caring for a baby is stressful and exhausting, and enlisting family members or others to help is a good idea.

Breastfeeding

Breast-feeding is recommended for most women with epilepsy. Breast-feeding has health benefits for the mother, and breast milk confers a variety of benefits to the baby, including protection against infection. However, the benefits of breast-feeding must be weighed against the risks when the mother takes antiepileptic drugs.

Table 10 shows the approximate percentages of the mother's blood drug level found in breast milk. The amount of drug found in breast milk is related to the proportion of the drug that is not bound to proteins. The more a drug is bound to proteins in the blood, the lower the amount that is free and the lower the amount found in breast milk.

TABLE 10
PERCENTAGE OF MOTHER'S BLOOD DRUG LEVEL
FOUND IN BREAST MILK

Antiepileptic Drug	% in Breast Milk
Valproate	10
Phenytoin	30
Carbamazepine, phenobarbital, zonisamide	50
Lamotrigine	65
Primidone	80
Ethosuximide, gabapentin, levetiracetam	90

Phenobarbital and primidone, both barbiturates, cause the most problems with breast-feeding. The baby's digestive system is particularly good at absorbing these drugs, and they linger for an unusually long time in the baby's blood. A single dose of phenobarbital may last more than 15 days. Because of the high amount of ethosuximide, gabapentin, and levetiracetam found in breast milk, these may also cause problems. The antiepileptic drugs in babies who are breast-fed *may* cause fussy feeding habits, sleepiness, and irritability. Some irritability and gas pains are normal, however, and should not be interpreted as medication effects. The mother should contact the pediatrician if she has any doubts.

If a breast-feeding woman takes two antiepileptic drugs, or takes barbiturates or ethosuximide, the baby should be watched for signs of adverse reactions to the drugs. The baby of a woman who breast-feeds and then stops taking a barbiturate should be observed for signs of drug withdrawal such as increased irritability, insomnia, or sweating. If these signs are observed, the pediatrician should be contacted.

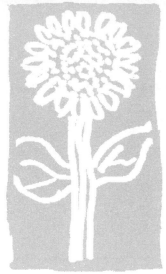

Employment for People with Epilepsy

A productive and satisfying work life is important to a person's overall quality of life and self-esteem. Most people with epilepsy are capable of productive and gratifying employment, but they may face severe discrimination in the job market. Employers have discriminated against them because of the stigma associated with epilepsy, misconceptions about its medical and social aspects, unfounded fears of legal and medical liability, and the misconception that people with epilepsy are not as productive as others. These biases have led to considerable hardship, but new laws have begun to change the landscape of employment opportunities in America for people with epilepsy and other disabilities.

Some employers still discriminate against those with epilepsy, although such discrimination generally is illegal under the Americans with Disabilities Act (ADA), which was passed in 1990. Therefore, before applying for a job, it may be helpful for a person with epilepsy to speak with a representative of the local affiliate of the Epilepsy Foundation (EF) about the relevant laws and restrictions preventing employers from asking questions about a job applicant's health. It also may be helpful to visit EF's website (www.efa.org) to read fact sheets that explain the ADA and permissible employer inquiries. The applicant also could speak with the protection and advocacy staff of the state human rights commission, the Equal Employment Opportunities Commission (EEOC), or a social worker who specializes in employment issues.

Protection Against Job Discrimination

The ADA makes discrimination based on disability illegal in employment, activities of state and local governments, public and private transportation, public accommodations, and telecommunications. In the 1980 census, 20% of Americans were found to be disabled in some way.

Epilepsy is a disability, but not all people with epilepsy are protected by the ADA. To be protected by the ADA, one must show that one's epilepsy substantially limits one or more major life activities (e.g., caring for oneself, sleeping, working, or reproduction) even when the condition is medically treated. Alternatively, the person must be able to show a record of such a limitation or of being regarded as being substantially limited in one or more major life activities.

Because of the side effects of medication and the effects of epilepsy itself on one's ability to reproduce, care for oneself, sleep, and work, many people with epilepsy should be able to claim the protections of the ADA. Although many lower court decisions suggest that the courts are taking a conservative approach to such claims, a recent Eighth Circuit Court of Appeals decision suggests that courts may abandon this approach in the future. In *Otting v. J.C. Penney Department Store, Inc.*, the Eighth Circuit found that a woman with epilepsy was disabled under the ADA. Title I of the ADA provides that people with disabilities cannot be excluded from employment unless they are unable to perform the essential requirements of the job. An employer may *not* discriminate on the basis of disability in:

- Recruitment, advertising, and job application procedures
- Hiring, upgrading, promotion, demotion, tenure, transfer, layoff, termination, return from layoff, and rehiring
- Rates of pay or other compensation and changes in compensation
- Job assignment, job classification, position descriptions, lines of progression, structures, and seniority lists
- Leaves of absence, sick leave, or other leave
- Fringe benefits, whether or not administered by the employer
- Selection and financial support for training, including apprenticeships, professional meetings, conferences and other related activities, and selection for leaves of absence to pursue training
- Activities sponsored by the employer, including social and recreational programs
- Any other term, condition, or privilege of employment

The ADA applies to all employers, employment agencies, labor organizations, and joint labor-management committees in which at least 15 employees work for each working day in each of 20 or more calendar weeks. The ADA excludes the federal government or other employers that receive a certain level of federal support (because they are subject to other similar regulations) as well as Indian tribes and private-membership clubs that are exempt from taxation.

In the following sections, the use of the term "employers" refers only to employers covered by the ADA. State and local laws against employment discrimination may provide protection equal to or better than the ADA and cover a wider range of employers.

CRITERIA FOR EMPLOYMENT

People with epilepsy or other disabilities must be both qualified and able to perform the *essential* job functions, even if they require some change in the work environment or procedures (that is, a "reasonable accommodation") to do so. The ADA does not require employers to change the fundamental duties of jobs to meet the needs of individuals with disabilities. Removing an essential function would fundamentally alter the position, according to the EEOC (www.eeoc.gov), which ensures equality of opportunity by enforcing federal laws prohibiting discrimination in employment.

The word "essential" is often critical in determining whether or not there is discrimination. For example, if a job description for a department store stock person requires that the person work in high places, but no one in this position has actually had to work in high places during the past several years, this function is not essential. If a person was fired for being unable to work in high places, then this would be illegal discrimination.

Driving privileges are essential for some jobs, such as pizza delivery, traveling salesperson, or taxi driver. Some positions may require applicants to have a driver's license, but further examination may show that driving is not an essential part of the job. Some jobs have driving requirements that are marginal and can be accommodated through job sharing. Because driving privileges are often restricted for people with epilepsy, such distinctions can be key.

DISCRIMINATION AND SEGREGATION

In the past, job applicants with epilepsy have often experienced discrimination because of the stigma attached to their disorder. Current laws, however, forbid employers from discriminating against people with disabilities because of fears and myths. Discrimination includes limiting, segregating, or classifying an applicant or employee in a negative way based on his or her disability. Each case must be viewed separately to determine what constitutes discrimination, especially because the type and frequency of seizures in epilepsy vary from person to person.

Employment decisions must be based on facts, not on presumptions and hearsay about people with a certain disability. For example, a department store could not categorically deny the position of salesclerk to a person with epilepsy because they are "afraid that seizures will frighten off the customers."

Employees must not be segregated on the basis of their disability. For example, it would be illegal for a company to sponsor an office party on a boat and not invite an employee who has epilepsy because it fears the liability if the person were to have a seizure on the boat and get hurt. Similarly, it would be illegal for a company to deny use of facilities such as an employees' exercise room to an employee with epilepsy, although it may be reasonable for the company to obtain medical clearance from the employee's doctor.

CONTRACTUAL ARRANGEMENTS

The ADA requires employers to provide equal benefits and privileges to all employees regardless of disability. Even indirect discrimination through an outside contractual arrangement is illegal. For example, if a company signs a contract allowing its employees to use a certain health club, but that club excludes people with epilepsy, the employer is violating the ADA's provision requiring equal benefits and privileges to all employees. Furthermore, the health club is unfairly discriminating against people with epilepsy under the ADA's public accommodations provisions. It is also illegal for employers to use an employment agency to screen out applicants with epilepsy or other disabilities.

REASONABLE ACCOMMODATIONS

The ADA requires that covered employers make reasonable accommodations for people with disabilities unless the employer can show that the individual poses a direct threat to the health and safety of others or that the accommodation would impose an "undue burden" on the employer. *Reasonable accommodation* is "any change in the work environment or in the way things are customarily done that enables an individual with a disability to enjoy equal employment opportunities." It is illegal for an employer to hire an individual who does not have a disability over an equally qualified disabled individual simply to avoid having to make a reasonable accommodation for the disabled person.

There are three categories of reasonable accommodations. These provide accommodations for (1) equal opportunity in the application process, (2) performing essential functions of the position held or desired, and (3) enjoying equal benefits and privileges of employment as are enjoyed by employees without disabilities.

A broad range of reasonable accommodations could apply to people with epilepsy. The following are some examples:

- Providing extended time to take an entrance examination
- Restructuring a job (redistributing nonessential or marginal job functions, such as driving, to other employees)
- Making temporary changes in job responsibilities or time required to perform certain tasks while someone is adjusting to new medications or to changes in an existing drug regimen
- Replacing a flickering light or loud banging noise if it could provoke a seizure
- Installing a safety shield around a piece of equipment
- Installing carpet on a concrete floor
- Asking a supervisor for written, as opposed to oral, instructions for someone with memory loss caused by antiepileptic medications
- Allowing an employee who experiences fatigue as an adverse effect of medications to take more frequent breaks
- Allowing an employee to take an extended break after a seizure

Determining what accommodation is reasonable can be difficult. The applicant or employee should notify the employer of his or her need for accommodation. The employer may require that the need for the accommodation be documented by a letter from the doctor. The employer and the qualified person with a disability are required to undertake a "flexible, interactive process" in determining what accommodation is reasonable. Because epilepsy affects each person differently, the input of both the employer and the employee is essential to provide the most helpful and efficient accommodations. When there are questions about what types of accommodations are best, employers may obtain useful information from the EEOC, EF (800-EFA-1000), their state vocational rehabilitation agency (for the one nearest you, call 800-222-JOBS), or the Job Accommodation Network (800-526-7234 Voice/TDD; for calls within West Virginia, 800-526-4698).

EMPLOYEE BENEFITS

The ADA does not require an employer to offer health benefits or other forms of insurance. Employers who do offer benefits to employees may not exclude people with disabilities and must offer the same plans or policies to all individuals. Employers may not refuse to hire people with disabilities because of a feared or actual increase in insurance costs. Similarly, an employer cannot refuse to hire the parent of a child with a disability because the cost of insurance benefits for dependents may increase. However, the employer may not be required to provide the employee the same benefits if it can prove that including the individual in the group's plan would increase the premiums so much that the plan would become unaffordable for the rest of the group's members.

The ADA does not affect the preexisting-condition clauses included in many insurance policies. Employers may continue to subscribe to health insurance plans that do not cover preexisting conditions. This exclusion may be permanent (that is, they will never cover the condition) or temporary (e.g., the condition could be covered after 1 year of employment).

BRINGING A CLAIM OF DISCRIMINATION

A person who believes that he or she has been discriminated against in the workplace should file a complaint with the EEOC (for an employment claim) or the Department of Justice (for claims regarding public access and government services). These government agencies will then investigate. If they believe that the facts support the person's claim, they will issue a "right to sue" letter. Although you do not need an attorney to file a complaint, it may be helpful to have had an attorney from the beginning if you later sue in court.

For a claim of discrimination to be valid, the ADA requires that the individual with a disability must establish that (1) the disability is covered under the act, (2) the employer in question is covered by the law, (3) the individual is qualified to perform the essential functions of the job, and (4) the employer violated one or more of the prohibitions of the ADA.

The employer has the burden of proof to show a valid defense to the employee's claim of discrimination. Various defenses can be used by the employer, including these two:

(1) *Direct threat:* The employer must show that the applicant or employee with a disability presents "a significant risk of substantial harm to the health or safety of the individual or others that cannot be eliminated or reduced by reasonable accommodation." The risk must be significant—not just slightly increased.

(2) *Undue hardship:* The employer must show that an accommodation required for the employee or applicant to do the job would be "unduly costly, extensive, substantial or disruptive, or would fundamentally alter the nature or operation of the business."

Application Process

The ADA makes it illegal for an employer to use any job application that requires individuals to disclose their disability. For example, applications cannot list medical, neurologic, or psychiatric disorders and ask people to check off those that apply to them. Also, a question such as, "Do you have a health condition that would affect your ability to do the job?" is prohibited by the ADA because it is overly broad. Similarly, application forms cannot ask if someone has previously filed a workers' compensation claim. An application can ask questions about the applicant's ability to perform essential job duties, however, and can request that the applicant list any type of reasonable accommodation that may be necessary during the application process. For example, an applicant may need more time to complete a written examination.

Applicants with epilepsy may choose not to disclose that they have the disorder if it is under good control, but seizures that interfere with consciousness or control of movement are potentially dangerous if the person drives, works on ladders or in high places, works as an electrician, works as a plumber with very hot water, or has a position (such as a ski-lift operator or lifeguard) with responsibility for the safety of others. Someone with epilepsy is not necessarily prevented from holding these jobs, but special consideration must be given to the person's specific seizure condition and the essential duties of the specific position.

The doctor is often asked to write a letter regarding the safety of the person with epilepsy in a specific situation. Unfortunately, no one can guarantee safety. Depending on the specific case and job, however, the doctor's letter can state that the person is able to work at the job and that the epilepsy does not represent a significant risk for injury.

JOB INTERVIEW

As with the application form, the ADA prohibits employers from asking any interview question that would require individuals to reveal their disability. The employer may ask about the applicant's ability to perform both essential and marginal job-related functions, but these questions cannot be phrased in terms of disability. For example, a flower shop owner who needs a delivery person can ask whether the applicant has a driver's license, which is essential for the job. If the response is no, the employer cannot ask if the applicant has epilepsy or a visual impairment. Although the employer can ask about the applicant's ability to perform marginal or nonessential job functions, the employer cannot refuse to hire someone with a disability because he or she is unable to perform these functions.

During the interview, the employer may ask if an accommodation will be needed during the application process. If the applicant tells the employer that he or she has epilepsy and that the medications affect the ability to respond quickly to written questions, then the employer may ask how much extra time is needed during an examination. However, the employer cannot probe and ask, "How long have you had epilepsy? How many medications do you take? What caused your epilepsy?" or other such questions.

If a disability is known or disclosed during the course of the interview, then the employer is limited in questions that can be asked about how the applicant's disability would interfere with performance of essential job functions. However, the employer may ask how the applicant would perform an essential function, with or without a reasonable accommodation.

If it becomes necessary to discuss one's epilepsy during the interview, the applicant should be honest and direct and should not argue or become defensive. If questioned as to how the epilepsy might have an impact on the job, the applicant should pause to collect his or her thoughts and answer the question in a calm but assured manner. Applicants should be familiar with the ADA because such questions before a job offer may be illegal, and they may not have to respond. The individual should know:

- His or her type of seizures
- How often they occur
- If there are certain times when seizures are especially likely to occur
- If there is a consistent warning (aura) that allows him or her to go to a safe place
- The types of supportive measures that may be needed
- How long it takes to recover after a seizure

It might be helpful to mention one's own "seizure safety" history; that is, during past jobs or schooling, did seizures ever cause physical injury or require special treatment? It is worth emphasizing that epilepsy is a common disorder (approximately 3% of the population will have epilepsy and 9% will have a single seizure), that people with epilepsy are effective in all segments of society and in workplaces as varied as the Congress of the United States and professional sports, that epilepsy does not affect the intellect or everyday behavior of most people who have it, and that injuries at work related to epilepsy are rare. Indeed, most people with epilepsy have no increased risk of work-related injuries.

MEDICAL EXAMINATIONS

The ADA's rules about medical examinations differ depending on the employment status of the individual. *Before* offering a job, employers are not allowed to conduct any type of medical examination. *After* a conditional offer of employment has been given (that is, once it has been determined that the applicant is qualified for the job), the ADA allows employers to require medical examinations of its employees with disabilities if medical examinations are required for all employees in that particular job. If a disability, such as epilepsy, is disclosed during the medical interviews and examination, the employer cannot use the disability to refuse to hire the applicant if essential job functions can be performed, with or without reasonable accommodation.

The ADA requires that all information obtained during a medical examination remain confidential. Such information can be disclosed to supervisors and managers only if accommodations or restrictions on the work or duties of the employee are needed. The information can also be disclosed to first aid and safety personnel and to government officials investigating compliance with the ADA.

TESTING FOR ILLEGAL DRUGS

Employers are allowed to test for use of illegal drugs during any stage of the application process or during employment if all employees are required to take a drug test as part of company policy. The ADA does not consider drug testing a medical examination. However, the employer cannot use the results of a drug test to discriminate against a person with a disability. The EEOC's regulation emphasizes that if the results of a drug test "reveal information about an individual's medical condition beyond whether the individual is currently engaging in the illegal use of drugs, the additional information is to be treated as a confidential medical record."

Tests for illegal drugs may be required before a conditional offer is made, but the employer cannot refuse to hire an individual based on information about drugs taken for medical conditions, such as epilepsy. Depending on the specific test, antiepileptic drugs can show up in standard drug testing, so applicants with epilepsy may want to disclose voluntarily that they are taking a prescription medicine to treat a medical condition. The employer is not allowed to ask what the condition is.

Drug tests that show illegal use should be repeated because laboratory errors do occur.

Explaining Seizures to Coworkers

A person with epilepsy whose seizures are not well controlled should prepare for the possibility that a seizure may occur at work. The preparation will depend on the type and frequency of seizures. The first and most important step is to discuss the seizures with the supervisor and coworkers. They likely will be the first ones to see the seizure and to administer first aid. Depending on the work environment, the people, the relationships with coworkers, and the nature of the seizures, a person with epilepsy may choose to tell only a few people or everyone in the workplace. The person with epilepsy should never rely entirely on one coworker, however, especially if the seizures are frequent or intense, because that person may be on vacation or out of the office when a seizure occurs.

People can be told individually or in a group. It is often a good idea to review first aid measures in a group setting. Coworkers need to know what happens during a seizure. The explanation should be reassuring. It is normal for them to be frightened when first watching a seizure. They should be told that the risk of serious injury is small and that the seizure does not cause pain. The employees should know what is going to happen when a seizure occurs: how their coworker may behave before, during, and after the seizure and what they should and should not do if one occurs. They should be told not to stick something in the person's mouth because the belief about swallowing the tongue is a myth. They should know when to call for medical personnel or an ambulance, but it should be emphasized that this is rarely necessary for a person with epilepsy who has a single seizure.

The local EF affiliate may be able to provide in-service education in the workplace. First aid cards, a videotape, and other educational materials are available from the EF.

Complex partial seizures may cause some work-related problems. Although the pattern of activity (e.g., staring, rubbing the hands, or mumbling a phrase) stays fairly constant from one seizure to the next, marked changes in behavior can occur during a seizure. The coworkers need to know that complex partial seizures usually last 1 to 2 minutes and that automatic acts are common. These automatisms can be misinterpreted. For example, someone having a complex partial seizure might crumple a sheet of paper or bang on a desk without being aware of it. The period after the seizure should be discussed. Many well-intentioned people try to restrain a person who has had a seizure. Restraint—even gentle restraint such as holding a hand—can occasionally produce agitation. Coworkers should know that a person may be confused after a seizure, but should be left alone if he or she is in a safe place and seems to be all right. They should not hold or restrain the person unless it is absolutely necessary for safety. It is always helpful for the person with epilepsy to have a clear description of what has happened during a seizure. A coworker may be willing to write a brief description of the event. There may also be some question as to whether consciousness was impaired. A coworker might be asked in advance to test the person's responsiveness (e.g., by saying, "Show me your left thumb") and memory (e.g., by asking the person to remember a particular word) during the seizure. When the person has fully recovered from the seizure and returned to work, he or she should acknowledge what happened, thank the people who were helpful, and ask if they have any questions.

Vocational Rehabilitation

A productive and fulfilling work life is an important component to overall quality of life. Most people with epilepsy have the potential to achieve satisfying employment, but they may have problems with employment as the result of recurrent seizures and their aftereffects, adverse effects of antiepileptic drugs on memory and attention, associated neurologic or medical disorders, and the negative feeling that some people still have about epilepsy. Vocational rehabilitation services can help those who have never held a job or who have been out of the work force for some time to train for and get employment that meets their individual needs. It provides specialized training to help them develop skills, confidence, and strategies to help make up for problems and enhance their chances for employment.

The Rehabilitation Act of 1973, a landmark law, provides employment rights for people with disabilities. This law changed the face of federal and state vocational rehabilitation programs, making services to people with disabilities a national priority. Many vocational rehabilitation services are available that address a range of needs. These services *may* include, but are not limited to:

- *Diagnostic evaluation* to assess any disability and determine eligibility for appropriate vocational training based on current skills and to help establish a career development plan
- *Counseling* to set goals, make choices, determine job-skill training needed, and provide support
- *Psychological, physical, or occupational therapies*

- *Training* to teach specific and general job skills, compensatory techniques to improve memory and concentration, job-search strategies, interviewing skills and job coaching, resume writing, and legal rights
- *Referral* to on-the-job training programs and other supported job experiences and employer education
- *Transportation*
- *Job placement* in the competitive work force, in supported community employment or in sheltered workshops, or in the home and arranging for independent-living services, personal assistance, and transition services
- *Post-employment services,* including short-term and long-term support during employment to help employees keep their jobs, and job accommodation assistance
- *Assistance in working with related agencies* such as the Social Security Administration, the Department of Social Services, the Office of Mental Health, the Veterans Administration, and the Office of Mental Retardation and Developmental Disabilities

The Workforce Investment Act of 1998 offers new opportunities for successful employment to people with epilepsy as well as to those without any disability. The law is designed to coordinate and improve access to job training, adult education, and literacy and vocational rehabilitation programs. It requires states to establish "one-stop shopping" centers in a single neighborhood location where people will have access to all such job training, education, and related employment services.

At this center, jobseekers can get evaluations of their individual abilities, skill levels, and training needs. The center will offer information about local training opportunities, help with filing claims for unemployment insurance, and assist with job searches and placement. The center will also offer information about job openings and local employment trends and provide access to special vocational rehabilitation services as authorized by the Rehabilitation Act.

ELIGIBILITY

Vocational rehabilitation programs are administered at the state level and vary by state, although the federal Rehabilitation Act authorizes the granting of federal funds to the states for these programs. The Department of Labor, Department of Education, Office of Mental Health, Office of Mental Retardation and Developmental Disabilities, and the Social Security Administration are examples of some of the agencies that can administer vocational rehabilitation programs. Many nonprofit organizations also offer specific vocational rehabilitation services, and others may be available in university medical centers.

To be eligible for a federally funded vocational rehabilitation program, a person must meet two criteria: (1) there must be a substantial barrier to employment and (2) the person must be able to benefit from the program and achieve a better employment outcome.

The first criterion requires that there be a mental or physical disability that impairs occupational performance. The nature of such a "substantial" handicap is not precisely defined and must be determined on an individual basis. There is now a presumption that even individuals with severe disabilities will meet the second criterion and benefit from services. The law requires that those with severe disabilities be given the highest priority.

There is an appeal process to be followed if vocational rehabilitation is denied or if the range of services provided is believed to be inadequate. The initial appeal is conducted by a state agency's supervisory staff and is known as the informal or administrative appeal. If the decision is not favorable, the person can request a hearing with an impartial hearing officer. If this decision is not favorable, a final appeal can be made to the director of the state vocational rehabilitation agency. Every state has a Client Assistance Program, which informs and assists all clients and applicants regarding their benefits and protections under the law.

INDIVIDUALIZED WRITTEN REHABILITATION PLAN

The person with a disability and the vocational rehabilitation counselor must jointly develop an individualized written rehabilitation plan. The disabled person may be joined by a parent, guardian, or someone else who can assist in developing the plan. The plan must identify the goals, services, and goods that are needed to obtain and continue with employment. As part of the planning process, the client must be clearly informed that he or she can challenge any agency decision.

VOCATIONAL REHABILITATION DILEMMA

People with epilepsy sometimes fall through the cracks in the current system. They may unfairly be in a "Catch 22" situation, in which the alternatives actually cancel each other out. If the level of seizure control is the only factor used to establish the relative severity of a person's disability, the counselor has an incomplete view of why the epilepsy presents a barrier to employment. As a result, people with good seizure control may be deemed ineligible for vocational rehabilitation services because their disability is not considered to be severe. Other difficulties—

like memory loss and adverse effects of medication—should be included so that the picture is clearer. If seizures persist despite treatment, however, the reviewer may consider the person with epilepsy to be unemployable (although recent changes in the law may make this less likely). To ensure that people with epilepsy are given fair consideration, it is critical that all the details of the individual case be clearly presented.

Even if seizures are fully or partially controlled, the stigma associated with epilepsy and the effects of medications can be significant barriers to employment. Nevertheless, many people with seizures can be success-fully employed in a wide range of positions, and it is important that the vocational rehabilitation counselor understand the full context of the person's condition to establish the severity of the disability and the potential for benefits through the vocational rehabilitation system.

The "one-stop shopping" centers authorized by the Workforce Invest-ment Act should offer useful alternatives for people with epilepsy who are not eligible for other vocational rehabilitation services. These centers are designed to serve all jobseekers, and they offer a variety of testing, training, and placement services. They also offer intensive services for those who do not get a job after using the core services.

Many nonprofit private organizations and public agencies also offer vocational rehabilitation services. Many of these programs work in partnership, and others stand alone. Not all programs offer all services, not all programs specialize in services for those with chronic and disabling conditions, and not all programs are available everywhere. It can be a confusing and frustrating process to sort through all the options and find the right program.

Workers' Compensation

Every state has laws that guarantee compensation for job-related injuries. Employers must either be self-insured or insured through the state workers' compensation program. Employers pay premiums to cover the cost of this insurance. Workers' compensation laws protect both employees and employers. For employees, an injury that results from performing their job will be covered and compensated, even if they were negligent. For employers, these laws serve to limit liability and costs because employees cannot receive anything more than workers' com-pensation. The rates set by workers' compensation for medical care are often low, and many doctors and surgeons do not accept the reimburse-ments paid by workers' compensation.

Work-related injuries are only covered if the injury occurred during work (not while getting ready to go to work or traveling between home and work) and was clearly a result of the employment. Therefore, if someone with epilepsy falls at work and is injured—whether or not the fall is related to a seizure—the accident could be viewed as independent of the employment and dependent only on the person's medical disorder. In the past, claims for falls because of seizures were denied. However, there has been a trend toward liberalization of workers' compensation coverage to include falls even if the conditions at work had little or nothing to do with the fall.

Work-related factors could cause or contribute to seizure-related injuries. For example, excessive overtime and stress can lead to sleep deprivation or exhaustion, which can make seizures more likely to occur. In such a case, the seizures could be viewed as "arising from the employment."

Some states and territories allow employers to demand that an employee waive his or her right to workers' compensation. Other states permit employees to waive benefits "voluntarily." Laws that allow employers to eliminate an employee's compensation rights should be abolished. These laws discriminate against people with disabilities by incorrectly assuming that their disability would be the cause of any injuries at work.

PREMIUM RATES

People with epilepsy do not have higher rates of accidents or absenteeism, and their overall work performance does not differ from the performance of other employees. Nevertheless, employers often fear that if they hire a person with epilepsy, their premiums for workers' compensation will go up. There is little evidence to support this fear. Premiums for workers' compensation do not increase because of a new employee's medical history and are rarely affected by a seizure-related work injury. For most employers, especially large companies, workers' compensation premiums are based on the class of employees in a specific industry, not on the medical history or work history of individual employees.

SECOND-INJURY FUNDS

Second-injury funds guarantee employers that hiring a person with a disability will not increase their workers' compensation premiums. For example, if an employee with epilepsy falls and is injured at work, that person may make a workers' compensation claim and cause the employer's premiums to rise. If the fall results from a preexisting condition (epilepsy) and not from the conditions of employment, however, the second-injury fund would compensate the employee for the fall, so neither the employer nor the workers' compensation fund must pay. These funds have been adopted in many states and encourage employers to hire people with disabilities. Applications, criteria for coverage, and types and amounts of coverage vary from state to state.

In most states, second-injury funds provide coverage for employees with a "permanent preexisting impairment" that could interfere with obtaining employment. Epilepsy may or may not be included in this category, depending on the state. In many states, the second-injury fund will provide coverage only if the employer is informed of the epilepsy at the time of hiring or it is proved that the employer kept the employee in the job after learning of the epilepsy.

Armed Services

The United States armed services (Army, Navy, Air Force, Coast Guard, and state National Guard) are not subject to the anti-discrimination requirements of the ADA and the Rehabilitation Act of 1973. The armed services require that members be available for duty 24 hours a day and have no condition that could impair their performance under adverse conditions. Because sleep deprivation and lack of medication are considered adverse conditions and can cause seizures in people with epilepsy, there are relatively strict regulations regarding the enlistment of people with epilepsy.

Currently, the armed services require those enlisting to be seizure-free without medications for at least 5 years. Cases are reviewed on an individual basis, and an appeal can be made for those who have been seizure-free for a shorter period, depending upon their medical history, outlook, and the specific position for which they are applying. For example, an appeal could be made for a young woman with benign rolandic epilepsy who applies to the military at age 18. Her last seizure was a nocturnal simple partial motor seizure at age 14, and she had stopped all antiepileptic drugs at 13. She has had normal electroencephalograms (EEGs) during the past 3 years. The likelihood that she will remain seizure-free is excellent, and she should be able to serve successfully in a variety of positions.

People with disorders of any kind that can cause a sudden loss of consciousness or motor control are excluded from flight training. The only exception is for individuals who had febrile seizures before age 5 and now have a normal EEG.

When a member of the armed services develops seizures or epilepsy, he or she may be discharged because of the disorder, but the regulations do not require automatic dismissal unless the person's seizures are not fully controlled by antiepileptic drugs. The military retains a limited number of people with disabilities who cannot actively serve under all conditions. The number of such positions is restricted, however, and members of the armed services have no legal or constitutional right to be retained in the service. Furthermore, the armed services have no obligation to accommodate an individual's disability by changing the work environment or position.

Because behavior during and after some seizures may be mistaken for intentional actions, people with epilepsy in the armed services may, on occasion, be less than honorably discharged. The military has review boards to which the discharge status may be appealed. It is up to the applicant to prove that the discharge was unfair or improper.

Acknowledgment

This chapter is based largely on *The Legal Rights of People with Epilepsy: An Overview of Legal Issues and Laws,* 6th ed. Epilepsy Foundation of America, Landover, MD, 1992.

Mental Health of Adults with Epilepsy

People with epilepsy are often subject to depression, anxiety, irritability, and more serious mental disorders. The behavioral disturbances may be unrelated to epilepsy, or they may be related to the person's emotional reactions to having epilepsy, the effect of medications, or the epilepsy itself. They also may be caused by the same thing that causes the person's epilepsy. Although people with epilepsy are often said to display more aggressive behavior than other people, there is little evidence for this difference, except in unusual cases such as when the person is restrained after a seizure. Experiencing unusual and bizarre episodes is a problem for some people with epilepsy, but these spells are often simple partial seizures preceding other seizures.

Personality Changes

Throughout history, a variety of derogatory labels have been applied to the personality and behavior of people with epilepsy. There used to be a widespread notion that most or all individuals with epilepsy had an "epileptic personality." Fortunately, that idea is now a historical relic.

Studies have shown, however, that some individuals may undergo behavioral changes. Most of the changes are undesirable, but sometimes they are for the better.

Certain behavioral traits continue to be associated with epilepsy, especially temporal lobe epilepsy. These include increased emotionality, "social stickiness" (a tendency toward prolonged interpersonal contact), circumlocution (talking around a point), excessive writing (hypergraphia), greater than usual religiousness or moral or philosophical interests, a sense of personal destiny, altered sexual interest (usually decreased libido), irritability, and anger. These traits are more common among people with epilepsy than in the general population, but they are also more frequent among people with various psychiatric disorders.

Other studies suggest that these traits may be just as common among patients with frontal lobe epilepsy or generalized epilepsy as among those with temporal lobe epilepsy. For example, absence epilepsy has been considered to have few behavioral effects. In one study, children with typical absence epilepsy were compared to children with juvenile rheumatoid arthritis (a disorder that affects physical function and requires long-term medication) at a follow-up after age 18. Those with typical absence epilepsy had greater difficulties with academic, personal, and behavioral functioning.

The study of personality and epilepsy has raised more questions than it has answered. It seems clear that behavioral changes and personality disorders are more frequent among people with epilepsy than in the general population. The relative roles of epilepsy, genetics, family and socioeconomic background, medications, brain abnormalities, and other factors remain uncertain. When behavioral changes interfere with personal, family, or professional life, professional help should be sought.

Depression

Depression causes feelings of sadness, helplessness, hopelessness, and guilt and makes the person unable to experience happiness. Other problems include difficulty with sleeping (insomnia or sleeping excessively), decreased sexual desire, and appetite disturbances (loss of appetite or overeating).

Depression is a common experience of people in the general population and people with epilepsy, but it occurs more often in those who have epilepsy. All people feel sad at some time in their life, and the depth of sadness varies. The borderline between sadness and depression is not precise, but, at some point, when sadness is prolonged and impairs a person's ability to work and enjoy life, there is a problem.

The most serious complication of depression is suicide. Just as the rate of depression is increased in people with epilepsy, there is also an increased rate of suicide. Patients, family members, and doctors often fail to recognize the presence or severity of depression. If there is any question, seek help. Anyone who expresses thoughts about hurting himself or herself should be taken extremely seriously. If someone who is depressed discusses a specific plan to hurt himself or herself or gives away treasured items, a psychiatrist should be consulted *immediately*.

CAUSES

In people with epilepsy, depression can result from:

- A psychological reaction to having the disorder or being treated differently because of it
- Medication effects
- The cause of the epilepsy, such as head injury or stroke
- The epilepsy itself

The relative importance of each of these factors is controversial, and often several factors contribute. In some cases, the depression is related to loss of a job or a loved one or to a flurry of seizures. Depression related to the psychological effects of living with epilepsy and other problems of life can be effectively treated in most cases by therapy and counseling. Discussion of troublesome feelings with a psychiatrist, psychologist, or counselor can be extremely helpful.

Antiepileptic drugs, especially the barbiturates phenobarbital and primidone, can cause depression. This kind of depression is often dose-related; that is, the higher the dose, the greater the risk of depression. Taking one or more other antiepileptic drugs in combination with a barbiturate can also increase the risk. It is rare that only a barbiturate can control epilepsy, however, so if a person who is taking a barbiturate is feeling depressed, he or she should ask the doctor about a medication change. Other antiepileptic drugs, especially the benzodiazepines topiramate and vigabatrin, also can occasionally contribute to depression.

Injury to the brain, whether from a stroke, oxygen deprivation, head injury, or infection, can cause depression. This is not surprising because the brain controls our emotions and moods. Studies suggest that people with injury to the left side of their brain, especially in the front portions (frontal and temporal lobes), are more prone to depression. Depression can also occur with injuries to other parts of the brain. However, most people with brain injuries do not become depressed.

The role that epilepsy itself plays in directly causing depression remains controversial. As more information accumulates, however, it appears that epilepsy does contribute to the problem in some cases. In some patients, depression occurs hours or days before or after a seizure. More frequently, depression occurs between seizures (in the interictal period).

TREATMENT

When possible, the cause or causes of depression should be treated. Serious depression requires antidepressant medication. Some psychiatrists and neurologists fear that antidepressants can aggravate the seizure disorder. Some evidence supports this concern, but most people with epilepsy who are treated with antidepressant medications do not experience more frequent seizures. Newer antidepressants, such as the selective serotonin reuptake inhibitors (SSRIs), appear safe for almost all epilepsy patients. These drugs include fluoxetine (Prozac), paroxetine (Paxil), sertraline (Zoloft), and citalopram (Celexa). Other new antidepressant drugs that are safe and well tolerated by most patients with epilepsy include nefazadone (Serzone), a serotonin antagonist and reuptake inhibitor, and venlafaxine (Effexor), a serotonin and norepinephrine reuptake inhibitor. These drugs also can be helpful in treating obsessive-compulsive disorder and anxiety disorder.

Besides counseling and medications, very severe depression may be treated with electroconvulsive shock therapy. Patients with epilepsy can safely undergo this procedure.

Anxiety

Anxiety disorders are quite common in the general population and are more common among people with epilepsy. We all experience feelings of anxiety and nervousness. Anxiety becomes a disorder when the feelings are frequent or intense, are produced by trivial things or nothing at all, and interfere with daily functioning. As with depression, several factors can be part of the cause of anxiety disorders, including psychological stress related to the epilepsy, medication effects, associated neurologic or psychiatric disorders, and the epilepsy itself.

Anxiety disorders can be effectively treated with counseling, therapy, and medications. A new medication to treat anxiety—buspirone (Buspar)—is safe for almost all patients with epilepsy and anxiety. SSRIs, listed in the section on depression, also can be helpful in treating anxiety.

Benzodiazepines are very effective in the short-term treatment of anxiety and insomnia, but they should be avoided if possible because they are among the most habit-forming (addictive) drugs legally available.

They include clobazam (Frisium; not available in the United States); clonazepam (Klonopin), diazepam (Valium), alprazolam (Xanax), chlordiazepoxide (Librium), clorazepate (Tranxene), estazolam (Prosom), lorazepam (Ativan), and triazolam (Halcion). These drugs also may temporarily reduce seizure frequency and intensity, but after someone takes the same dose for weeks, the effect on anxiety, insomnia, and seizure control diminishes. As the original anxiety or seizures return, there is a strong tendency for the patient and doctor to increase the dose, which again briefly reduces troublesome symptoms. This cycle leads to a buildup of the dose to levels that can cause memory impairment, depression, tiredness, and other problems. If the dose is then reduced, the real trouble begins: anxiety, insomnia, and seizures become more severe.

Irritability

We all get irritable. People vary considerably with regard to how often they get irritable and what triggers it. Only a few studies have compared irritability in people with and without epilepsy. Most of the studies suggest that some people with epilepsy may be more prone toward irritability than are people without the condition. Irritability in people with epilepsy usually has the same causes as in people without epilepsy, but it may also be related to medications (especially the barbiturates phenobarbital and primidone), brain abnormalities in areas that regulate emotions, or the epilepsy itself. Irritability can precede or follow seizures in a few individuals.

In some people, a change in medications or improved control of the seizures is associated with a reduction in anxiety and irritability. For the few people with epilepsy in whom irritability is a serious problem, it would be worthwhile to discuss the problem with the doctor. A new antiepileptic medication, a change in dosage of the present drugs, treatment of an underlying depression or sleep disorder, or some form of counseling or therapy may be beneficial. Buspirone (Buspar) and SSRIs, such as citalopram (Celexa) and sertraline (Zoloft), also can be helpful.

Psychosis

Psychosis is a serious mental disorder with various characteristics. Thoughts may be disorganized and the person may experience delusions or disturbances of perception (hallucinations and distortions of sensation). The person may feel a lack of emotions or inappropriate emotions. The sense of self can be disturbed. The person may display decreased drive and motivation, social withdrawal and detachment, or extreme levels of physical activity (becoming either hyperactive or immobile).

Psychosis can occur as a psychiatric disorder (such as schizophrenia) without any associated neurologic disorder. Psychosis can also result from brain injuries, such as viral encephalitis, or can be caused by the use of certain medications, such as amphetamines (stimulants). People with epilepsy have an increased rate of interictal psychosis (psychosis "in between" seizures, not only around the time of seizures). Overall, the chances that someone with epilepsy will develop an interictal psychosis are approximately 7%. Patients with temporal lobe epilepsy appear to be at the greatest risk.

The best-documented form of psychosis in epilepsy occurs after seizures, usually after a cluster of complex partial or tonic-clonic seizures. These individuals often appear well for a few hours or days and then express disordered thoughts, delusional ideas (e.g., paranoid thoughts that someone is going to hurt him or her), and aggressive behavior. Such psychoses are usually relatively brief and can be effectively treated with medications (antipsychotic and tranquilizing drugs). Prompt recognition and treatment of this disorder are most important.

Some older antipsychotic drugs, such as chlorpromazine (Thorazine) and thioridazine (Mellaril), can occasionally cause seizures and should be used at the lowest effective dosage. Newer antipsychotic drugs, however, have minimal risk of worsening seizure control. These drugs include rispiridone (Risperidal), olanzapine (Zyprexa), and molindone (Moban).

Aggression

The false association between epilepsy and aggressive behavior is one of the most damaging stigmas cast on people with epilepsy. There is some evidence that a few children and adults with epilepsy show aggressive behavior that may be related to antiepileptic drugs, underlying brain abnormalities, or the confused (postictal) state after certain seizures. But there is no clear evidence that people with epilepsy as a group are more likely than other people to commit violent crimes or to be involved in other types of criminal activity. Unfortunately, the stigma still lingers in social and medical communities.

Children are less able to control their impulses than adults. They translate thoughts into actions more readily. Control over social behavior and aggressive impulses is acquired relatively late in childhood as the brain develops and matures. Some children with epilepsy, and those with other neurologic disorders such as mental handicap, are reported to have higher rates than other children of aggressive behaviors. In part, this results from injury to brain areas that are important in developing social skills and learning to control impulses. Similar aggressive behaviors may develop in adults who have suffered brain injuries in motor-vehicle accidents, even if they have never had a seizure.

Taking certain medications can make aggressive behavior more likely to occur, especially in people with a preexisting injury in areas that regulate aggressive behavior. Barbiturates (phenobarbital and primidone) are most likely to cause aggressive behaviors. Although barbiturates usually have tranquilizing effects, they may cause agitation in elderly people. Other antiepileptic drugs and some stimulants, such as methylphenidate or dextroamphetamine, also can trigger aggressive behaviors in susceptible individuals.

During a complex partial seizure, directed aggressive behavior is exceedingly rare. Aggressive behavior can occur during the period of confusion after a tonic-clonic seizure, usually because someone tries to restrain the person. The best response to such a reaction is to remove the restraint.

Unusual Seizures

Some people with epilepsy, especially those with partial seizures, may experience unusual and bizarre phenomena during seizures. The experiences can be fascinating, frightening, or both. Very often, people are reluctant to discuss strange symptoms or experiences for fear of being considered odd or crazy. However, symptoms that begin suddenly and last for a brief time can be a seizure, no matter how strange they seem.

The following are descriptions of unusual seizures. These descriptions often were provided only after specific questions were asked:

- I had a feeling of extreme embarrassment, as though I had made a very foolish remark.

- I feel that someone else is in the room behind me, that I am not alone.

- Looking into the mirror, I noticed that the right side of my face was missing.

- On the left half of space there were colored balls of light. As I looked at them, they changed to multiple figures of small men. On later occasions, I recognized these as myself—tiny replicas that would approach and then recede.

- I have a flood of thoughts. I don't know where they come from. I can't shut them off.

Scenes appear in my mind's eye. I have never lived them. They must be imaginary, not real memories, but they appear real. During this time I sort of know what is going on around me, but I am also a bit tuned out.

My seizures start with a warning of fear, and then I feel as if I am a character in the Pac-Man video game and the monster is going to eat me. I am actually in the machine, running away from the Pac-Man.

It is the most frightening feeling, as if I know the worst thing in the world is about to happen. I don't know what, just that something horrible is imminent.

There is a forced recollection of childhood memories that flash in front of me like a slide show in fast motion. They are all real memories—things that happened that I haven't thought about for decades. It's like what people describe before they die.

The next thing I knew I was floating just below the ceiling. I could see myself lying there. I wasn't scared—it was too interesting. I saw myself jerking and overheard my boss telling someone to "punch the timecard out" and that she was going with me to the hospital. Next thing, I was in space and could see Earth. Next thing, I woke up in the emergency room.

These experiences are not typical seizure symptoms. The range of seizure symptoms is so broad, however, that almost any emotion or experience is possible. Although most seizure symptoms are brief, lasting less than 3 minutes, on rare occasions they can last more than 10 or 15 minutes. The important feature is the sudden onset, although obviously many symptoms and experiences unrelated to epilepsy also begin suddenly.

Patients who experience phenomena such as the ones described should mention them to their doctor. If the symptoms precede definite complex partial or tonic-clonic seizures, then they are almost certainly part of the seizure (a simple partial seizure).

Epilepsy in the Elderly

Epilepsy spares no age group. Although epilepsy is often considered a disorder of childhood, it can begin at any age. In some people it persists from childhood to old age. The rate of newly diagnosed epilepsy is higher in elderly people than in middle-aged adults. As in younger people, the cause of epilepsy that begins in an elderly person cannot be determined in about half of the cases. Of those in whom the cause can be determined, the largest number of cases (about 33%) are caused by stroke, often a small one that did not cause other symptoms. Degenerative disorders such as Alzheimer's disease cause about 11%, tumors (either benign or malignant) lead to about 5%, head injury causes about 2%, and infection gives rise to 1% of cases of epilepsy in older people. Although alcohol abuse is not considered a major cause of epilepsy in the United States, a study in Denmark found that it was very often associated with newly diagnosed epilepsy in adults.

The elderly are more sensitive than younger people are to a variety of mental, physical, and environmental stressors. They are also more likely to develop many medical, neurologic, and psychiatric disorders, some of which can make seizures more likely to occur. These disorders include metabolic changes such as very high or very low blood sugar, very low sodium levels, and endocrine disorders (e.g., diabetes, thyroid or parathyroid disorders).

Elderly people are also prone to falls. Approximately one-third of people older than age 65 years will fall at least once each year. Many of these falls are associated with head injury, which can make seizures more likely and contribute to cognitive and behavioral problems. Because nearly 25% of elderly individuals take between four and six medications, drug side effects and interactions are another prominent problem. Drug side effects are more than twice as likely to occur in patients older than age 60 years than in younger people. Some drugs (see Appendix 3) can cause or contribute to the occurrence of seizures. Memory problems, financial limitations, and side effects also commonly prevent elderly patients from taking their medications in the prescribed dosages.

Diagnosis

The diagnosis and classification of seizures is often difficult in elderly people. Many older individuals live alone or with partners whose memory and observational skills are limited, so the descriptions of seizures and seizure patterns provided by the patient and witnesses may be less reliable than from younger people. Many elderly individuals also are prone to other disorders that may resemble seizures. For example, it can be very difficult to determine if an episode of loss of consciousness results from a simple faint, a disturbance of the heart rhythm, or a seizure. In most cases, the cause is fainting; heart disturbances or seizures are less likely. Similarly, an episode with brief speech difficulty, confusion, or change in sensory function (e.g., numbness or disturbance of vision) could result from a seizure, a transient ischemic attack (often a sign of an upcoming stroke), or a variety of other disorders.

Effects

There are special concerns about the effects of seizures on older people. The body becomes less resilient with age, so the effects of tonic-clonic seizures can be more severe. Tonic-clonic seizures cause stress on the heart and potential problems for people with heart disease. Similarly, breathing is affected during a tonic-clonic seizure, which poses potential problems for people who have lung disorders. Bones also are more fragile in elderly people, so the risk of neck or back pain, or even a fracture, during a tonic-clonic seizure is increased. Despite these and other potential problems, most older people who suffer tonic-clonic or other seizures have no serious aftereffects.

Effects of Antiepileptic Drugs and Other Medications

▌ A 74-year-old woman began to experience twitching movements on the right side of her face. A computed tomography (CT) scan showed a benign tumor—a meningioma that grows from the membrane that covers the brain—on the surface of the left frontal lobe. She was treated with phenytoin, and the seizures stopped. An operation was performed to remove the tumor. She had no seizures for 6 months after the operation, during which time she continued to take 400 mg of phenytoin each morning. Then the twitching movements began to recur, usually in the late evening or awakening her from sleep at night. Around lunchtime, she would complain of tiredness and unsteadiness, which she attributed to the drug. Because of the seizures, her doctor increased the dose to 500 mg a day, but the adverse effects became worse. Two months later, her internist prescribed sucralfate (Carafate) for a stomach problem, and she had a brief tonic-clonic seizure during sleep several weeks later. The next day, the neurologist measured the blood phenytoin level early in the morning, before she took her five phenytoin pills, and found it was low. The blood phenytoin level was measured again around lunchtime, when the adverse effects were most severe. The blood level then was at the high end of the therapeutic range. The phenytoin was divided into two doses and eventually adjusted to 200 mg in the morning and 230 mg at night. Sucralfate, which can lower the blood phenytoin level, was discontinued, and another medication that did not interact with phenytoin was prescribed. The patient's blood phenytoin level became much steadier, the adverse effects almost completely disappeared, and the seizures were fully controlled.

This case report illustrates several important aspects of therapy for epilepsy in older patients. People become more sensitive to the effects of medications as they grow older. The adverse effects that occurred in this woman while the blood phenytoin level was in the therapeutic range are common for older people using all types of antiepileptic drugs and other medications. Older people (and sometimes younger ones) may need to take their doses of phenytoin or other antiepileptic drugs more frequently during the day to "smooth out" their blood levels of the drugs, thereby reducing the chances of seizures and adverse effects. Drug interactions also can be a problem (see Appendix 3). It is important that doctors treating an older person know of all the prescription and over-the-counter medications he or she is taking.

The way elderly people metabolize medications and eliminate them from the body differs greatly from how it happens in younger people.

Reduced functioning of the liver and kidneys is part of the aging process. For example, kidney size and the flow of blood to the kidneys decline by 40% to 50% between young adulthood and the ninth decade of life. Elderly people, therefore, should be given lower doses of drugs that are largely eliminated through the kidneys (e.g., gabapentin). For instance, one 79-year-old man was treated with gabapentin for seizures related to a brain tumor. While taking a standard adult dosage he became unsteady, fell several times, and developed slurred speech and confusion. His blood level was found to be twice the recommended upper limit of normal. When his dose was reduced by two-thirds, his seizures were controlled and he felt fine. People vary considerably with most biological functions, however, and not all elderly individuals have a marked decline in liver or kidney function.

Some of the side effects of antiepileptic drugs in the elderly are not easily noticed. For example, someone who takes carbamazepine or phenytoin for many years may become progressively less steady in walking. Because the dose of medication has not changed in many years, a neurologist may attribute the disorder to another cause, such as a head injury or a degenerative disorder. Reducing the dosage or changing the medication could completely end the unsteadiness. In other cases, a side effect resulting from an increased dose of an antiepileptic drug may not appear until weeks or months later; therefore, it may not be readily identified.

In certain cases, some medications that are often used to treat the elderly may provoke seizures. These medications include drugs used to treat behavioral and psychiatric problems, asthma, heart disorders, and infections. Therefore, all people with epilepsy or with a history of epilepsy should make it known to their doctors because a medication prescribed for an unrelated problem could make seizures more likely.

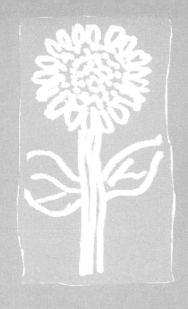

part five

LEGAL AND FINANCIAL ISSUES IN EPILEPSY

Legal Rights of People with Epilepsy

Unfortunately, discrimination against people with disabilities, and especially epilepsy, continues in public accommodations and housing. A variety of state and federal laws have been enacted to protect people with disabilities against discrimination. At the federal level, there are two major laws (also discussed in Chap. 27) that protect the rights of people with disabilities. They are the Americans with Disabilities Act (ADA) of 1990 and the Rehabilitation Act of 1973. Most states also have laws prohibiting discrimination in public places, housing and real estate, and credit transactions.

People with epilepsy or other disabilities also may face unjust accusation of antisocial or criminal behavior after a seizure in public, denial of adequate medical care in correctional facilities, and problems in child adoption or custody cases. In many of these areas, the rights of disabled people are secured by federal or state laws prohibiting discrimination. In other cases, such as false arrest, people with epilepsy can take precautions to avoid mistreatment or unfair judgments.

Medical Care

In the United States, no one has a legal right to medical care. However, most hospital emergency departments do not refuse medical care to someone who has a serious medical problem. The greatest obstacle for many people is availability of insurance to cover nonemergency office visits, outpatient tests, and hospitalizations. Individuals and families whose incomes are low may apply for Medicaid benefits, which will be discussed further in Chapter 31. Some states also provide health care to all children whose parents cannot afford it.

Public Services

Federal law requires state and local governments to provide public services in a nondiscriminatory manner. Some states protect people with disabilities as part of their civil rights laws. Other states have separate laws specifically addressing the rights of those with disabilities. In some states, protection against discrimination for people with disabilities extends both to services rendered directly by the state and those that are regulated or funded by the state. Thus, state laws may also provide protection in areas such as education, insurance, licensing, and access to transportation.

Public Accommodations

The ADA prohibits places of public accommodation (excluding religious organizations and private clubs) from discriminating against individuals with disabilities. Such people are entitled to full and equal enjoyment of goods, services, facilities, privileges, advantages, or accommodations. To enforce the ADA, individuals may bring a private lawsuit or file a complaint with the U.S. Attorney General through the Department of Justice.

People with epilepsy are sometimes unfairly prohibited from entering public places such as hotels, doctor's offices, and restaurants. Although such instances are rare, seizures may recur when a person has previously had a seizure in that place. There are legal remedies, but it may be easiest for the individual to inform the supervisor or manager of the place about his or her disorder and to describe the type and frequency of the seizures and any first aid measures that may be helpful. It is also worth reminding them that they must comply with the ADA and any applicable state law.

Housing

The Fair Housing Amendments Act (FHAA) of 1988 prohibits discrimination in the sale, rental, or financing of housing because of a disability. The FHAA mandates that housing providers make "reasonable accommodations" in rules, policies, and services to allow people with disabilities an equal opportunity to use and enjoy housing. Multifamily housing built after March 13, 1991, must meet minimum standards allowing access so that the housing can be used by people with disabilities.

Complaints of housing discrimination can be filed with the U.S. Department of Housing and Urban Development or in federal district court.

Airline Travel

People with epilepsy can be passengers on airplanes because there is no evidence that seizures are more likely to occur during or shortly after airplane flights than at other times. For people who have uncontrolled seizures, it may be worthwhile to consider special precautions. If the person is traveling alone, it may be helpful to inform flight attendants about the disorder and provide first aid information. Then, if a seizure occurs during the flight, they will be much less likely to overreact. When a tonic-clonic seizure occurs in someone without a known history of epilepsy, the airline may divert a long-distance flight to have the person treated in the closest city.

False Arrest

After having a complex partial or tonic-clonic seizure, some people will appear to be confused or under the influence of alcohol or illegal drugs. In this situation, they may be unfairly arrested and charged with being drunk and disorderly or creating a public disturbance. Similarly, during complex partial seizures, some people may perform automatic acts that are misinterpreted as willful and criminal. For example, they may undress in public, grab someone's arm, or pick up something in a store and break it or place it in their pocket. In these cases, a careful description of the act and of the person's behavior before, during, and after it, as well as a statement from family members or friends about the person's behavior during previous seizures, can be extremely helpful.

Unfortunately, a person may be unjustly accused of criminal behavior for something done during his or her first seizure. In such a case, a doctor can usually determine whether the behavior occurred during or after a seizure, and his or her report can lead to dismissal of the charges.

Restraint after seizures should be avoided because even relatively mild restraint can lead to violent reactions. During and after a seizure that impairs consciousness, the person is in a confused state, may interpret physical contact as an aggressive act, and may respond in a combative manner. The person with epilepsy may then be charged with assault or resisting arrest or the person may be injured. If he or she is then more aggressively restrained by police officers or others, that can stimulate even more violent behavior. In the worst case, because some police officers and other public employees are unfamiliar with epilepsy, seizures and their aftereffects are mistaken for criminal behavior, and the person with epilepsy is jailed, denied medication, and suffers additional seizures.

People with epilepsy can do several things to help avoid mistreatment and possible unjust arrest. They should wear a bracelet or necklace identifying them as having a seizure disorder, and it should include the telephone numbers of their doctor and the person to call in case of an emergency (see Chap. 9). In addition, people with epilepsy should carry their medications in the bottle from the pharmacy or carry a copy of the prescription or a doctor's note. If stopped by police or security personnel (e.g., at an airport during the search of carry-on bags), problems may arise if prescription drugs are not in their original containers. Your local police department or a local attorney can tell you about your state's laws governing possession of controlled substances. Because these laws vary from place to place, caution should be used when traveling outside your state or the country.

Rights of Inmates of Correctional Facilities

Epilepsy is more common among prisoners than in the general population. This is largely the product of sociological factors, including a higher rate of epilepsy in impoverished groups, which tend to be the people who are more likely to be imprisoned. Prisoners also have an increased incidence of head trauma, alcoholism, and drug abuse—problems that can cause seizures and epilepsy.

Prisoners have grave health care problems. Although their need for better medical care is well recognized, the delivery of that care is still lacking. The health care in many federal and state prisons has improved, but it is still inadequate in many ways. The greatest problems are in local jails, where people with epilepsy may be denied medication or are given medication in unreasonable ways so that they needlessly suffer additional seizures.

The simplest solution for inmates who believe they have been denied adequate medical care may be to have their own doctor contact the prison doctor or nurse. If this is impossible or unsuccessful, the attorney who represented them in their trial or an attorney recommended by the local Legal Aid office or the American Civil Liberties Union may be helpful in obtaining better health care.

Child Adoption

People with epilepsy can adopt children. Laws concerning adoption are generally written with safeguards to ensure the child's best interests. The fitness of a potential adoptive parent who has seizures may be questioned. Although no state law specifically mentions epilepsy, many states have adoption laws that require consideration of the mental and physical health of prospective parents. If the seizures are fully or partially controlled, however, there should be no restrictions on the ability of a person to be a parent.

Children with epilepsy may face great difficulty finding an adoptive home. State or federal assistance programs may provide financial assistance to people who adopt a child with epilepsy.

Child Custody

People with epilepsy can obtain custody of their children. Courts deciding custody matters should primarily consider the best interests of the child. A parent's epilepsy should not affect most custody decisions. Some state courts have recognized that epilepsy should not be the sole basis for denying custody to a parent, but it can be considered in determining the child's best interests.

If a parent's seizures are completely or partially controlled, epilepsy should not influence the custody decision. Unfortunately, negative attitudes toward epilepsy still persist, and some courts may unfairly deny custody on the basis of perceptions, not facts.

The parent with epilepsy should be ready to provide detailed information about the type, duration, and frequency of seizures and about medications taken. If the seizures impair consciousness or control of movement, it may be helpful to discuss specific safeguards that will be taken to protect the child. If the other person seeking custody claims that the child was injured while the parent was having a seizure, the event should be carefully investigated and the direct relevance of the seizure should be examined. It may be worthwhile to refer to articles and guides on parenting with epilepsy. (Contact the Epilepsy Foundation or see Appendix 4.)

If epilepsy has been a factor in making a custody decision, but the disorder later comes under better control, the parent can present a doctor's statement of the improvement and request a change in the custody decision. Some may claim that even if the parent's seizures cause no physical harm to the children, they will be psychologically harmful. There is no evidence to support this claim (see Chap. 26). No study has found that children of parents with epilepsy have more psychological problems than children in the general population.

Acknowledgment

Much of this chapter is based on *The Legal Rights of People with Epilepsy: An Overview of Legal Issues and Laws,* 6th ed. Epilepsy Foundation of America, Landover, MD, 1992.

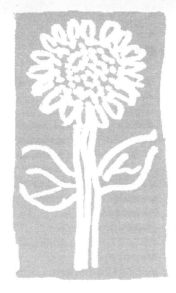

31

Insurance and Government Assistance

People with epilepsy, like most people in our society, have to be concerned with health insurance to cover the cost of medical care as well as with the many other kinds of insurance, such as life insurance, mortgage insurance, and disability insurance, that are available to provide security for themselves and their families. In addition to the financial protection afforded by private insurance, the federal government offers health insurance to people who meet certain eligibility requirements through programs called Medicare and Medicaid. These types of federal insurance and income maintenance programs are also available to those who qualify.

Health Insurance

Lack of affordable health care is one of our nation's gravest problems. Despite a concerted effort by state and national regulatory agencies, insurance companies, and hospitals, health care costs are increasing. As the costs increase, private health insurance moves further from the reach of individuals, families, and businesses.

Health insurance policies are expensive, especially for people with preexisting conditions (such as epilepsy). Although people with epilepsy have always had trouble obtaining affordable health care, the problem is growing more acute. One cost-cutting tactic used by many health insurance providers is to limit coverage for certain conditions, such as epilepsy.

People with epilepsy who have health insurance may find that certain diagnostic procedures and treatments are not covered. For example, some plans do not cover expensive outpatient tests such as ambulatory electroencephalograms (EEGs) and magnetic resonance imaging (MRI) scans. Other policies deny coverage for specialized inpatient services, such as video-EEG monitoring. Sometimes the resistance of insurers can be overcome if both the patient and the doctor persist in documenting the need for specialized services. The process of getting approval for these specialized services is often unduly prolonged, however, and sometimes coverage is ultimately denied.

There are different categories of health insurance. Commercial or private indemnity insurance policies are the most expensive, but they provide the most comprehensive coverage of hospital, doctor, and outpatient services. They allow the patient to choose the doctor and hospital. These plans typically pay all or a large portion of the hospital and doctor bills. Some plans pay a large percentage of outpatient charges as well.

Health maintenance organizations (HMOs) and preferred provider organizations (PPOs) are alternative health care delivery systems formed by groups of doctors and hospitals. Medical care is usually rendered only by the individuals and institutions within the system. In these organizations, as well as in managed health care plans (see the following), a single doctor often acts as a "gatekeeper." He or she must approve all tests and referrals to other doctors within or outside the group. Usually no fee or only a small fee is charged for medical services, but patients have to select a doctor or hospital from a specified list. Further, to help reduce costs, these organizations can limit the number of diagnostic procedures. If the HMO or PPO does not have an epileptologist, a neurologist with expertise in treating epilepsy, or a facility that performs studies such as video-EEG monitoring, the organization may approve consultation with one. The financial incentives for the HMO or PPO to restrict the number of patients who receive health care outside its system are strong, but if seizures remain poorly controlled, the adverse effects of medication are intolerable, or the epilepsy has a significant impact on the quality of life, a consultation with an epileptologist should be considered.

Managed group health care plans are also becoming more common. These plans are administered by companies that use a network of doctors, laboratories, and hospitals. These networks are often large, including facilities and staff at both community hospitals and university-related medical centers. The picture is becoming even more complex because many managed health care companies include their traditional plans, point-of-service plans, HMOs, PPOs, Medicare+Choice plans, and third-party administration of employer-funded benefit plans.

Group health plans may offer greater protection for people with epilepsy because of the Health Insurance Portability and Accountability Act (HIPAA) of 1996. This act states that group health plans cannot exclude a preexisting condition from coverage for more than 12 months, provided the condition is one that is generally covered in the policy.

The Comprehensive Omnibus Benefits Reform Act (COBRA) of 1984, a federal law, helps people maintain insurance coverage when they leave group health plans. People who are no longer eligible for group health coverage can purchase COBRA coverage for up to 18 months. COBRA and HIPAA can work together to (1) maintain coverage while a person finds or starts a new job and (2) limit the exclusion period for a preexisting condition that may apply to a new insurance plan.

MEDICARE

Medicare, administered by the federal Health Care Financing Administration, is health insurance for all members of our society aged 65 or over and for people who receive Social Security Disability Insurance (SSDI) benefits for at least 2 years. Medicare benefits are divided into two parts: Part A and Part B. Part A covers hospital services and skilled nursing services, except for a modest deductible paid by the patient. Part B covers doctor services, home health services, outpatient hospital services, and nondisposable equipment.

MEDICAID

Medicaid, a federal-state program administered by the states, provides health insurance to individuals older than 65 years of age and people with disabilities who meet specific income and medical criteria. Eligibility and benefits vary from state to state. Most states provide coverage for hospital and doctor services; inpatient and outpatient services and prescription drugs are usually included. In many states, a person who is eligible for Supplemental Security Income (SSI) is automatically eligible for Medicaid.

Although Medicaid covers doctor services, most private practice ("fee-for-service") doctors do not accept Medicaid. The reimbursement from Medicaid often does not cover the doctor's expenses for maintaining the office (rent, utilities, staff, malpractice insurance). However, many private practice doctors are willing to see a limited number of patients who have Medicaid. If a patient consults a doctor who does not accept Medicaid, the patient may use Medicaid to help with inpatient hospital costs, outpatient tests, and medications, but will have to pay the doctor's fee out of his or her own pocket.

Life Insurance

There are few things as complicated as life insurance. The buyer faces aggressive salespeople, a smorgasbord of policy types and levels of coverage, and a variety of companies offering slight variations on the same themes. Before buying a life insurance policy, buyers need to define their goals in obtaining life insurance, determine the type of policy and the amount of insurance they need, and do comparative shopping. All forms of life insurance get more expensive as the insured person gets older, so it is worth considering purchasing a policy sooner rather than later. It pays to be careful, however; it is easy to buy life insurance that is not needed.

Most people want life insurance to provide financial security for their family when they die, so it is most important to insure family members who provide significant income. People (such as children) who have little or no income have little need for life insurance. Also, individuals with no dependents may not need life insurance. After meeting with one or two insurance salespeople, however, initial goals may become clouded with terms like "investment," "cash value," and "retirement planning." Buyers must never lose sight of their goals.

The two main types of life insurance are term and whole-life. A third type, universal (flexible) life, has become popular in recent years. Term insurance is the least expensive; it is pure insurance and has no growth potential as an investment. Whole-life insurance is more expensive, but it accumulates value; the insured can withdraw money after a certain time depending on the specific policy. Some universal-life policies may allow the policy owner to direct how the cash value of the policy is invested; in others the investments are controlled by the insurance company, but the yearly premium varies more depending on the prevailing interest rates and other economic factors. One should be cautious in using life insurance policies as investments. Insurance sales people are often aggressive in promoting these policies, for which they receive their commission early on. If one is looking for an investment, life insurance is probably not the best choice, based on historical returns of other options such as a balanced stock portfolio.

Epilepsy can influence a person's eligibility for life insurance and the size of the premiums to be paid. Insurance companies rely on statistics regarding lifestyle, habits, and life span in different diseases and disorders when deciding on whether to offer life insurance and how much to charge for it. For example, people who smoke or have a history of heart disease pay higher rates. Because epilepsy does not follow the same course for everyone, it is unfair for insurance companies to lump together everyone with a history of epilepsy. Most insurance companies are aware of this and ask for a medical history, usually from the doctor.

Lying about a history of epilepsy on a life insurance application can backfire badly. If the insurance company investigates after the insured person's death and finds that the disorder had been concealed, the company may be able to deny any benefits, even if death was in no way related to the epilepsy.

Mortgage Insurance

Mortgage insurance is a kind of life insurance. In case of the insured person's death, it will pay off the remainder of the mortgage. It provides another form of security for the family and is worth considering. As with life insurance, mortgage insurance can be more difficult to obtain and more expensive for people with epilepsy. However, providing accurate medical information is critical to ensure that the policy is valid.

Disability Insurance

For people younger than 45 years old, chances are greater that they will be disabled in the near future than that they will die. People whose income is critical for their own support or their family's support should consider disability insurance. Unfortunately, it is expensive although it resembles term insurance; that is, you pay as you go and build no savings in the process. Furthermore, disability insurance gets more expensive as a person gets older. People with epilepsy may find disability insurance more difficult to obtain and more expensive than it is for people without epilepsy because some of them have a greater chance of becoming disabled.

Disability insurance policies vary considerably. Some of the most important questions a buyer should ask include:

- How long do I have to be disabled before benefits begin?
- Can I renew the disability insurance without another physical examination at the end of the term period?
- Do I have to be completely disabled or only unable to work at my current job to obtain benefits?

- What amount of benefits will I receive?
- Will future payments be adjusted for changes in the cost of living?
- Are the benefits lifelong or only until a certain age?
- Is the cost of the insurance stable for the duration of my coverage, or does it increase?

It is also important to make sure that the insurance company is well rated (AAA is the highest rating).

Government Financial Assistance*

SOCIAL SECURITY DISABILITY BENEFITS

The federal government's Social Security Administration (SSA) sponsors two programs that provide monthly income payments to individuals whose disabilities are expected to prevent them from working for at least 12 months. For these programs, disability is defined by the inability of the person "to engage in any substantial gainful activity by reason of any medically determinable physical or mental impairment which can be expected to result in death or which has lasted or can be expected to last for a continuous period of not less than 12 months."

Establishing eligibility for Social Security disability benefits can be a difficult process. Criteria are strictly enforced, and many deserving applicants are initially denied benefits, but are later approved on appeal. People who believe that their benefits were wrongfully denied can file an appeal with the help of an attorney. If the appeal is successful, payments are retroactive to the date of the initial application.

The first program, Social Security Disability Insurance (SSDI), pays benefits to eligible workers under age 65 (and their dependents or survivors) who have worked for a minimum period and have paid Social Security taxes. Generally, there is a 5-month waiting period between the determination that one is disabled and the initial payment.

The second program, Supplemental Security Income (SSI), is based on need and does not require prior payment of Social Security taxes. To qualify, the applicant must have no more than $2000 in assets, which includes cash or other property that could be converted to cash and used to help support that individual, and the monthly income cannot exceed $572 per month. For a couple, the asset level is $3000 and the income ceiling is $769 per month. (These criteria are subject to change. For the latest information, check www.ssa.gov or call 800-772-1213.)

---

*This portion of the chapter is based largely on *The Legal Rights of People with Epilepsy: An Overview of Legal Issues and Laws*, 6th ed. Epilepsy Foundation of America, Landover, MD, 1992.

Disabled children under age 18 years who live at home are considered to have their parents' income and assets and are therefore usually not eligible for SSI, but special rules may apply to some children. SSI payments begin as soon as the person is determined to be eligible and are retroactive.

APPLYING FOR BENEFITS

An application should be filed, in person if possible, at the local SSA office. The applicant should be prepared for lots of questions about his or her disability, medical history, work history, and financial status. When applying, the applicant should bring the following information:

- Social Security card or record of the number
- A list of all doctors, clinics, and hospitals where the applicant has been treated
- A detailed letter from the applicant's doctor on the nature of the disability and how it prevents the applicant from working; if there is more than one physical or mental disability, the doctor should describe all of them
- A list of activities of daily living (e.g., cooking, cleaning, and grocery shopping) that the applicant cannot do
- A list of past jobs that the applicant can no longer perform; if possible, a letter from a previous employer concerning inability to continue at the previous job
- Names, addresses, and telephone numbers of all social workers and counselors the applicant has consulted
- Birth certificate or other proof of age
- Information about the applicant's home, such as lease or mortgage
- Pay stubs, bankbooks, insurance policies, car registration, burial fund records, and any other documents establishing the applicant's financial situation
- Proof of U.S. citizenship or resident alien status

SOCIAL SECURITY ADMINISTRATION CRITERIA FOR ELIGIBILITY

The SSA considers epileptic seizures in two broad groups:

- *Major motor:* tonic-clonic (grand mal)
- *Minor motor:* absence (petit mal), complex partial (psychomotor), and focal motor

Major motor seizures must occur at least once a month despite at least 3 months of treatment. There must be either daytime seizures with loss of consciousness or convulsive seizures, or there must be seizures during sleep with residual effects that interfere significantly with daytime function. Minor motor seizures must occur more often than once a week despite at least 3 months of treatment. According to the SSA, there must be "alteration of awareness or loss of consciousness and transient postictal manifestations of unconventional behavior or significant interference with activity during the day."

If epilepsy is the cause of the disability, the SSA requires documentation of the disorder with an EEG and a detailed description of a typical seizure. To help document the seizure history, the applicant may want to keep a written diary recording the date and time of seizures, medication changes, and side effects. Although the SSA requires an EEG, it is recognized that a normal EEG does not rule out the diagnosis of epilepsy. If the EEG is normal, however, it may be helpful to have the neurologist write a note confirming that normal EEGs occur in people with epilepsy and also to submit a statement from a textbook confirming that fact. Detailed documentation of a typical seizure is essential. The description should include whether there is a warning or an aura (and the features of the aura, if present), tongue biting, loss of bladder or bowel control, injuries caused by the seizure, and postseizure symptoms such as confusion or sleepiness. The doctor who provides the seizure description should state the source of the information and whether corroboration was obtained from more than one person. If a health professional has witnessed a seizure, those observations should be included and the source should be noted. Although the patient's doctor will provide information about the seizures and the patient's examination, the SSA has the right to request that the applicant see an agency-paid doctor.

Several other issues may be relevant to the determination of disability benefits on the basis of epilepsy:

- Although the actual seizure count for the last 2 months may not fulfill the SSA criteria, the average seizure frequency over the past 6 to 12 months can be used because seizures often occur in clusters. This point must be emphasized because a cluster of three seizures in 2 days can be extremely disabling. Although this criterion is not yet recognized, it could be argued that this seizure frequency is equivalent to the one currently used and has a similar meaning for determining the presence of a disability.

- If seizures can only be controlled with very high dosages of medications, then the disabling effects of these drugs must also be considered.

- Documentation of the levels of antiepileptic drugs in the person's blood is requested and helps to confirm that he or she is taking the prescribed medications. If the levels are below the therapeutic range although the medication is being taken as prescribed (see Chap. 10), then the person's doctor should note that the low levels are not the result of failure to take the drugs, but may be due to problems with absorption or rapid metabolism or to the person's inability to tolerate higher levels because of adverse effects.

Because the SSA regulations regarding epilepsy may change, the agency should be contacted for current regulations and requirements.

REVIEW AND TERMINATION OF BENEFITS

After Social Security disability benefits have been granted, the SSA conducts periodic reviews to determine whether the condition has improved and the person is now able to be gainfully employed. The SSA may request documentation from both the person and the doctor regarding the current status of the disability. Benefits may be stopped (terminated) if the SSA finds that the impairment is gone, did not exist, or is no longer disabling.

If a person believes that his or her benefits have been terminated unfairly, he or she should immediately file a request to have the decision reconsidered. The person may also want to make a separate request to have benefits continue while the appeal is pending. This request must be made within 10 days of receiving the notice of termination.

If the termination is based on medical factors, a disability hearing must be requested within 10 days of receiving notification of benefits termination. If the termination is based on new information regarding income or assets, reconsideration is made only by review of the file. If a disability hearing is not requested or if it is determined that the person is no longer disabled, the person still can request a full hearing before an administrative law judge. This hearing must be requested within 60 days of the disability hearing decision or notification of the termination of disability benefits. The request that benefits be continued must also be renewed while waiting for the decision of the administrative law judge.

RETURNING TO WORK

New rules affecting Social Security coverage were established by the Ticket to Work and Work Incentives Improvement Act of 1999. Under the act, those receiving government financial assistance and health benefits (such as Medicare or Medicaid) can continue to receive financial support as part of their disability benefits for a limited time even after they return to work. Many people receiving SSDI can get their full benefits for as long as 1 year after they return to work. Those receiving

SSI payments may continue to get benefits as long as their monthly income does not exceed the maximum income allowed. In determining how much assistance a person will receive under SSDI or SSI, the SSA excludes from the person's gross income any work expenses related to the impairment, such as equipment or assistants.

Those who participate in Vocational Rehabilitation programs may be eligible to continue to receive benefits, regardless of income, until the program is completed. Those receiving SSDI or SSI who return to work may also be eligible for free rehabilitation services, job training, and educational programs through the SSA's Ticket to Work and Self Sufficiency Program.

Those receiving Medicare benefits can continue to get them for up to 39 months after returning to work, and those getting Medicaid can continue to receive benefits as long as their monthly income falls below the maximum allowed to be eligible for SSI and their employer does not provide similar health insurance or prescription coverage. The income level and extended period of eligibility is determined by each state. More specific information can be obtained from local Medicare or Medicaid offices.

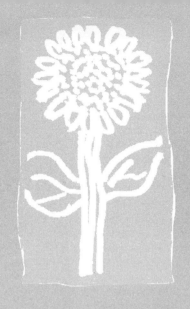

part six

RESOURCES
FOR PEOPLE
WITH EPILEPSY

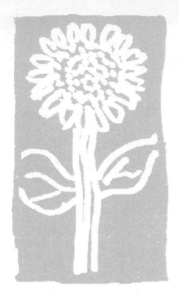

The Epilepsy Foundation

The Epilepsy Foundation (EF) is the national voluntary health organization committed to the prevention and cure of seizure disorders, the easing of their effects, and the promotion of independence and the best possible quality of life for people with these disorders. The EF seeks to accomplish its mission through support of research, education, advocacy, and service. It is a voice for people with epilepsy nationwide, and it works to promote legal rights and provide information and assistance in a variety of areas. Its growth in size and scope during more than 30 years has been dramatic.

Advocacy for People with Epilepsy: The Formation of the Epilepsy Foundation

People with epilepsy have faced severe stigma, isolation, and discrimination since ancient times (see Chap. 1). The misunderstandings and misconceptions that formed the image of epilepsy in earlier times have been proved wrong, but the damage from these false views persists. Members of older generations may still believe that epilepsy is a curse and a shame—a disorder that should be shrouded in secrecy and never revealed to the outside world. Some of these false views survive in old medical textbooks as well as in folklore. The misrepresentation of epilepsy has exacted a bitter price in the form of job bias, discrimination, and restrictive legislation directed against people with epilepsy. During the first half of the 20th century, laws in several states forbade people with epilepsy from marrying, permitted sterilization of people with epilepsy, and barred children with epilepsy from attending regular schools.

At the end of World War II it became clear that many wounded veterans had developed epilepsy as a result of serious head injury, and there was renewed interest in rehabilitation and fairer treatment. The late 1940s and the 1950s saw the emergence of a movement to help people with epilepsy. Public education campaigns began to demystify epilepsy and remove the stigma and discrimination. Local groups formed to provide information, medical referrals, and emotional support. Some of them established clinics. They raised funds for vital equipment, such as electroencephalograph (EEG) machines, and provided medications for people in need. Individual and group efforts combined to repeal many of the laws that restricted and discriminated against people with epilepsy, and efforts were made to improve their acceptance in schools.

The EF was established in 1968 as the Epilepsy Foundation of America, formed by a series of mergers of local and regional epilepsy advocacy groups. Its initial task was to obtain greater recognition for the problems faced by people with epilepsy, to help direct public opinion away from misinformation and misunderstanding to a more realistic and open view of epilepsy, and to stimulate increased federal funding for research and other programs.

As the epilepsy advocacy groups grew in strength and number during the 1950s and 1960s, so did federal interest in epilepsy and other neurologic disorders. A special institute was formed to fund research in these areas. Today, the National Institute of Neurological Disorders and Stroke (NINDS), a part of the National Institutes of Health, supports research on epilepsy at its own clinics and laboratories and at universities across the nation. With the active encouragement of the EF, the NINDS has played a critical role in the establishment of comprehensive epilepsy centers and the development of new antiepileptic drugs.

In 1975, Congress responded to pressure from the EF and passed a law calling for the establishment of a commission to study the treatment of epilepsy in the United States. The Commission for the Control of Epilepsy and Its Consequences concluded that:

1. Epilepsy was widely misunderstood throughout society.
2. There was a chronic lack of information about it.

3. People with epilepsy wanted to be more involved in their own care.
4. People with epilepsy wanted to become as independent as possible.

The commission's findings were based on many hours of testimony by people with epilepsy and their families, dozens of papers by leading experts in the field, and the active participation of the EF. Its report helped prepare the groundwork for the funding of many important federal initiatives, including the increased growth of epilepsy centers to evaluate the whole patient while providing state-of-the-art medical care. These came to be known as comprehensive epilepsy centers. The commission also made important recommendations to the executive branch of the federal government, urging that people with epilepsy be included in key programs and services, such as those provided through the Education of All Handicapped Children Act (Public Law 94-142) and by the Rehabilitation Services Administration.

The commission's recommendations provided a blueprint for action, and the EF responded enthusiastically. It pushed successfully for Food and Drug Administration approval of a new drug that the commission believed should be available in the United States, and it strengthened its own programs to provide information about epilepsy to individuals and families and to stimulate research in key areas of inquiry, especially regarding some of the social problems associated with epilepsy.

In 1982, the EF fulfilled a commission recommendation when it established the National Epilepsy Library at its offices in Landover, Maryland. Since then it has built its library into the world's largest single source of information on the social and medical aspects of epilepsy.

The EF has worked tirelessly to remove barriers that prevent the entry of people with epilepsy into the mainstream of American life. Its representatives have testified in legislatures across the country; it has filed friend-of-the-court briefs in lawsuits that test legal issues of importance to people with epilepsy; and it was a major force in the campaign to secure passage of the 1990 Americans with Disabilities Act, which opened new doors of opportunity in many areas of life for people with seizure disorders.

Studies have shown that the more than 30 years of public education sponsored by the EF and its affiliates have begun to pay off. Its annual campaigns on television and radio to change the negative image so long associated with the condition are beginning to have an effect. Public opinion about epilepsy has changed. There is greater acceptance of people with epilepsy and greater recognition that it can be effectively treated in many cases.

Today, the EF wants to build on that understanding by helping the public to see that there is a wide range of disability and that, although some people can now do very well, the disorder is by no means conquered. For those with severe seizures or associated disabilities, or those who have to take so much medication that their lives are severely limited, epilepsy is still a major barrier to a normal life.

Programs and Activities

The EF supports programs at the national and local levels to improve the lives of people with epilepsy and their families. It works closely with international and national organizations—including the American Epilepsy Society, the professional association of doctors and other health care workers. The Foundation also works with government agencies and organizations at the federal, state, and local levels. The EF has affiliates in most states. The affiliates are independently organized state and local groups that are bound to the national organization by an affiliation agreement.

The national office of the EF works with its affiliates to provide local services and a variety of educational, research, legislative, and other programs. It is led by an all-volunteer board of directors and a professional advisory board of leaders in the scientific community who provide expertise, guidance, and oversight for the Foundation's programs and services. The number of programs offered by the affiliates varies depending on the local needs and the level of support from the surrounding community. They often include community education, camping for children, support groups, and case management.

INFORMATION AND REFERRAL SERVICES

The national office of the EF receives more than 30,000 calls and letters each year requesting information about epilepsy. Since a toll-free number (see Appendix 4) was installed in 1986, the number of requests has increased dramatically. The calls come from people with epilepsy, their family members, doctors, and others in search of information. The Foundation provides current information on a wide range of epilepsy-related topics and on resources in each person's local area.

The EF's affiliates also distribute basic information about epilepsy and local services. Although pamphlets usually contain answers to most of the basic questions, a personal explanation is often more gratifying. Referrals to local medical, psychological, social, and other services can be provided.

NATIONAL EPILEPSY LIBRARY

Requests for technical information are referred to the EF's National Epilepsy Library. The library provides doctors, research scientists, nurses, people with epilepsy and their family members, and others with the most up-to-date information on medical and other aspects of epilepsy. Literature searches on the latest developments in research and clinical aspects of epilepsy are provided for doctors and other health care professionals. The National Epilepsy Library has a large database of its own and is linked with other major research collections.

The National Epilepsy Library responds to thousands of requests for information each year. For information, call the library's toll-free number (see Appendix 4).

INFORMATION AND EDUCATION

The EF produces and distributes a variety of educational materials about epilepsy. These materials include pamphlets, videotapes, posters, and books. More than 750,000 pamphlets are distributed annually by the national office. People can choose from more than 30 pamphlets, covering topics such as basic information, medicines, legal rights and issues, employment, first aid for seizures, information for babysitters of children with epilepsy, parenting children with epilepsy, and epilepsy and learning disabilities.

The EF actively promotes epilepsy education and the spreading of information through the media. Public-service messages are sent to magazines and radio and television stations nationwide. Through its educational campaigns, the EF seeks to improve the public's understanding of epilepsy and issues faced by people who live with seizure disorders.

THE INTERNET

The EF's Website (www.epilepsyfoundation.org) offers yet another opportunity for individuals, families, and the general public to learn more about seizure disorders. There are more than half a million visits a year, and the average time spent on the site is more than 12 minutes. The site, which has won acclaim from several sources, is divided into a series of channels, including advocacy, research, and an information section called the Answer Place. An online version of the EF's publication, *EpilepsyUSA,* is part of the site. A Gene Discovery Project to recruit families in which there is a history of epilepsy and seizures is also accessible through the Website. The goal of this program is to promote genetic research and to help identify epilepsy-producing genes.

ADVOCACY PROGRAMS

The EF's advocacy program helps fight discrimination; promotes access to health care, education, and employment; and supports independent living. Through position papers, congressional testimony, and legal briefs, the EF attacks the inequities and barriers that people with epilepsy face. As already noted, in 1990 the EF worked with other national health agencies to support passage of the Americans with Disabilities Act, which was discussed in previous chapters of this book.

Each year, representatives testify in support of essential government programs related to the needs of people with epilepsy. These include medical research, improved quality of medical care, better access to insurance, financial assistance for the disabled and ill, and employment and rehabilitation programs.

Legal advocacy is another important program. Staff attorneys provide general information about epilepsy-related legal issues. Staff lawyers work with local attorneys and, in some cases, file friend-of-the-court briefs in cases that have far-reaching significance for people with epilepsy. Such cases are ones in which a precedent or point of law may be established that can advance the well-being of others with epilepsy. Advocacy programs of the local affiliates are designed to support the interests of people with epilepsy, by speaking up on their behalf and getting the message out to those in a position to affect their lives. The advocacy can be on a personal level to solve a dispute or misunderstanding. In one instance, a woman with absence seizures was accused of being on drugs because she was "so spacey." An explanation to her supervisor from the doctor on the local affiliate's professional advisory board not only resolved her employment problem, but, for the first time, made her own doctor aware that her absence seizures were frequent. With adjustments of her medications, she gained better seizure control and a more secure job.

Advocacy can also help people with epilepsy pass through the bureaucracy and red tape that pervades society. The "Catch 22s" of life—problems in which the solutions create new problems or make the original one worse—can often be resolved through advocacy efforts. In some cases, advocacy programs provide experts to write a letter to legislators or agencies or to testify in support of better services or a needed facility, such as additional disability benefits or a living unit for young adults learning independence for the first time.

In some instances, advocacy simply provides recognition for people with epilepsy. One local affiliate recently secured a letter of recognition from New York's governor to a boy who was graduating from high school. Despite uncontrolled epilepsy, cerebral palsy, and serious learning disabilities, the boy persisted and graduated from his public high school. When his name was called, he received a standing ovation. When the letter from the governor was presented, the crowd could not stop applauding.

EMPLOYMENT PROGRAMS

Employment remains a major challenge for people with epilepsy, with an unemployment rate of at least 25% among people living in the community. The EF's employment service programs have helped thousands of people with epilepsy find work each year. Local affiliates provide job counseling, job clubs, and employer outreach services to improve opportunities. In some instances, follow-up services after employment are also available.

RESEARCH GRANTS

Advancing knowledge about the prevention, diagnosis, and treatment of epilepsy through research is one of the EF's primary goals. Research can provide new insights into the causes of epilepsy, help discover new drugs to stop seizures, and promote a better understanding of the medical and social disorders that occur in people with epilepsy. Every year the organization funds research projects by both young and established investigators. This support helps to uncover new information, stimulates the interests of young scientists and doctors in epilepsy research, and moves us closer to a cure.

PROFESSIONAL EDUCATION

The EF sponsors educational programs and materials about epilepsy for health care professionals. It devotes a section of its Website to information on clinical care for primary care doctors, doctors in training, nurses, and other health care professionals. It also funds training and fellowships for students and doctors. Special emphasis in recent years has been given to educational programs on the effects of epilepsy on women.

Local affiliates, together with local medical centers, coordinate educational programs to bring up-to-date information about epilepsy to professionals in the community. These programs may include full-day courses for doctors, seminars for nurses, lectures to police officers and firefighters about recognition of seizures and first aid for them, and in-service presentations for personnel directors. These educational services help keep professionals knowledgeable and help them do a better job of serving people with epilepsy.

NATIONAL CONFERENCE

The EF's annual conference brings together volunteers and staff of its local affiliates, national staff, health care professionals, and people with epilepsy and their families. Each conference has a theme and includes lectures and workshops on specific aspects of epilepsy. Experts present information about new developments in treatment, medications, surgery, quality-of-life concerns, and the occurrence of epilepsy in select populations.

WINNING KIDS PROGRAM

The Winning Kids program was designed to change the negative stereotypes that children with epilepsy face, but it has broadened to honor children's courage in coping with epilepsy's challenges. The program promotes self-esteem and rewards achievements large and small. Every year, EF affiliates enter their Winning Kids. Although only one of them is chosen to represent the others as the national Winning Kid, in the EF's view, they are all winners.

COUNSELING PROGRAMS AND SUPPORT GROUPS

Professionally staffed counseling programs or peer-group support programs involving people with epilepsy or their parents are offered by many of the affiliates. Counseling sessions may cover such issues as adjusting to and living with epilepsy and parenting a child with epilepsy.

Support groups allow people to gain strength from shared experiences and provide the recognition that their feelings, frustrations, and joys are not unique. Depending on local resources, support groups may be provided for adults, teenagers, parents, or even children. If one is not available, anyone can work to generate interest and get one started.

SCHOOL ALERT PROGRAM

The School Alert program is a locally conducted, national educational program to improve the school environment for children with epilepsy. Information about epilepsy is made available to teachers, school nurses, other school personnel, and students through videotapes, manuals, pamphlets, and in-person presentations of the EF's curriculum on seizure recognition and first aid. For young children, the "Kids on the Block" puppet show is offered by many affiliates; these shows present the information in a way young children can understand, and they have been warmly received. The goal of the program is a safer school environment for children with seizures.

SPEAKERS' BUREAU

The Speakers' Bureau is an educational service through which local affiliates provide trained speakers to talk to groups and clubs about epilepsy.

EPILEPSY MONTH

November is Epilepsy Month, a time devoted to providing the public with information about epilepsy. An intensive education campaign may include press and publicity materials, radio and television messages and stories, and fund-raising events. This campaign is nationwide.

ASSISTED LIVING

Some EF affiliates offer residential programs for adults with epilepsy who need some assistance with activities of daily living, but who are not so disabled that they need more care. Other affiliates work with agencies that operate independent living centers and can be helpful in getting places in such facilities. Such facilities range from large houses in which residents have individual bedrooms to individual apartments to day-care centers.

CAMPING AND RECREATIONAL PROGRAMS

EF affiliates in many parts of the country offer camping experiences, often combined with epilepsy education, for children with epilepsy. Parents whose children go to these camps frequently find they are more independent and self-confident afterward. Other recreational programs include day camps and weekend retreats for the whole family.

RESPITE CARE

When a child has severe seizures or associated disabilities, parents may need an occasional time out. Some EF affiliates offer respite care in the form of trained people to relieve parents and other family members for predetermined periods.

Getting Involved

The EF was created and has grown through the efforts of people with epilepsy, their families, and others who want people with seizure disorders to achieve success and the best possible quality of life.

Anyone who has epilepsy or who is the parent or other family member of someone with epilepsy should consider contacting the EF and becoming active at the local level. Volunteers can help in various efforts, such as speaking at school gatherings, fund-raising, and organizing and participating in support groups.

The Epilepsy Foundation Today and in the Future

The EF continues to grow and serve people with seizure disorders and their families in innovative ways. The positive changes in public perception about epilepsy need to be reinforced. The struggle to end discrimination because of epilepsy is not over yet. Most of all, we must work together to prevent seizure disorders, to find a cure for them, and to pursue activities that will improve opportunities for people with epilepsy to be independent and employed and to enjoy their lives. Research is also an important part of the EF's mission for the future. Only through research can we achieve our ultimate goal of no seizures and no adverse medication effects for people with a diagnosis of epilepsy.

Other Resources

Although the Epilepsy Foundation (EF) is the national organization for people with epilepsy (see Chap. 32), other resources may also be helpful. People with epilepsy often face specific individual challenges. No matter how unique or difficult the problem, there are successful solutions. Identifying the resources available is often the first step in overcoming the problem.

The Internet

The Internet is a vital source of information regarding epilepsy and related medical, neurologic, and psychiatric disorders. Information can also be obtained on topics as wide-ranging as medical research, drug interactions, patient and family experiences, special education, vocational rehabilitation, and alternative therapies. *Epilepsy.com* is a site dedicated to enhancing the lives of people with epilepsy through information and interaction. The information is presented at several levels of sophistication (both basic and more advanced knowledge), with a humanistic side (magazine type articles, personal anecdotes of patients and doctors), a research component (latest advances in trying to better understand and cure epilepsy), and an on-line nurse practitioner and physicians who can answer questions and provide guidance through the maze of epilepsy information. Many other valuable Internet sites are listed in Appendix 4.

National Resources

A variety of national organizations serve certain groups. In many cases, information, services, and advocacy by these organizations are relevant to people with epilepsy who have special needs. When a person has more than one disability, the challenges are often greater. In such cases, tapping into the resources of related organizations can be beneficial. For example, blind people who have uncontrolled epilepsy have special challenges, some of which can be met through organizations that serve the blind.

OFFICE OF VOCATIONAL AND ADULT EDUCATION

The federal Office of Vocational and Adult Education (OVAE) supports a wide range of programs and activities that help young people and adults obtain the knowledge and skills they need for successful careers and productive lives. Although it deals primarily with non-profit and government agencies rather than with individuals directly, people can use its Website or office as an additional resource to identify programs that may be located in their communities. Its Website (www.ed.gov/offices/OVAE/) provides information about programs, grants, events, and federal legislation and policy. This office helps coordinate the distribution of federal funds provided to each state for vocational-technical education for students with special needs. It also conducts research and provides technical assistance to educators in career or technical education and adult education.

MEMBERS OF CONGRESS

Elected representatives in the Senate and House of Representatives also may be helpful. For example, a young man from Iran with refractory partial seizures who lives with his father and brother in the United States was scheduled to undergo epilepsy surgery. His mother was unable to obtain a visa to enter the United States from Iran. With the support of doctors at the epilepsy center, the local congressional representative was able to secure the visa through the U.S. Department of State.

Community Resources

People, organizations, agencies, and other resources available at state or local levels can provide information, advocacy, and services to people with epilepsy and their family members. In many cases, the greatest challenge is identifying these resources. The resources range from financial assistance for food, shelter, and medical care to respite-care programs for parents with severely disabled children. Some of the most important local resources are as follows. Others can be found by calling the EF's national office or local affiliate, the local or state government, or a comprehensive epilepsy center. Consulting some of the many Websites run by these and other organizations also is helpful. See Appendix 4 for more specific information.

STATE DEPARTMENT OF EDUCATION

Each state has a Department of Education, which establishes educational standards for regular and special education programs and services. Depending on the state, the Department of Education may also provide funding for special education and for services needed by students with disabilities to help them attend school. Although the local school district (in some states run by the county and in others by the town or city) provides education to each child and is responsible for determining whether a child needs special services or instruction, the state Department of Education can provide information about special education programs and services. This office can also be helpful in determining whether a child is receiving the needed services to which he or she is entitled.

BOARD OF EDUCATION

Each school district has a board of education that sets local policies. The person who coordinates special education or other programs of the local school district can be found there.

PROTECTION AND ADVOCACY OFFICES FOR INDIVIDUALS WITH DISABILITIES

The protection and advocacy office (the exact title varies from state to state) can provide information on the state's services for people with disabilities. Depending on the state, services may include education, recreational activities, respite programs, residential housing, and legal representation. To locate the protection and advocacy office for your state, visit the Website of the National Association of Protection and Advocacy Systems (http://www.protectionandadvocacy.com) or call the Consumer Services Division of the national office of the EF (see Appendix 4).

DEVELOPMENTAL DISABILITIES AGENCY

Each state's developmental disabilities agency (the name varies by state) allocates federal funds to nonprofit private and public organizations to assist people with developmental disabilities. Some of the services include medical care (evaluation, diagnosis, and treatment), information, social services, protection, social activities, group homes, and advocacy.

STATE VOCATIONAL REHABILITATION AGENCY

The state vocational rehabilitation agency has numerous local offices that coordinate medical, physical, and occupational therapy and provide program planning, education, and vocational programs to assist people in obtaining employment. "One-stop" employment assistance centers offer access to training and other services.

Comprehensive Epilepsy Centers

The growth of our understanding about epilepsy has led to the realization that, for some patients, the treatment of epilepsy involves the coordination of several disciplines and may require expertise beyond the capacity of general medical or neurologic care. Comprehensive epilepsy centers provide expert care for patients with epilepsy.

The principal doctors at comprehensive epilepsy centers are epileptologists. These are neurologists who, after they finish their training in general neurology, complete additional training in caring for people with epilepsy. This training includes exposure to a multidisciplinary approach to epilepsy-related problems; that is, training incorporates input from various health care workers. Most programs include extensive training in the interpretation of electroencephalograms (EEGs) and video-EEG recordings and also include training in the use of investigational drugs and epilepsy surgery.

Investigational drugs are those that have not been approved for general use by the Food and Drug Administration. All new drugs must go through extensive testing of their effectiveness and safety. The process includes clinical trials or testing of the drugs in patients. The clinical trials are supervised by both the drug company and the doctor who studies the patients. Before a study is begun, it must be approved by the center's Institutional Review Board. This board usually includes doctors and other health care professionals, a member of the clergy, a bioethicist (someone familiar with ethical issues in medicine), and others. If a patient's seizures have not been controlled by the standard antiepileptic drugs, investigational drugs or surgery may be considered. Comprehensive epilepsy centers are the only facilities with the teams and expertise to perform epilepsy surgery and implant and manage vagal nerve stimulators (see Chap. 12).

Most people with epilepsy do not require care at comprehensive epilepsy centers. A patient may be referred to an epilepsy center because the nature of the attack is uncertain (Is it epilepsy or something else?), because the type of epilepsy is difficult to classify (Are the seizures partial or primary generalized?) or because the seizures or adverse effects of medication are continuing despite the finest treatment. Referral can also be made because employment problems or social disabilities resulting from the epilepsy need expert attention, or because an investigational drug, epilepsy surgery, or vagal nerve stimulation is recommended. In most cases, patients are referred to a comprehensive epilepsy center by their neurologist or other doctor.

For some people, a single consultation at a comprehensive epilepsy center may be worthwhile. For example, a woman with epilepsy who is thinking about starting a family may benefit from speaking with an expert on epilepsy and pregnancy. Although the information provided by the woman's neurologist and the epileptologist may be quite similar, it can be comforting simply to hear the answers from another source. In other cases, the expert at the epilepsy center may be aware of more specific or new information before it is known by most doctors in the community.

The most common referral to a comprehensive epilepsy center is for people with poorly controlled seizures or troublesome adverse effects of medications. Epilepsy centers can help control seizures or avoid adverse effects of medication in these patients by recommending the best way to use antiepileptic drugs or prescribing changes in lifestyle, such as more sleep. All of these recommendations can be made by other doctors, but it may be helpful for patients with difficult-to-control seizures to have a fresh assessment.

There are differences among epilepsy centers. Some centers care predominantly for children or adults, and others care for patients of all ages. Some centers offer only consultation with an epilepsy specialist and certain diagnostic studies, such as video-EEG monitoring. Other centers conduct investigational drug trials or specialize in epilepsy surgery. The types of epilepsy surgery performed, the age of patients considered for surgery, and the costs of the surgery may vary considerably at different epilepsy centers. In some cases, one epilepsy center may offer advantages over other centers.

The EF can provide a list of comprehensive epilepsy centers in various parts of the country and their services. See Appendix 4 for contact information.

Toward a Cure for Epilepsy

In recent decades, our society has become much more aware of epilepsy and has expanded the health care resources available for those affected. New antiepileptic drugs are helping people with difficult-to-control seizures and providing alternatives for those suffering troublesome adverse effects from older medications. Diagnostic and surgical techniques have been improved and are more effective than ever, thanks to recent scientific advances that have enhanced our ability to map the region of the brain from which seizures arise and our ability to map areas that are critical for normal brain functions. Vagal nerve stimulation is the first new therapeutic technique for epilepsy in more than a century. Other new therapies for epilepsy are under investigation, and the mechanisms leading to seizures and epilepsy are the focus of intensive study.

Neuroscience in the New Millennium

The new millennium will see an explosion of information on how the brain works and on how to conquer neurologic disorders, based on research funded largely by federal grants. Epilepsy research is active in a wide spectrum of areas, including:

- Investigating changes in brain cells and chemicals associated with seizures and the tendency to have seizures

- Mapping genes linked to epilepsy
- Exploring gene therapy for epilepsy
- Studying changes of metabolism in cells during and after seizures
- Developing electrodes that can provide "early warning" of when seizures will occur
- Developing more effective antiepileptic drugs
- Developing and refining advanced techniques for mapping areas of the brain responsible for seizures to improve the results of epilepsy surgery
- Developing and refining new epilepsy surgery procedures, including stimulation of brain sites, transplantation of stem or fetal cells, and disrupting connections or nerve cells in deep brain areas of the thalamus where seizure activity may be synchronized
- Understanding the social impact of seizures on children
- Examining quality-of-life issues in epilepsy and identifying problems that place long-term quality of life at risk

GENETIC RESEARCH

The greatest potential for a cure for epilepsy lies in better understanding its genetics. Although most forms of epilepsy are not "genetic," genes influence many functions of the body that in turn deeply affect seizure activity. Unlocking the mysteries of the genes could help us in many ways control and possibly cure seizures.

Current genetic research has focused on epilepsy syndromes that are known to be inherited. DNA samples are obtained from several affected and nonaffected family members, and a comparison is made to identify which genes are found only in affected individuals. The next step is finding out what product this gene is responsible for and then understanding its function. Several genes have been successfully identified in specific, although relatively uncommon, epilepsy syndromes, such as benign familial neonatal convulsions. It appears that many of these genes are involved in mechanisms that regulate the flow of electrical charges into and out of nerve cells, thereby affecting their electrical excitability.

One target of this research will be to identify drugs that can counteract the negative effects of these genes. For example, if a gene produces a defective protein that is part of one of these mechanisms, it may be possible to create a drug that "fills in" for the defect or bypasses that mechanism. Another target of gene research is gene therapy—actually modifying the DNA. For example, in patients with genetic forms of epilepsy, one might be able to "splice" out bad genes and replace them with good genes. This kind of treatment could extend to many genetic disorders in which epilepsy commonly occurs, such as mitochondrial disorders and tuberous sclerosis. In patients with epilepsy that is not genetic, it may be possible to insert genes that will control abnormal electrical discharges, thereby treating the fundamental problem.

SEIZURE DETECTION

One of the most dangerous aspects of seizures is their unpredictability. For many patients, they can occur at any time of the day and in any setting. Although some patients have auras (simple partial seizures that warn them when a seizure is about to occur), they may not occur before all seizures. Unpredictability keeps many people with epilepsy away from activities such as driving and causes injuries from falls. For years we have known that there are often changes in brain waves that precede the initial symptoms of a seizure. Software programs are available that can identify rhythmic changes on electroencephalogram recordings that are associated with the early phase of a seizure. Several groups of researchers are now working on a device in which several electrodes, possibly implanted in a person's scalp, could provide early detection of seizure activity. If we could reliably identify the brain-wave changes and warn the person or their family member, it could greatly improve quality of life for many people with epilepsy. For example, patients who are prone to harmful falls could be placed in a safe position. Early warning also may offer new types of treatment: medications to stop seizures could be released "on demand" through a device implanted in the brain, or electrical stimulation of the brain or vagus nerve could be triggered to help stop the seizure.

Supporting Epilepsy Research

The largest source of financing for research is government grants, but individuals and small groups can have significant impact by writing to government representatives and strongly encouraging their support of epilepsy research. The Epilepsy Foundation (EF) provides grants to researchers studying epilepsy and supports a wide range of programs and services for people with epilepsy. Contributions to the EF and its local affiliates are important for advancing epilepsy research and support services for people with epilepsy.

Regional comprehensive epilepsy centers often conduct research studies on epilepsy as well as provide patient care. Support of these centers can be directed toward specific programs, such as treatment of children with epilepsy or basic science research studies on epilepsy.

EPILEPSY VENTURES

Epilepsy Ventures is a venture fund that seeks to bridge the gap between "pure research" and commercial development. Although epilepsy is the tenth largest pharmaceutical market, it was recently termed the "stepchild of pharmaceutical development" by a pharmaceutical company CEO. Many larger pharmaceutical companies only do epilepsy projects if there is the potential to also address larger, related, CNS opportunities like neuropathic pain, bipolar disorder, migraine, anxiety, and depression.

By bringing financial resources together with strong scientific know-how and industry experience, Epilepsy Ventures will try to add value to the development process of promising new therapies. The focused expertise in epilepsy can help Epilepsy Ventures achieve attractive financial returns and help stimulate new epilepsy therapies in a self-sustaining model.

Several strategies will be pursued. First, they will co-invest with independent companies in therapies in the early stages of commercial development. Second, they will invest in promising new biotechnology companies at the corporate level in return for a commitment to make epilepsy an early clinical focus. The fund will launch with $10 million and plans will be to start a second, larger Epilepsy Ventures Fund.

Individuals interested in Epilepsy Ventures should contact: *warren. lammert@epilepsyventures.com*.

Future Advances in Understanding Epilepsy

Despite the enormous efforts of the medical and scientific communities to shed light on the causes, diagnosis, and treatment of epilepsy, a cure is not on the horizon, and it is unlikely that significant advances in treatment will occur very soon. We are likely to see an increase in our understanding of the causes of epilepsy, however, and this will lay the foundation for breakthroughs in treatment.

Perhaps the greatest obstacle to finding a cure for epilepsy is the fragmented nature of medical research. Some of man's greatest achievements, such as walking on the moon, were the result of very focused and intensive resources aimed at a specific goal. We need to bring our resources together to cure this disorder.

Appendixes

APPENDIX 1

Glossary of Terms

Absence seizure: A primary generalized epileptic seizure, usually lasting less than 20 seconds, characterized by a stare sometimes associated with blinking or brief automatic movements of the mouth or hands; formerly called *petit mal* seizure. Absence seizures usually begin in childhood, are usually easily controlled with medication, and are outgrown by approximately 75% of children. *See* Atypical absence seizure.

Accommodation (*or* Reasonable accommodation): Any change in the work environment or in the way things are customarily done that enables an individual with a disability to have equal employment opportunities.

ADA: *See* Americans with Disabilities Act.

ADD: *See* Attention deficit disorder.

ADHD: Attention deficit/hyperactivity disorder.

Adjunct: Something added to another thing in a subordinate position or use; for example, an adjunct drug is one used in addition to another drug, not alone (*add-on therapy*).

Adverse effects: The undesirable or unfavorable effects of something; for example, the adverse effects of an antiepileptic drug cause troublesome and, occasionally, serious problems for patients.

Ambulatory EEG monitoring: A system for recording the electroencephalogram for a prolonged period (typically 18 to 24 hours) in an outpatient; the electrodes are connected to a small cassette tape recorder.

Americans with Disabilities Act: A law that makes discrimination against people with disabilities illegal; the act applies to employment, access to public places, and places of accommodation.

Antiepileptic drug: A medication used to control both convulsive and nonconvulsive seizures; sometimes called an *anticonvulsant*.

Atonic seizure: An epileptic seizure characterized by sudden loss of muscle tone; may cause the head to drop suddenly, objects to fall from the hands, or the legs to lose strength, with falling and potential injury; usually not associated with loss of consciousness.

379

Attention deficit disorder (ADD): An impairment in the ability to focus or maintain attention.

Atypical absence seizure: A staring spell characterized by partial impairment of consciousness; often occurs in children with the Lennox-Gastaut syndrome; the EEG shows slow (less than 3 per second) spike-and-wave discharges.

Aura: A warning before a seizure; a simple partial seizure occurring within seconds or minutes before a complex partial or secondarily generalized tonic-clonic seizure, or it may occur alone; also a warning before a migraine headache or a primary generalized seizure.

Autoinduction (of metabolism): A process in which continued administration of a drug leads to an increase in the rate at which the drug is metabolized.

Automatism: Automatic, involuntary movement during a seizure; may involve mouth, hand, leg, or body movements; consciousness is usually impaired; occurs during complex partial and absence seizures and after tonic-clonic seizures.

Autonomic: Pertaining to the autonomic nervous system, which controls bodily functions that are not under conscious control (e.g., heartbeat, breathing, sweating); some partial seizures may cause only autonomic symptoms; changes in autonomic functions are common during many seizures.

Autosomal dominant: A mode of inheritance in which a gene is passed on by either parent; in most cases, the child has a 50% chance of inheriting the gene; the *expression* of the gene (that is, the development of the physical trait or the disorder) can vary considerably among different individuals with the same gene.

Autosomal recessive: A mode of inheritance in which an individual has two copies of a gene that requires both copies for *expression*, or development, of the trait. Both parents must be *carriers* (that is, they have only one copy of the gene and, therefore, do not have the physical trait that the gene confers) or have the trait (that is, have two copies of the same gene).

Axon: The part of the nerve cell (neuron) that communicates with other cells, similar to a telephone wire; the axon is often covered with myelin, an insulating fatty layer, which functions similarly to plastic around a copper wire.

Benign: Favorable for recovery.

Benign rolandic epilepsy: An epilepsy syndrome of childhood characterized by partial seizures occurring at night and often involving the face and tongue; the seizures may progress to *tonic-clonic* seizures, have a characteristic EEG pattern, are easily controlled with medications but may not require treatment, and are outgrown by age 16 years.

Blood drug level: The concentration, or amount, of circulating drug in the bloodstream, measured in micrograms (µg) or nanograms (ng) per milliliter (mL). The concentration may be measured as the free or total level because some of the drug is bound to the protein in the blood and some is not; the *free level* is the amount of drug that is "free" (unbound); the *total level* is the amount of drug that is both bound and unbound to the blood protein; the drug that is free (unbound) is the portion that reaches the brain and exerts an effect on the disorder.

Brand-name drug: Medication manufactured by a major pharmaceutical company; the drugs are often expensive, but tend to be uniform in the amount of drug and the method of preparation.

Breath-holding spells: Episodes in children in which intense crying or an emotional upset is followed by interruption of breathing and sometimes loss of consciousness; the episodes are not harmful, but when prolonged, slight jerking movements may occur.

Catamenial: Referring to the menses or to menstruation; with regard to women with epilepsy, a tendency for seizures to occur around the time of the menses.

Cerebral hemisphere: One side of the cerebrum (upper brain); each hemisphere contains four lobes (frontal, parietal, occipital, and temporal).

Cerebral palsy: A condition with various combinations of impaired muscle tone and strength, coordination, and intelligence.

Clonic seizure: An epileptic seizure characterized by jerking movements and involving muscles on both sides of the body.

Cognitive: Pertaining to the mental processes of perceiving, thinking, and remembering; used loosely to refer to intellectual functions as opposed to physical functions.

Complex partial seizure: An epileptic seizure that involves only part of the brain and impairs consciousness; often preceded by a simple partial seizure (aura, or warning).

Computed tomography (CT): A scanning technique that uses x-rays and computers to create pictures of the inside of the body; shows the structure of the brain; not as sensitive as MRI.

Consciousness: State of awareness; if consciousness is preserved during a seizure, the person can respond (either in words or actions, such as raising a hand on command) and recall what occurred during the spell.

Controlled study: An experiment in which two groups are the same except that only one receives the drug, treatment, etc. being tested.

Convulsion: An older term for a tonic-clonic seizure.

Convulsive syncope: A fainting episode in which the brain does not receive enough blood, causing a seizure; the episode is not an epileptic seizure, but a result of the faint.

Corpus callosotomy: A surgical technique that disconnects the cerebral hemispheres and is most effective in reducing atonic and tonic-clonic seizures.

Cortical dysplasia: An abnormality in the development and organization of the cerebral cortex that can cause seizures and other neurologic disorders. These disorders can result from abnormal migration of nerve cells during development or can occur with disorders such as tuberous sclerosis or Sturge-Weber syndrome.

CT scan: *See* Computed tomography.

Daily dose: The average amount of medication taken over the course of the day to achieve a therapeutic blood level of the drug, usually measured in milligrams (mg) per kilogram (kg) of the patient's body weight (1 kg = 2.2 pounds).

Deficit: A lack or deficiency of an essential quality or element; for example, a neurologic deficit is a defect in the structure or function of the brain.

Deja vu: Feeling as if one has lived through or experienced this moment before; may occur in people without any medical problems or immediately before a seizure (i.e., as a simple partial seizure).

Development: The process of physical growth and the attainment of intelligence and problem-solving ability that begins in infancy; any interruption of this process by a disease or disorder is called *developmental delay.*

Dose-related effects: Adverse effects that are more likely to occur at times of peak blood levels of a drug.

EEG: *See* Electroencephalogram.

EEOC: Equal Employment Opportunity Commission.

EF: Epilepsy Foundation.

Electrode: A conductor through which electrical current enters or leaves. When used to record the electroencephalogram, a small metal disc attached to a wire is usually used.

Electroencephalogram (EEG): A diagnostic test of brain electrical activity; helpful in diagnosing epilepsy.

Elimination: The removal of waste products from the body.

Encephalitis: An inflammation of the brain, usually caused by a virus.

Epilepsia partialis continua: A continuous or prolonged partial seizure that causes contraction of the muscles; usually restricted to the muscles of the face, arm, or leg; usually not associated with impairment of consciousness.

Epilepsy: A disorder characterized by transient but recurrent disturbances of brain function that may or may not be associated with impairment or loss of consciousness and abnormal movements or behavior.

Epilepsy syndrome: A disorder defined by seizure type, age of onset, clinical and EEG findings, family history, response to therapy, and prognosis.

Epileptiform: Resembling epilepsy or its manifestations; may refer to a pattern on the EEG associated with an increased risk of seizures.

Epileptogenic: Causing epilepsy.

Epileptologist: A neurologist with specialty training in epilepsy.

Equilibrium period: *See* Steady state.

Excitatory: Stimulating or increasing brain electrical activity; causing nerve cells to fire.

Febrile seizure: A seizure associated with high fever in children aged 3 months to 5 years, usually a tonic-clonic seizure; benign in most cases.

Fit: An older term for a seizure, usually a tonic-clonic seizure; still used in some places.

Focal seizure: An older term for a partial seizure.

Focus: The center or region of the brain from which seizures begin; used in reference to partial seizures.

Generalized seizure: A seizure that involves both sides of the brain and causes tonic and clonic movements (primary or secondary generalized) or another type of primary generalized epilepsy (e.g., absence or atonic seizure).

Generic drug: A drug that is not sold under a brand name; for example, carbamazepine can be obtained as a generic drug or as Tegretol, its brand name.

Grand mal: An older term for a tonic-clonic seizure.

Half-life: The time required for the amount of a drug in the blood to decline to half of its original value, measured in hours; a drug with a longer half-life lasts longer in the body and, therefore, generally needs to be taken less often than a drug with a shorter half-life.

Hemispherectomy: A surgical procedure to remove a cerebral hemisphere (one side of the brain); the operation is now often modified to remove a portion of the hemisphere and to disconnect the remaining portions.

Hereditary: Passed from one generation to the next through the genes.

Hydrocephalus: A condition associated with obstruction of the cerebrospinal fluid pathways in the brain and accumulation of excess cerebrospinal fluid within the skull.

Hyperventilation: Increased rate and depth of breathing; may be done during the EEG to increase the chances of finding epileptiform or other abnormal activity.

Hypsarrhythmia: An abnormal EEG pattern of excessive slow activity and multiple areas of epileptiform activity; associated with infantile spasms.

Ictal: Referring to the period during a sudden attack, such as a seizure or stroke.

Idiopathic: Referring to a disorder of unknown cause.

Idiosyncratic: Pertaining to an abnormal susceptibility to some drug or other agent, peculiar to the individual.

Incidence: The number of new cases of a disorder occurring in a population during a specified period.

Individuals with Disabilities Education Act (IDEA): A U.S. federal law ensuring that all handicapped children receive appropriate education at no cost and in the least restrictive environment.

Infantile spasm: A sudden jerk followed by stiffening; spasms usually begin between age 3 and 12 months and usually stop by age 2 to 4 years, although other seizure types often develop; in some spells, the arms are flung out as the body bends forward ("jackknife seizures"), but in others the movements are more subtle.

Inhibitory: Shutting off or decreasing brain electrical activity; causing nerve cells to stop firing.

Intensive monitoring: *See* Video-EEG monitoring.

Interictal: Referring to the period between seizures.

Intractable: Difficult to alleviate, remedy, or cure; for example, intractable seizures are difficult to control with the usual antiepileptic drug therapy.

Intravenous infusion: Administering a drug or other substance as part of a liquid solution injected directly into a vein (usually in the arm) at a prescribed rate.

Investigational drug: A drug available only for experimental purposes because its safety and effectiveness have not yet been proven.

JME: *See* Juvenile myoclonic epilepsy.

Juvenile myoclonic epilepsy (JME): A primary generalized epilepsy syndrome, usually beginning between ages 5 to 17 years, characterized by myoclonic (muscle-jerk) seizures and possibly also absence and tonic-clonic seizures; responds well to valproate.

Ketogenic diet: A high-fat, low-carbohydrate diet used to control seizures.

Kindling: A process (demonstrated by experiments using animals) in which electrical abnormalities become more intense over time; for example, small electrical shocks are delivered to the brain once a day to cause a progressive tendency toward seizures; eventually, seizures may occur without the electrical shocks.

Landau-Kleffner syndrome: A disorder of childhood characterized by the regression of language milestones in association with frequent epilepsy waves on the EEG.

Lennox-Gastaut syndrome: A disorder beginning in childhood, characterized by developmental delay or mental retardation, multiple seizure types that do not respond well to therapy, and slow spike-and-wave discharges on the EEG.

Magnetic resonance imaging (MRI): A scanning technique that creates pictures of the inside of the body and the brain; uses a strong magnet (does not use x-rays); more sensitive than CT.

Magnetic resonance spectroscopy (MRS): A scanning technique that examines the atoms hydrogen and phosphorus to glean information about chemical activity in small areas of brain.

Magnetoencephalography (MEG): Recording the brain's magnetic activity, which is generated by its electrical activity.

Mainstream: Regular (public, private, or parochial) school or classes.

Medical history: The account of a patient's disorder.

MEG: *See* Magnetoencephalography.

Meningitis: A bacterial infection of the membranes surrounding the brain; often diagnosed by a spinal tap (lumbar puncture).

Metabolism: The physical and chemical processes by which substances are produced or transformed (broken down) into energy or products for the uses of the body.

Metabolite: Chemical product derived from breakdown (metabolism) of another chemical; may be biologically *active* or *inactive;* an active metabolite of an antiepileptic drug can be effective in controlling seizures or can cause or contribute to the drug's adverse effects.

Migraine: A headache characterized by throbbing head pain, often greater on one side; may be preceded by a warning (aura) and accompanied by nausea, vomiting, and sensitivity to light and sound; in rare cases, weakness, language problems, or other neurologic disorders are associated with migraine.

Minor (motor) seizure: An older term for seizures that cause contraction of muscles but do not become tonic-clonic seizures; mostly used in certain laws and acts.

Monotherapy: Treatment with a single medication.

Motor: Of, pertaining to, or designating nerves carrying impulses from the nerve centers to the muscles; of or relating to movements of the muscles.

MRI: *See* Magnetic resonance imaging.

MRS: *See* Magnetic resonance spectroscopy.

Muscle tone: The level of muscle contraction present during the resting state; with *increased tone* there is stiffness and rigidity; with *decreased tone* there is looseness or floppiness of the limbs and trunk.

Myoclonic jerk: Brief muscle jerk; may involve muscles on one or both sides of the body; may be normal (e.g., as one falls asleep) or caused by a seizure or other disorders.

Myoclonic seizure: A brief muscle jerk resulting from an abnormal discharge of brain electrical activity; usually involves muscles on both sides of the body, most often the shoulders or upper arms.

Narcolepsy: A condition characterized by sudden and uncontrollable attacks of sleep.

Neuron: A nerve cell.

Neurotransmitter: A chemical substance produced by nerve cells, transported in the axon, and released at the synapse; causes chemical and electrical changes in adjacent cells.

Paroxysmal: Pertaining to a sudden outburst, such as the sudden recurrence or intensification of symptoms or epileptiform activity on the EEG.

Partial complex seizure: An alternative term for complex partial seizure.

Partial seizure: A seizure that involves or arises from part of the brain.

Peak blood level: The highest concentration of a drug in the bloodstream.

PET: *See* Positron emission tomography.

Petit mal: An older term for absence seizure; sometimes used incorrectly by the general public to refer to any kind of seizure that is not a convulsion.

Pharmacology: The study of drugs, including their effectiveness, adverse effects, metabolism, interaction with other drugs, and other actions.

Photic stimulation: Shining, flashing (strobe) lights in the eyes (which may be closed) of a person; used during the EEG to detect photosensitive epilepsy.

Photosensitive epilepsy: A form of reflex epilepsy in which certain lights, especially flashing lights, can provoke seizures.

Positron emission tomography (PET): A diagnostic test that uses a very low and safe dose of a radioactive compound to measure metabolic activity in the brain; can identify areas of decreased metabolism corresponding to the area from which seizures arise; helpful in planning epilepsy surgery.

Postictal: Referring to the period immediately after a seizure; the person may be tired and confused or may immediately return to an awake, attentive state after the seizure.

Predisposition: Tendency or inclination.

Premonitory: Serving as a warning.

Prevalence: The number of cases of a disorder present in a population at a specified time.

Primary drug: A drug that has stood the test of time in terms of its efficacy and safety in treating a particular disorder; for example, phenytoin and carbamazepine are primary drugs for partial seizures because they have been demonstrated to have very good safety and effectiveness in well-designed and well-controlled studies.

Prognosis: The outlook for a medical condition; the chances the condition will improve, remain unchanged, or worsen.

Progressive: Increasing in scope or severity over time.

Progressive myoclonic epilepsy: A rare group of epilepsies, often with a hereditary component, characterized by myoclonic and other types of seizures and progressive neurologic impairment; medications help control the seizures, but there is no cure.

Psychic: Pertaining to intellectual or emotional (affective) functions.

Psychogenic (nonepileptic; pseudo) seizure: A behavioral episode that resembles an epileptic seizure, but does not result from abnormal brain electrical activity; psychological in origin, but not resulting from conscious actions; video-EEG monitoring is often used to make the diagnosis.

Psychomotor seizure: An older term for a complex partial seizure with automatism.

Rasmussen's syndrome: A disorder with frequent or continuous partial seizures and a progressive abnormality in the brain, possibly the result of a virus.

Reasonable accommodation: *See* Accommodation.

Reflex epilepsy: Seizures precipitated by certain conditions or stimuli, such as flashing lights or jazz music.

Refractory: A condition that does not respond easily to treatment.

Secondary drug: A drug whose efficacy and safety are not as clearly defined as those of a primary drug, usually because it has not been used for as long or as extensively as the *primary*, or first-line, drug or because it was found to be less effective or less safe in controlled studies; some secondary drugs are used in *adjunct*, or *add-on*, therapy.

Seizure: A sudden, excessive discharge of nervous-system electrical activity that usually causes a change in behavior.

Seizure threshold: Minimal conditions necessary to produce a seizure.

Sensory: Pertaining to the senses (touch, vision, hearing, taste, smell).

Sharp wave: An EEG pattern indicating the potential for epilepsy; "benign" sharp waves are not associated with seizures.

Sibling: A brother or sister.

Simple partial seizure: An epileptic seizure that involves only part of the brain and does not impair consciousness.

Single-photon emission computed tomography (SPECT): A diagnostic test that uses a very low and safe dose of a radioactive compound to measure blood flow in the brain; not as sensitive as PET for baseline (interictal) studies, but can more readily be obtained during a seizure.

Slowing: A term used to describe a group of brain waves on the EEG that have a lower frequency than expected for the subject's age and level of alertness and the area of the brain recorded; slow waves can result from drowsiness or sleep, drugs, or brain injuries and occur during or after seizures.

Social Security Disability Income (SSDI): A federal assistance program for disabled people who have paid Social Security taxes or are dependents of people who have paid these taxes.

SPECT: *See* Single-photon emission computed tomography.

Spell: A period, bout, or episode of illness or indisposition; refers to seizures or other disorders that produce brief episodes of behavioral change.

Spike: An EEG pattern strongly correlated with seizures; "benign" spikes are not associated with seizures.

SSA: Social Security Administration.

SSDI: *See* Social Security Disability Income.

SSI: *See* Supplemental Security Income.

Status epilepticus: A prolonged seizure (usually defined as lasting longer than 30 minutes) or a series of repeated seizures; a continuous state of seizure activity; may occur in almost any seizure type.

Steady state: A state in which equilibrium has been achieved. In reference to antiepileptic drugs, steady state is achieved when a constant daily dose of a drug produces consistent blood levels of the drug (takes at least five times the half-life of the drug in question).

Sturge-Weber syndrome: A disorder of blood vessels affecting the skin of the face, eyes, and brain; brain involvement is associated with seizures.

Supplemental Security Income (SSI): A federal assistance program.

Symptomatic: Referring to a disorder with an identifiable cause; for example, severe head trauma can cause symptomatic epilepsy.

Synapse: The junction between one nerve cell and another nerve cell; the axon of one nerve cell releases a neurotransmitter, which diffuses across the synapse and causes changes in the membrane of the adjacent cell.

Syncope: Fainting.

Syndrome: A group of signs and symptoms that collectively define or characterize a disease or disorder; signs are objective findings such as weakness, and symptoms are subjective findings such as a feeling of fear or tingling in a finger.

Temporal lobe epilepsy: An older term for partial epilepsy arising from the temporal lobe of the brain.

Temporal lobe seizure: A simple or complex partial seizure arising from the temporal lobe of the brain.

Therapeutic blood level: The amount of drug circulating in the bloodstream that brings about seizure control without troublesome adverse effects in most patients. "Subtherapeutic" (lower) levels are effective in some patients, and "supratherapeutic" or "toxic" (higher) levels are tolerated by others.

Threshold: The level at which an event or change occurs *(see* Seizure threshold).

Tic: Repeated involuntary contractions of muscles, such as rapid head jerks or eye blinks, as in Tourette's syndrome; may be under partial voluntary control (e.g., can be temporarily suppressed); nonepileptic.

Time to Peak Blood Level: The interval between the time a drug is taken and the time it reaches the highest concentration in the blood.

Todd's paralysis: Weakness after a seizure; originally used to describe muscle weakness on the side of the body opposite the side in which the seizure began (in the brain), but now used to describe a variety of temporary problems after seizures, such as blindness, loss of sensation, or loss of speech.

Tolerance: Decreased sensitivity to the effects of a substance, such as a drug.

Tone: *See* Muscle tone.

Tonic seizure: An epileptic seizure that causes stiffening; consciousness is usually preserved. The seizure involves muscles on both sides of the body, and electrical discharge involves all or most of the brain.

Tonic-clonic seizure: A convulsion; newer term for grand mal or major motor seizure; characterized by loss of consciousness, falling, stiffening, and jerking; electrical discharge involves all or most of the brain.

Trauma: An injury or wound caused by external force or violence.

Tuberous sclerosis: A disease in which benign tumors affect the brain, eyes, skin, and internal organs; associated with mental retardation and seizures; inherited as an autosomal dominant trait.

Vagus nerve stimulator (VNS): A pacemakerlike device, implanted in the upper chest, which stimulates a nerve in the left neck and can reduce seizure activity.

Video-EEG monitoring: A technique for recording the behavior and the EEG of a patient simultaneously; changes in behavior can be correlated with changes in the EEG; useful for making the diagnosis of epilepsy and localizing the seizure focus.

West's syndrome: An epileptic syndrome characterized by infantile spasms, mental retardation, and an abnormal EEG pattern (hypsarrhythmia); begins before 1 year of age.

APPENDIX 2

Glossary of Drugs Used Against Epilepsy

Generic Name	Brand Name	Seizure Types for which Drug is Used
Acetazolamide (ah-seet-ah-**zole**-ah-myd)	Diamox (**dye**-ah-mox)	Myoclonic seizures, ?catamenial seizures
Adrenocorticotropic hormone (ACTH)	Cortrosyn (**cor**-tro-sin)	Infantile spasms
Carbamazepine (kar-bah-**maz**-ah-peen)	Tegretol (**teh**-greh-tol) Carbatrol (**car**-bah-trol)	Partial seizures, tonic-clonic seizures
Clonazepam (kloh-**na**-zeh-pam)	Klonopin (**klah**-ni-pin)	Myoclonic seizures, absence seizures
Clorazepate (klor-**a**-zeh-pate)	Tranxene (**tran**-zeen)	Absence seizures, partial seizures
Diazepam (dye-**ah**-zah-pam)	Valium (oral) (**va**-lee-um) Diastat (rectal) (**dye**-ah-stat)	Seizure clusters, status epilepticus
Ethosuximide (eth-o-**sux**-i-mide)	Zarontin (za-**ron**-tin)	Absence seizures, myoclonic seizures
Felbamate (**fel**-bah-mate)	Felbatol (**fel**-bah-tol)	Partial seizures, tonic-clonic seizures, atonic seizures, tonic seizures
Gabapentin (**gab**-ah-pen-tin)	Neurontin (nur-**on**-tin)	Partial seizures, tonic-clonic seizures

(continued)

(continued)

Generic Name	Brand Name	Seizure Types for which Drug is Used
Lamotrigine (lah-**mo**-tri-jeen)	Lamictal (lah-**mi**-ktal)	Partial seizures, tonic-clonic seizures
Levetiracetam (lehv-i-tir-**a**-si-tam)	Keppra (**kep**-pra)	Partial seizures, generalized seizures
Lorazepam (lor-**a**-zeh-pam)	Ativan (**ah**-ti-van)	Status epilepticus, seizure clusters
Mephobarbital (meh-fo-**bar**-bi-tal)	Mebaral (**meh**-bah-ral)	Partial seizures, tonic-clonic seizures, myoclonic seizures
Oxcarbazepine (ox-car-**bah**-zeh-peen)	Trileptal (try-**lep**-tal)	Partial seizures, tonic-clonic seizures
Phenobarbital (fee-no-**bar**-bi-tal)	Luminal (and others) (**lu**-mih-nall)	Partial seizures, tonic-clonic seizures
Phenytoin (**fen**-i-toe-in)	Dilantin (dye-**lan**-tin)	Partial seizures, tonic-clonic seizures
Prednisone (**pred**-nih-sone)	—	Infantile spasms
Primidone (**pri**-mi-done)	Mysoline (**my**-soh-leen)	Partial seizures, tonic-clonic seizures
Tiagabine (ti-**ah**-gah-been)	Gabitril (**gab**-ih-tril)	Partial seizures, tonic-clonic seizures
Topiramate (toh-**peer**-ah-mate)	Topamax (**toh**-pah-maks)	Partial seizures, tonic-clonic seizures; infantile spasms, myoclonic seizures
Valproate (valproic acid; divalproex sodium)	Depakene (**deh**-pah-keen) Depakote (**deh**-pah-kote)	Absence seizures, tonic-clonic seizures, myoclonic seizures, partial seizures
Zonisamide (zoh-**nih**-sah-mide)	Zonegran (**zon**-ah-gran)	Partial seizures, tonic-clonic seizures, myoclonic seizures

APPENDIX 3

Drug Interactions

INTERACTIONS OF ANTIEPILEPTIC DRUGS	
Drug	**Drug Affected**
Acetazolamide	⇑ Carbamazepine ⇑ Phenobarbital ⇑ Phenytoin, in children
Carbamazepine	⇑ Clobazam ⇓ Clonazepam ⇓ Ethosuximide ⇓ Felbamate ⇓ Lamotrigine ⇓ Methsuximide ⇑/⇓ Phenytoin ⇓ Primidone (but increases phenobarbital metabolite) ⇓ Topiramate ⇓ Valproate ⇓ Zonisamide
Clobazam	⇑ Carbamazepine ⇑ Phenytoin ⇑ Valproate
Clonazepam	⇓ Carbamazepine ⇑ Primidone Valproate: prolonged absence seizures developed in 5 of 12 patients studied
Clorazepate	None
Ethosuximide	⇓ Carbamazepine ⇓ Primidone ⇑ Valproate

⇑, Blood level of drug is increased; ⇓, blood level of drug is decreased; ⇑/⇓, blood level of drug may be increased, decreased, or remain unchanged.

(continued)

391

INTERACTIONS OF ANTIEPILEPTIC DRUGS *(continued)*

Drug	Drug Affected
Ethotoin	⇓ Carbamazepine ⇓ Valproate
Felbamate	⇓ Carbamazepine (but increases metabolite) ⇑ Ethotoin ⇑ Phenytoin ⇑ Phenobarbital ⇑ Valproate
Lamotrigine	⇑ Carbamazepine metabolite ⇓ Clonazepam ⇓ Lamotrigine ⇓ Valproate
Levetiracetam	None
Lorazepam	None
Methsuximide	⇓ Primidone
Oxcarbazepine	⇑ Phenytoin ⇑ Valproate ⇓ Zonisamide
Phenobarbital	⇓ Carbamazepine ⇑ Clobazam ⇓ Felbamate ⇓ Lamotrigine ⇑ Methsuximide (active metabolite) ⇓ Oxcarbazepine ⇑/⇓ Phenytoin ⇓ Valproate ⇓ Zonisamide
Phenytoin	⇓ Carbamazepine ⇑ Clobazam ⇓ Felbamate ⇓ Lamotrigine ⇑ Methsuximide (active metabolite) ⇓ Oxcarbazepine (⇑ metabolism but not formation of active metabolite) ⇑ Phenobarbital ⇓ Primidone (⇑ phenobarbital level) ⇓ Topiramate ⇓ Valproate ⇓ Zonisamide
Tiagabine	None

(continued)

INTERACTIONS OF ANTIEPILEPTIC DRUGS (continued)

Drug	Drug Affected
Topiramate	⇑ Phenytoin (⇓ Carbamazepine) (⇓ Valproate)
Valproate	⇑/⇓ carbamazepine (⇑ active metabolite) Clonazepam: prolonged absence seizures developed in 5 of 12 patients studied ⇑ Ethosuximide ⇑ Ethotoin ⇑ Felbamate ⇑ Lamotrigine ⇑ Lorazepam ⇑ Phenobarbital ⇑ Primidone ⇓ Phenytoin (total) ⇑ Phenytoin (free) ⇑ Zonisamide
Vigabatrin	⇓ Phenytoin
Zonisamideslight	⇑ Carbamazepine slight ⇑ Phenytoin

⇑, Blood level of drug is increased; ⇓, blood level of drug is decreased; ⇑/⇓, blood level of drug may be increased, decreased, or remain unchanged.

EFFECTS OF ANTIEPILEPTIC DRUGS ON OTHER DRUGS

Antiepileptic Drug	Other Drug Affected
Acetazolamide	⇑ Aminophylline ⇑ Cyclosporine ⇓ Lithium
Carbamazepine	⇓ Acetaminophen ⇓ Bupropion ⇓ Cyclosporine A ⇓ Desipramine ⇓ Doxycycline ⇓ Felodipine ⇓ Haloperidol ⇓ Itraconazole ⇓ Ketoconazole ⇓ Methylphenidate ⇓ Miconazole ⇓ Neuroleptics ⇓ Olanzapine ⇓ Rispiridone ⇓ Steroid hormones ⇓ Tricyclic antidepressants (e.g., amitryptiline) ⇓ Theophylline ⇓ Warfarin
Ethotoin	⇓ Cyclosporine ⇓ Steroid hormones
Lorazepam	⇑ Moxonidine
Oxcarbazepine	See carbamazepine
Phenobarbital and primidone	⇓ Acetaminophen ⇑ Alcohol (increased sedation, unsteadiness) ⇓ Amidopyrine ⇓ Chlorpromazine ⇓ Cimetidine ⇓ Cyclosporin ⇑ Dexamethasone ⇓ Digitoxin ⇓ Doxorubicin ⇓ Doxycycline ⇓ Felodipine ⇓ Fenoprofen ⇓ Furosemide ⇓ Haloperidol ⇓ Metronidazole ⇓ Methadone ⇓ Metoprolol ⇓ Neuroleptics (e.g., clozapine) ⇓ Nifedipine (primidone only) ⇓ Paroxetine

(continued)

EFFECTS OF ANTIEPILEPTIC DRUGS ON OTHER DRUGS *(continued)*

Antiepileptic Drug	Other Drug Affected
Phenobarbital and primidone *(continued)*	⇓ Propranolol ⇓ Quinidine ⇓ Steroid hormones ⇓ Tricyclic antidepressants ⇓ Theophylline ⇓ Warfarin
Phenytoin	⇓ Acetaminophen ⇓ Amiodarone ⇓ Aminophylline ⇓ Cholecalciferol ⇓ Cyclosporine ⇓ Dicoumarol ⇓ Digoxin ⇓ Disopyramide ⇓ Doxycycline ⇓ Felodipine ⇓ Folic acid ⇓ Furosemide ⇓ Levodopa ⇓ Metronidazole ⇓ Mexiletine ⇓ Misonidazole ⇓ Nisoldipine ⇓ Paroxetine ⇓ Praziquantel ⇓ Psoralens ⇓ Quinidine ⇑ Risperidone ⇓ Steroid hormones ⇓ Theophylline ⇓ Topotecan ⇓ Tirilazad ⇓ Tricyclic antidepressants ⇓ Vitamin K ⇓ Warfarin
Topiramate	⇓ Steroid hormones
Valproate	⇑ Amoxepine ⇑ Doxepine ⇑ Nimodipine ⇓ Tricyclic antidepressants
Zonisamide	?

⇓, Blood drug level is decreased; ⇑, blood drug level is increased.

EFFECTS OF OTHER DRUGS ON ANTIEPILEPTIC DRUGS

Other Drug	Antiepileptic Drug Affected
Acetaminophen	mild ⇓ Lamotrigine
Alcohol	⇑ Clobazam ⇓ Phenytoin (prolonged alcohol intake) ⇑ Phenytoin (moderate or heavy intake in person who does not often consume alcohol) ⇑ Phenobarbital (active metabolite of primidone*)
Aminophylline	⇓ Phenytoin
Amiodarone	⇓ Phenytoin
Amitryptiline	⇑ Carbamazepine
Antacids	⇓ Phenytoin ⇑ Valproate
Maalox TC	+/- ⇑ Gabapentin
Aspirin	⇑ Free phenytoin ⇑ Free valproate ⇑ Acetazolamide
Caffeine	Carbamazepine half-life in blood doubled
Cimetidine	⇑ Carbamazepine ⇑ Clobazam ⇑ Clorazepate ⇑ Diazepam ⇑ Phenytoin
Ciprofloxacin	⇓ Phenytoin
Cisplatin	⇓ Carbamazepine
Clarithromycin	⇑ Carbamazepine
Coumadin	+/-⇑ Phenytoin
Danazol	⇑ Carbamazepine
Desipramine	⇑ Carbamazepine
Diltiazem	⇑ Carbamazepine +/- ⇑ Phenytoin
Disulfiram	⇑ Phenytoin ⇑ Diazepam
Doxepin	⇑ Carbamazepine
Doxycycline	⇓ Carbamazepine
Erythromycin	⇑ Carbamazepine

(continued)

EFFECTS OF OTHER DRUGS ON ANTIEPILEPTIC DRUGS (continued)

Other Drug	Antiepileptic Drug Affected
Fluconazole	⇑ Clorazepate (when fluconazole is stopped) ⇑ Phenytoin
Fluoxetine	⇑ Carbamazepine ⇑ Phenytoin ⇑ Valproate
Fluvoxamine	⇑ Carbamazepine
Flurithromycin	⇑ Carbamazepine
Folic acid	⇓ Phenytoin
Grapefruit juice	⇑ Carbamazepine
Haloperidol	⇑ Carbamazepine +/- ⇓ Valproate
Isoniazid (INH)	⇑ Carbamazepine ⇑ Phenytoin ⇑ Primidone +/- ⇑ Valproate
Itraconazole	⇑ Phenytoin
Ketoconazole	⇑ Carbamazepine
Methotretxate	⇓ Phenytoin
Metronidazole	⇑ Phenytoin ⇑ Carbamazepine
Miconazole + flucytosine	⇑ Phenytoin
Nefazadone	⇑ Carbamazepine
Nicotinamide	⇑ Carbamazepine ⇑ Primidone
Nortryptiline	⇑ Carbamazepine
Omeprazole	⇑ Diazepam +/- ⇑ Phenytoin
Panipenem-betamipron	⇓ Valproate

⇑, Blood level of drug is increased; ⇓, blood level of drug is decreased; +/-, variable or mild effect not seen in all patients, and rarely affects how patients feel or their condition
*The drug primidone is metabolized by the liver. One of the main products of this reaction is phenobarbital, which is also an active compound and an antiepileptic drug. Some drugs can increase the amount of phenobarbital that is made from primidone, which influences the overall effectiveness of primidone.

(continued)

EFFECTS OF OTHER DRUGS ON ANTIEPILEPTIC DRUGS *(continued)*

Other Drug	Antiepileptic Drug Affected
Phenylbutazone	⇑ Free phenytoin ⇓ Phenobarbital
Propoxyphene	⇑ Carbamazepine +/- ⇑ Phenobarbital with high dosage ⇑ Phenytoin
Pyridoxine	⇓ Phenobarbital from primidone metabolism*
Quinine	⇑ Phenobarbital
Ranitidine	+/- ⇑ Phenytoin
Rifampin	⇓ Clonazepam ⇓ Clorazepate ⇓ Ethosuximide ⇓ Phenobarbital from primidone metabolism* ⇓ Phenytoin
Risperidone	May react with valproate to cause swelling
Sertraline	⇑ Lamotrigine ⇑ Phenytoin
Sucralfate	⇓ Phenytoin
Sulfa drugs	⇓ Phenytoin
Theophylline	⇓ Carbamazepine
Ticlopidine	⇑ Carbamazepine ⇑ Phenytoin
Trimethoprim	⇑ Phenytoin
Troleandomycin	⇑ Carbamazepine
Verapamil	⇑ Carbamazepine
Viloxazine	⇑ Carbamazepine ⇑ Phenytoin
Vinblastine	⇓ Phenytoin
Warfarin	⇑ Phenytoin

⇑, Blood level of drug is increased; ⇓, blood level of drug is decreased; +/-, variable or mild effect not seen in all patients, and rarely affects how patients feel or their condition

*The drug primidone is metabolized by the liver. One of the main products of this reaction is phenobarbital, which is also an active compound and an antiepileptic drug. Some drugs can increase the amount of phenobarbital that is made from primidone, which influences the overall effectiveness of primidone.

SELECTED OVER-THE-COUNTER DRUGS AND FOODS THAT CAN AFFECT SEIZURE CONTROL OR DRUG SIDE EFFECTS

Drug/Food	Effect	Common Products*
Acetaminophen	May decrease level of **lamotrigine** in the blood	Alka-Seltzer Drixoral Excedrin Midol Robitussin Sudafed TheraFlu Tylenol
Aspirin or other salicylates[†]	May decrease total level of **phenytoin** in the blood, but increase free level (effects variable) May increase levels of **valproate** in the blood, causing adverse side effects	Alka-Seltzer Anacin Bayer Aspirin Bufferin Excedrin
Diphenhydramine	Can lower seizure threshold (minimum conditions necessary to produce a seizure)	Alka-Seltzer PM Pain Reliever and Sleep Aid Benadryl Goody's PM Powder Nytol Sominex Tylenol PM
Grapefruit juice	Increases level of **carbamazepine** in the blood, causing adverse side effects	

*These are not all inclusive lists. Refer to ingredient lists when determining whether a product may affect seizure control or contribute to side effects of drugs.
[†]Low to moderate doses of aspirin (less than 1500 mg per day) are generally very safe for people who take antiepileptic drugs. Higher doses should only be taken after discussion with a doctor, especially if phenytoin or valproate is used. Aspirin-free versions of some products listed are available.

APPENDIX 4

Resources for People with Epilepsy

General—Adult and Teen

BRAIN TALK (BULLETIN BOARD)
(run by Massachusetts General Hospital)
www.braintalk.org

EPILEPSY.COM
(Internet site for patients and families affected by epilepsy. Includes information and videos and on-line nursing and medical support to answer questions)
www.epilepsy.com

THE EPILEPSY FOUNDATION
(general information and online community section)
4351 Garden City Drive
Landover, MD 20785
(800) 332-1000 or (301) 459-3700
www.efa.org or
www.epilepsyfoundation.org

EPILEPSY INFORMATION SERVICE
Medical Center Boulevard
Winston-Salem, NC 27157-1078
(800) 642-0500

HEALTHWATCH100
(Medical Reminder Watch)
ReCall Services, Inc
Medical Reminder Systems
95 Main Street
Maynard, MA 01754
(800) 732-2592
www.epil.com

400

INTELIHEALTH
(linked with Harvard University School of Medicine)
www.intelihealth.com (General site)
www.intelihealth.com/IH/ihtIH/WSIHWOOO/8803/8803.html (Epilepsy)
www.intelihealth.com/IH/ihtIH/WSIHWOOO/8124/
8124.html?k=menux8803x8124 (Drug information)

THE JOSEPH P. KENNEDY, JR. FOUNDATION
(services for those with mental retardation)
1325 G Street, NW, Suite 500
Washington, DC 20005-4709
(202) 393-1250 voice
(202) 824-0351 fax
www.familyvillage.wisc.edu/jpkf

NATIONAL ASSOCIATION OF PROTECTION AND ADVOCACY INC.
900 Second Street, NE, Suite 211
Washington, DC 20002
(202) 408-9514
www.protectionandadvocacy.com

NATIONAL EPILEPSY LIBRARY
The Epilepsy Foundation of America
4351 Garden City Drive
Landover, MD 20785
(800) EFA-4050

NATIONAL LIBRARY OF MEDICINE
8600 Rockville Pike
Bethesda, MD 20894
www.nlm.nih.gov
www.ncbi.nlm.nih.gov/PubMed (Excellent site for abstracts of medical articles)

General–Child

CHILDREN'S DEFENSE FUND
25 E Street, NW
Washington, DC 20001
(202) 628-8787
www.childrensdefense.org

THE COUNCIL FOR EXCEPTIONAL CHILDREN
1110 North Glebe Road, Suite 300
Arlington, VA 22201-5704
(888) CEC-SPED or (703) 620-3660
(703) 264-9446 TTY (text only)
(703) 264-9494 fax
www.cec.sped.org

DANMAR PRODUCTS, INC.
(custom head protection)
221 Jackson Industrial Drive
Ann Arbor, MI 48103
(800) 783-1998
www.danmarproducts.com

INTERNET RESOURCES FOR SPECIAL CHILDREN (IRSC)
www.irsc.org

KIDS ON THE BLOCK, INC.
(educational puppet programs)
9385-C Gerwig Lane
Columbia, MD 21046-1583
(800) 368-KIDS (5437) or 410-290-9095
(410) 290-9358 fax
www.kotb.com

**THE NATIONAL INFORMATION CENTER
FOR CHILDREN AND YOUTH WITH DISABILITIES**
P.O. Box 1492
Washington, DC 20013-1492
(800) 695-0285 voice/TTY or (202) 884-8200 voice/TTY
(202) 884-8441 fax
www.nichcy.org/

THE SIBLING SUPPORT PROJECT
Dedicated to the interests of brothers and sisters of
people with special health and developmental needs.
Peer support groups, publications, other resources.
www.thearc.org/siblingsupport

Related Neurologic and Metabolic Disorders

THE ARC OF THE UNITED STATES
(formerly Association for Retarded Citizens)
National Headquarters Office
1010 Wayne Ave., Suite 650
Silver Spring, MD 20910
(301) 565-3842
www.thearc.org

AUTISM SOCIETY OF AMERICA
7910 Woodmont Avenue, Suite 300
Bethesda, Maryland 20814-3067
(301) 657-0881 or (800) 3AUTISM
www.autism-society.org

AUTISM-PDD RESOURCES NETWORK
www.autism-pdd.net

LEARNING DISABILITIES ASSOCIATION OF AMERICA, INC.
4156 Library Road
Pittsburgh, PA 15234-1349
(412) 341-1515
www.ldanatl.org

NATIONAL ALLIANCE FOR THE MENTALLY ILL (NAMI)
Colonial Place Three
2107 Wilson Blvd., Suite 300
Arlington, VA 22201-3042
(800) 950-NAMI (6264) NAMI HelpLine
(703) 524-7600 main office
(703) 516-7227 TDD
www.nami.org

NATIONAL ANGELMAN SYNDROME FOUNDATION
414 Plaza Drive, Suite 209
Westmont, IL 60559
(800) 432-6435 or (630) 734-9267
www.angelman.org

THE NATIONAL FRAGILE X FOUNDATION
P.O. Box 190488
San Francisco, CA 94119
(800) 688-8765 or (510) 763-6030
www.nfxf.org

NATIONAL INSTITUTE OF NEUROLOGICAL DISORDERS AND STROKE
NIH Neurological Institute
P.O. Box 5801
Bethesda, MD 20824
(800) 352-9424
www.ninds.nih.gov

THE NATIONAL NEUROFIBROMATOSIS FOUNDATION, INC.
95 Pine Street, 16th Floor
New York, NY 10005
(800) 323-7938 or (212) 344-NNFF(6633)
www.nf.org

THE STURGE-WEBER FOUNDATION
P.O. Box 418
Mount Freedom, NJ 07970
(800) 627-5482 or (973) 895-4445
www.sturge-weber.com

TUBEROUS SCLEROSIS ALLIANCE
801 Roeder Road, Suite 750
Silver Spring, MD 20910
(800) 225-6872 or (301) 562-9890
www.tsalliance.org

UNITED CEREBRAL PALSY
1660 L Street, NW, Suite 700
Washington, DC 20036-5602
(800) 872-5827 or (202) 776-0406
(202) 973-7197 TTY
www.ucpa.org

UNITED MITOCHONDRIAL DISEASE FOUNDATION
P.O. Box 1151
Monroeville, PA 15146-1151
(412) 793-8077
www.umdf.org

WILLIAMS SYNDROME ASSOCIATION
P.O. Box 297
Clawson, MI 48017-0297
(248) 541-3630
www.williams-syndrome.org

Career and Rehabilitation

ACCESS AMERICA FOR PEOPLE WITH DISABILITIES
(Website established by Presidential Task Force on Employment of Adults with Disabilities, with extensive information and links to government services)
www.disAbility.gov

AMERICANS WITH DISABILITY ACT
Department of Justice
P.O. Box 66118
Washington, DC 20035
(202) 514-0301
www.usdoj.gov/crt/ada/adahom1.htm

DISABILITYRESOURCES.ORG
(information on employment discrimination)
www.disabilityresources.org/EMPLOYMENT.html
(state listing of agencies for people with disabilities)
www.disabilityresources.org/DRMreg.html

THE U.S. EQUAL EMPLOYMENT OPPORTUNITY COMMISSION (EEOC)
1801 L Street, NW
Washington, DC 20507
(202) 663-4900
To be connected to nearest field office, phone (800) 669-4000 or (800) 669-6820 TTY
www.eeoc.gov

THE JOB ACCOMMODATION NETWORK (JAN)
918 Chestnut Ridge Road, Suite 1
West Virginia University, P.O. Box 6080
Morgantown, WV 26506
(800) 526-7234
www.jan.wvu.edu

NATIONAL ORGANIZATION ON DISABILITY
910 Sixteenth Street, NW, Suite 600
Washington, DC 20006
(202) 293-5960 or (202) 293-5968 TTY
www.nod.org

NATIONAL REHABILITATION INFORMATION CENTER (NARIC)
8455 Colesville Road, Suite 935
Silver Spring, MD 20910
(800) 346-2742 or (301) 495-5626 TTY
www.naric.com/index.html

REHABILITATION SERVICES ADMINISTRATION (RSA)
OFFICE OF SPECIAL EDUCATION AND REHABILITATION SERVICE (OSERS)
U.S. Department of Education
Switzer Building
330 C Street, SW
Washington, DC 20202
(202) 205-5465 voice or TTY
www.ed.gov/offices/OSERS/RSA/rsa.html

SOCIAL SECURITY ADMINISTRATION
(800) 772-1213 or (800) 325-0778 TTY
www.ssa.gov/regions/regional.html (regional offices)
www.ssa.gov/disability (Social Security Disability Insurance [SSDI])
www.ssa.gov/notices/supplemental-security-income (Supplemental
Security Income [SSI])

YOUNG ADULT INSTITUTE (YAI)/NATIONAL INSTITUTE
FOR PEOPLE WITH DISABILITIES
Central Office
460 West 34th Street
New York, NY 10001-2382
(212) 563-7474
www.yai.org

Pharmacies—Mail-Order and Online

AARP PHARMACY SERVICE FROM RETIRED PERSONS SERVICES, INC.
(800) 456-2277
(800) 933-4327 TTY
www.rpspharmacy.com

ATHENA RX HOME PHARMACY
(specializing in neurologic disorders)
(800) 528-4362
www.athenarx.com

DRUGSTORE.COM
(800) 378-4786
www.drugstore.com

EXPRESS SCRIPTS
(800) 441-8976
www.express-scripts.com/prescriptions/prescriptions.htm

PREFERRED RX
P.O. Box 39368
Solon, Ohio 44139-0368
(800) 843-7038
(440) 247-9313 fax
www.preferredrx.com

WEBRX.COM
Customer Service Center
2924 Telestar Court
Falls Church, VA 22042
(877) DRUG411
www.webrx.com

APPENDIX 5

References and Suggested Readings

Chapter 4—Epileptic Syndromes

Dostoyevsky F: The Idiot. Translated by Eva M. Martin. No. 682 in Everyman's Library, Dent, London, 1970, pp 52, 213–214, 222.

Chapter 5—An Overview of Epilepsy

Hauser WA and Hesdorffer DC: Epilepsy: Frequency, Causes, and Consequences. Demos Publications, New York, 1990.

Chapter 6—Seizure-Provoking Factors

Ferber R: Solve Your Child's Sleep Problems. Simon & Schuster, New York, 1986.

Chapter 13—Other Therapies

Brake D and Brake C: The Ketogenic Cookbook. Pennycorner Press, 1997.

Freeman JM, et al: The Ketogenic Diet: A Treatment for Epilepsy, ed 3. Demos Medical, New York, 2000.

Chapter 18—Intellectual and Behavioral Development

Blank M, et al: Links to Language. Presented at the American Speech-Language, Hearing Association meeting, Atlanta, GA, November 1991.

Bridwell, N: Clifford's Manners. Scholastic, New York, 1990.

Gardner RA: MBD: The Family Book about Minimal Brain Dysfunction. Jason Aronson, New York, 1973.

Greenspan SI: The Essential Partnership: How Parents and Children Can Meet the Emotional Challenges of Infancy and Childhood. Viking Penguin, New York, 1990.

Greenspan SI: First Feelings: Milestones in the Emotional Development of Your Baby and Child. Penguin USA, New York, 1989.

Smith SL: No Easy Answers: The Learning Disabled Child at Home and at School. Bantam Books, New York, 1995.

Chapter 19—Telling Children and Others about Epilepsy

Moss DM: Lee, the Rabbit with Epilepsy. Woodbine House, Bethesda, MD, 1990.

Chapter 27—Employment for People with Epilepsy

Americans with Disabilities Act (ADA) 1990 (full 90 pages): Copies can be obtained free from U.S. Senate Subcommittee on Disability Policy, 113 Hart Senate Office Building, Washington, DC 20510. (202) 244-6265 or TTY (202) 244-3457.

INDEX

An "f" following a page number indicates a figure; a "t" indicates a table.